Advances in Laminitis, Part I

Guest Editor

CHRISTOPHER C. POLLITT, BVSc, PhD

VETERINARY CLINICS OF NORTH AMERICA: EQUINE PRACTICE

www.vetequine.theclinics.com

Consulting Editor

A. SIMON TURNER, BVSc, MS

April 2010 • Volume 26 • Number 1

SAUNDERS an imprint of ELSEVIER, Inc.

W.B. SAUNDERS COMPANY
A Division of Elsevier Inc.

1600 John F. Kennedy Boulevard • Suite 1800 • Philadelphia, Pennsylvania 19103

http://www.vetequine.theclinics.com

VETERINARY CLINICS OF NORTH AMERICA: EQUINE PRACTICE Volume 26, Number 1
April 2010 ISSN 0749-0739, ISBN-13: 978-1-4377-1882-9

Editor: John Vassallo; j.vassallo@elsevier.com
Developmental Editor: Theresa Collier

Veterinary Clinics of North America: Equine Practice (ISSN 0749-0739) is published in April, August, and December by Elsevier Inc., 360 Park Avenue South, New York, NY 10010-1710. Business and Editorial Offices: 1600 John F. Kennedy Blvd., Suite 1800, Philadelphia, PA 19103-2899. Subscription prices are $222.00 per year (domestic individuals), $339.00 per year (domestic institutions), $111.00 per year (domestic students/residents), $259.00 per year (Canadian individuals), $424.00 per year (Canadian institutions), $299.00 per year (international individuals), $424.00 per year (international institutions), and $151.00 per year (international and Canadian students/residents). To receive student/resident rate, orders must be accompanied by name of affiliated institution, date of term, and the signature of program/residency coordinator on institution letterhead. Orders will be billed at individual rate until proof of status is received. Foreign air speed delivery is included in all *Clinics* subscription prices. All prices are subject to change without notice. **POSTMASTER:** Send address changes to *Veterinary Clinics of North America: Equine Practice*, 3251 Riverport Lane, Maryland Heights, MO 63043. Customer Service (orders, claims, online, change of address): Elsevier Health Sciences Division, Subscription Customer Service, 3251 Riverport Lane, Maryland Heights, MO 63043. Tel: 1-800-654-2452 (U.S. and Canada); 314-447-8871 (outside U.S. and Canada). Fax: 314-447-8029. E-mail: journalscustomerservice-usa@elsevier.com (for print support); E-mail: journalsonlinesupport-usa@elsevier (for online support).

Reprints. For copies of 100 or more of articles in this publication, please contact the Commercial Reprints Department, Elsevier Inc., 360 Park Avenue South, New York, NY 10010-1710. Tel.: 212-633-3812; Fax: 212-462-1935; E-mail: reprints@elsevier.com.

Veterinary Clinics of North America: Equine Practice is covered in *MEDLINE/PubMed (Index Medicus), Excerpta Medica, Current Contents/Agriculture, Biology and Environmental Sciences, and ISI.*

Printed and bound in the United Kingdom
Transferred to Digital Print 2011

Contributors

CONSULTING EDITOR

A. SIMON TURNER, BVSc, MS
Diplomate, American College of Veterinary Surgeons; Professor, Department of Clinical Sciences, College of Veterinary Medicine and Biomedical Sciences, Colorado State University, Fort Collins, Colorado

GUEST EDITOR

CHRISTOPHER C. POLLITT, BVSc, PhD
Professor, Australian Equine Laminitis Research Unit, School of Veterinary Science, The University of Queensland, St Lucia, Queensland, Australia; Laminitis Institute, University of Pennsylvania School of Veterinary Medicine, New Bolton Center, Kennett Square, Pennsylvania

AUTHORS

GREGORY I. BALDWIN, BSc, BVSc
Research Master of Philosophy Candidate, Australian Equine Laminitis Research Unit, School of Veterinary Science, The University of Queensland, St Lucia; Senior Veterinary Steward, Harness Racing Queensland, Albion Park Raceway, Albion, Queensland, Australia

JAMES K. BELKNAP, DVM, PhD
Diplomate, American College of Veterinary Surgeons; Professor of Equine Surgery, Department of Veterinary Clinical Sciences, College of Veterinary Medicine, The Ohio State University, Columbus, Ohio

SIMON N. COLLINS, BSc (Hons), PhD
Orthopaedic Research Group, Centre for Equine Studies, Animal Health Trust, Lanwades Park, Kentford, Newmarket, Suffolk, United Kingdom

SUSAN C. EADES, DVM, PhD
Diplomate, American College of Veterinary Internal Medicine-Large Animal; Professor, Department of Veterinary Clinical Sciences, Equine Health Studies Program, Louisiana State University, Baton Rouge, Louisiana

JULIE B. ENGILES, VMD
Diplomate, American College of Veterinary Pathologists; Assistant Professor of Pathology, Department of Pathobiology, School of Veterinary Medicine, New Bolton Center-Murphy Laboratory, University of Pennsylvania; Adjunct Assistant Professor of Pathology, Department of Clinical Studies, New Bolton Center, School of Veterinary Medicine, University of Pennsylvania, Kennett Square, Pennsylvania

HENRY W. HEYMERING, CJF, RMF
Private Practice Farrier, Frederick, Maryland

ROBERT J. HUNT, DVM, MS
Diplomate, American College of Veterinary Surgeons; Hagyard Equine Medical Institute, Lexington, Kentucky

ATHOL V. KLIEVE, BAgSc, MRurSc, PhD
Associate Professor, Schools of Animal Studies and Veterinary Science, The University of Queensland, Gatton; Animal Research Institute, Agri-Science Queensland, Department of Employment, Economic Development and Innovation, Moorooka, Queensland, Australia

ATSUTOSHI KUWANO, DVM, PhD
Clinical Sciences and Pathobiology Division, Sports Science Research Centre, Equine Research Institute, Japan Racing Association, Utsunomiya-shi, Tochigi, Japan

GABRIEL J. MILINOVICH, BAgSc, PhD
Australian Equine Laminitis Research Unit, School of Veterinary Science, The University of Queensland, St Lucia, Queensland, Australia; Department of Genetics in Ecology, University of Vienna, Austria

JAMES A. ORSINI, DVM
Diplomate, American College of Veterinary Surgeons; University of Pennsylvania, Department of Clinical Studies, New Bolton Center, Kennett Square, Pennsylvania

CHRISTOPHER C. POLLITT, BVSc, PhD
Professor, Australian Equine Laminitis Research Unit, School of Veterinary Science, The University of Queensland, St Lucia, Queensland, Australia; Laminitis Institute, University of Pennsylvania School of Veterinary Medicine, New Bolton Center, Kennett Square, Pennsylvania

PATRICK RILEY
Chief, Farrier Services, University of Pennsylvania, Department of Clinical Studies, New Bolton Center, Kennett Square, Pennsylvania

AMY RUCKER, DVM
MidWest Equine, Columbia, Missouri

MICHEAL L. STEWARD, DVM
Private Practice Farrier, Shawnee, Oklahoma

DARREN J. TROTT, BVMS, PhD
Associate Professor, Australian Equine Laminitis Research Unit, School of Veterinary Science, The University of Queensland, St Lucia, Queensland, Australia

ANDREW VAN EPS, BVSc, PhD
Member of the Australian College of Veterinary Scientists, Diplomate, American College of Veterinary Internal Medicine, Senior Lecturer in Equine Medicine, School of Veterinary Science, The University of Queensland, St Lucia, Queensland, Australia

MICHELLE B. VISSER, PhD
School of Veterinary Science, Faculty of Natural Resources, Agriculture and Veterinary Science, The University of Queensland, St Lucia, Queensland, Australia

DONALD M. WALSH, BS, DVM
Director of Clinical Research, Homestead Veterinary Hospital, Pacific, Missouri

ROBIN E. WHARTON, DVM
Hagyard Equine Medical Institute, Lexington, Kentucky

JENNIFER WRIGLEY, CVT
University of Pennsylvania, Department of Clinical Studies, New Bolton Center, Kennett Square, Pennsylvania

Contents

the ultimate attachment unit of the SADP. Laminitis destroys and dislocates the BM and its components and without an intact, functional BM, the structure and function of the lamellar epidermis is pathologically compromised. Transcription and activation of constituent proteases occurs in normal hoof lamellae but in increased amounts during laminitis.

Overview of Current Laminitis Research **51**

Susan C. Eades

All cases of laminitis are characterized by failure of the attachment of the epidermal cells of the epidermal laminae to the underlying basement membrane of the dermal laminae despite the diversity of diseases that underlie the syndrome. The preponderance of evidence supports roles for inflammation, metabolic derangement, endothelial and venous dysfunction, and matrix degradation as causes of laminitis. Inflammation, oxidant stress, and matrix degradation may be factors common to each of these mechanisms that lead to the laminar damage of laminitis. The understanding of the pathophysiology and progression of the disease is incomplete, and this limits efforts to prevent and treat this devastating disease successfully. However, scientific investigations are occurring at a phenomenal rate and shedding light on the pathophysiologic events involved with laminitis.

Carbohydrate Alimentary Overload Laminitis **65**

Christopher C. Pollitt and Michelle B. Visser

In acute laminitis, the suspensory apparatus of the distal phalanx fails at the lamellar dermal/epidermal interface. A grading system for the histopathology of laminitis is based on the consistent pattern of histologic changes to the secondary epidermal lamellae, basal cells, and basement membrane that occur as carbohydrate-induced laminitis develops. The actual trigger factors of carbohydrate-induced laminitis remain unidentified.

Microbial Events in the Hindgut During Carbohydrate-induced Equine Laminitis **79**

Gabriel J. Milinovich, Athol V. Klieve, Christopher C. Pollitt, and Darren J. Trott

Equine laminitis is the most serious foot disease of the horse, often resulting in death or euthanasia. Laminitis has long been recognized as an affliction of horses, as has the association of this condition with the ingestion of carbohydrates. Research into the pathophysiology of this condition has been facilitated by the development of reliable models for experimentally inducing laminitis, and DNA-based techniques for profiling complex microbiomes have dramatically increased the knowledge of the microbiology of this disease. Recent studies have provided substantial evidence showing equine hindgut streptococcal species to be the most likely causative agent. Although these studies are not definitive, they provide the foundations for future work to determine the source of laminitis trigger factors and their mechanisms of action.

Black Walnut Extract: An Inflammatory Model 95

James K. Belknap

The black walnut extract (BWE) model was developed after the discovery that horses bedded on shavings from black walnut trees commonly developed laminitis. The first investigators that consistently induced laminitis with black walnut shavings established that it was only the heartwood of the tree that induced laminitis. The BWE model of laminitis has allowed investigators to determine many of the early pathologic signaling events likely to occur in the developmental and acute clinical stages of the disease process, and has brought inflammatory injury to the forefront of laminitis research. These events must also be assessed in the carbohydrate overload models, the models that more closely reflect the clinical case of laminitis.

Acute Laminitis: Medical and Supportive Therapy 103

Andrew van Eps

Acute laminitis is a serious complication of many primary conditions in the horse. This article summarizes the most appropriate approach to management of the horse with acute laminitis, based on current information.

The Pharmacologic Basis for the Treatment of Developmental and Acute Laminitis 115

James K. Belknap

The treatment of laminitis has been fraught with confusion and controversy for several decades, mainly because of a lack of understanding of the pathophysiology of the disease process. However, recent advances in laminitis research have greatly improved our understanding of the disease process. This article discusses the various treatment options for laminitis in the context of the findings of recent scientific investigations of laminitis pathophysiology.

Therapeutic Hypothermia (Cryotherapy) to Prevent and Treat Acute Laminitis 125

Andrew van Eps

Digital hypothermia successfully reduces the severity of experimentally induced laminitis. Continuous-distal limb cryotherapy may be a useful technique in clinical cases that are at risk of developing laminitis. This article examines the effects of hypothermia on tissue as well as the rationale, and suggested protocols for the usage of distal limb cryotherapy in the prevention and treatment of laminitis.

Progression of Venographic Changes After Experimentally Induced Laminitis 135

Gregory I. Baldwin and Christopher C. Pollitt

Venography (retrograde venous angiography) is a relatively simple and practical method for vascular assessment of the digits in the standing horse. The technique is a useful adjunct to routine radiography. The clinical use of the laminitis venogram has resulted in a more comprehensive understanding of the collateral pathology associated with distal phalanx displacement and abnormal hoof growth. The effectiveness of therapeutic procedures such as hoof wall resection, coronary band grooving, deep digital flexor tenotomy, and therapeutic shoeing can be assessed by serial venography. This article discusses the venographic appearance during the transition from the clinically normal hoof to the severe chronic laminitis cases similar to those seen in practice.

Clinical Presentation, Diagnosis, and Prognosis of Chronic Laminitis in North America **141**

Robert J. Hunt and Robin E. Wharton

Chronic laminitis involves laminar morphologic changes resulting in digital collapse and can vary greatly in its clinical manifestation depending on duration, severity of lameness, and stability of the distal phalanx/hoof wall interface. Accurate assessment of the whole patient is mandatory and consideration must be given to signalment, occupation, and owner expectations, as well as history and etiology, which often predict the broad course of the disease. Diagnosis is made via physical examination with adjunctive serial radiographic evaluation and possibly venography. Eventual functionality of the foot is determined by structural integrity, which is dictated by the degree of morphologic damage of the soft tissue and bone architecture of the foot. Structures involved include the digital vasculature, the laminar/hoof wall interface, and the distal phalanx. Patient outcome is largely determined by the degree of instability between the distal phalanx and hoof wall, and the ultimate prognosis is further influenced by owner expectation.

Pathology of the Distal Phalanx in Equine Laminitis: More Than Just Skin Deep **155**

Julie B. Engiles

The etiopathogenesis of laminitis is complex and involves multiple tissue types. It may be initiated by biomechanical, traumatic, inflammatory, vascular, toxic, and metabolic factors. Although histopathologic changes occurring within the lamellae of experimental models of laminitis are well described and reported, histopathologic changes occurring in the distal phalanx are not, even though gross and radiographic evidence of disease are often apparent and bony lesions could be considered a significant source of pain. Recent scientific evidence indicates that the microenvironment of bone is an important modulator of inflammatory processes that can both influence, and be influenced by components of other organ systems, including the immune, nervous, gastrointestinal, and integumentary systems. This article describes various laminitis-associated histopathological changes in the distal phalanx, introduces concepts of osteoimmunology with regards to equine laminitis, and provides a rationale for histopathological examination of the distal phalanx, as well as the soft tissue structures of the lamellae and corium in laminitis cases.

Equine Venography and Its Clinical Application in North America 167

Amy Rucker

The digital venogram uses contrast radiography to evaluate the soft tissues and vasculature of the foot, thus identifying pathology attributable to laminitis. Pathology can be detected before changes appear on plain-film radiographs. When used in conjunction with clinical and radiographic findings, information gained from a venographic study informs and directs treatment. Serial venograms assess the response to treatment and help determine prognosis early in the course of therapy. If the venographic contrast pattern does not improve, either the treatment needs to be altered, or the damage is so extensive that there can be no favorable response to treatment.

The Lamellar Wedge 179

Simon N. Collins, Andrew W. van Eps, Christopher C. Pollitt, and Atsutoshi Kuwano

In horses with chronic laminitis, an abnormal horn structure called the lamellar wedge develops within the lamellar region of the foot. This pathologic structure adversely affects normal foot function, and influences return to previous performance levels. Understanding the pathologic process that leads to the development of this structure is essential for correct supportive foot management of the horse with chronic laminitis. The ability to prevent or reduce the formation of the lamellar wedge may eventually lead to better outcomes in cases of laminitis.

Chronic Laminitis: Strategic Hoof Wall Resection 197

Amy Rucker

In the chronic-laminitic foot, severe soft-tissue compression and compromised circulation can result in osteitis and sepsis at the margin of the distal phalanx. Resultant inflammation and sepsis may cause the coronary corium to swell, drain, or separate from the hoof capsule, usually within 8 weeks of laminitis onset. Slow-onset cases of soft-tissue impingement can develop secondary to distal phalanx displacement due to lack of wall attachment. With either presentation, partial upper wall resection is required to reverse compression and vascular impingement by the hoof capsule. If the pathology is not overwhelming, the area reepithelializes and grows attached tubular horn. Firm bandaging and restricted exercise until tubular horn has regrown enhances recovery and the return of a strong hoof.

The Use of the Wooden Shoe (Steward Clog) in Treating Laminitis 207

Micheal L. Steward

This article describes the use of the wooden shoe in the treatment of chronic laminitis. The shoe, designed to provide a solid base and full roller motion, offers mechanical advantages and enables reduction and redistribution of forces within the hoof capsule.

Home Care for Horses with Chronic Laminitis **215**

James A. Orsini, Jennifer Wrigley, and Patrick Riley

Home care for horses with chronic laminitis has been discussed rarely in the veterinary literature even though, at any given time, most of us have at least 1 chronic laminitis case in our care that is being managed at home by the owner. Almost all of our knowledge on this aspect of laminitis treatment has been gleaned through experience, by individually working through the medical, ethical, financial, and emotional challenges these cases can present. Much has already been presented on the medical management of the laminitic horse and on strategies for trimming and shoeing the laminitic foot. This article focuses on the other challenges so often faced when directing the home care of a horse with chronic laminitis.

Index **225**

FORTHCOMING ISSUES

August 2010
Laminitis, Part II
Christopher Pollitt, BVSc, PhD,
Guest Editor

December 2010
Pain Management and Analgesia
William Muir, DVM, PhD,
Guest Editor

April 2011
Endocrine Diseases
Ramiro E. Toribio, DVM, PhD,
Guest Editor

RECENT ISSUES

December 2009
Practice Management
Reynolds Cowles, DVM
Guest Editor

August 2009
New Perspectives in Equine Colic
Frank M. Andrews, DVM, MS,
Guest Editor

April 2009
Clinical Nutrition
Raymond J. Geor, BVSc, MVSc, PhD,
Guest Editors

RELATED INTEREST

Veterinary Clinics of North America: Food Animal Practice
November 2007 (Vol. 23, No. 3)
Ruminant Diagnostic Medicine
Robert J. Callan, DVM, MS, PhD, *Guest Editor*

Preface

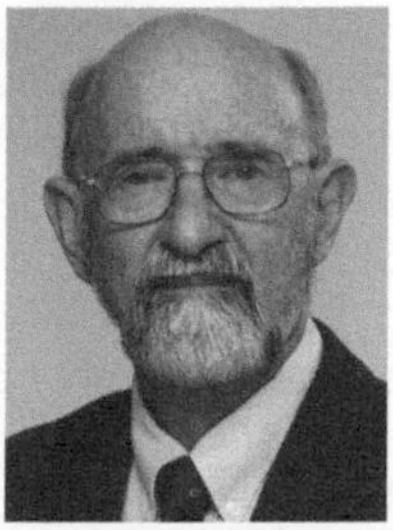

Christopher C. Pollitt, BVSc, PhD
Guest Editor

Despite centuries of close contact with mankind, horses still develop laminitis. This may cripple them, shorten their working lives, and euthanasia may be recommended because of the dreadful suffering. The causes of laminitis remain a mystery despite a considerable international research effort. With increasing intensity, teams of research scientists and postgraduate students have, for the past 70 years, studied the causes, prevention, and therapy for laminitis. As usual with research into difficult biologic problems, every question answered seems to generate more unknowns. Poor funding for laminitis research prevents rapid progress, but nevertheless some aspects of laminitis have become a little clearer although others seem more complex and unreachable. The current importance of laminitis is reflected in the decision by the editors of *Veterinary Clinics of North America: Equine Practice* to dedicate not just 1, but 2 issues to the topic of laminitis. The first issue deals mainly with laminitis associated with septic/inflammatory conditions and the second concentrates on metabolic and endocrinopathic laminitis. Both issues include articles on treatment/preventive strategies and how to cope with chronic laminitis, the aftermath of the acute stage.

Ten years have passed since David Hood edited the landmark edition in this series entitled *Laminitis*. Readers are encouraged to consult the 1999 issue, as much of the material is current and needs little revision. In particular, the terminology for the stages of laminitis, outlined in Fig. 1, p. 289,[1] has been universally adopted and is used throughout the current editions. Thus, there is an initial developmental phase when the inducing mechanisms begin to operate and lead to the onset of lameness. This is the phase when preventive strategies have the best chance of succeeding (see article by Andrew van Eps in this issue), but unfortunately, it is relatively asymptomatic and may not be recognized in clinical practice. All too frequently, a therapeutic opportunity is lost. In the second acute phase of laminitis, the clinical signs are clear and have never been better described than by Nils Obel in 1948.[2] Obel's 4 degrees of lameness range from mild to very severe. Part of the description of the first mild stage includes paddling or shifting weight from 1 foot to the other every few seconds while in the standing position. Although strictly speaking not a gait abnormality or true lameness, shifting weight while standing still is an important observation as even this early subtle

Vet Clin Equine 26 (2010) xv–xvii
doi:10.1016/j.cveq.2010.02.001 vetequine.theclinics.com
0749-0739/10/$ – see front matter

clinical sign is associated with histologic and ultrastructural lesions (see article by Pollitt and Visser in this issue).

As in the 1999 edition, Henry Heymering has provided a historical perspective on laminitis which is always salutary to read. Confronted by the same phenomenon of developing and then acute laminitis, the veterinary scientific minds of the distant and recent past have repeatedly developed opposing etiologic and pathophysiologic opinions. Understanding laminitis has yet to fall to the scientific method. Read Heymering' article from the beginning and you will be rewarded by this pearl at the end: "We have had nearly 2000 years of bleeding as treatment, 1700 years of exercise as treatment, and more than 40 years of phenylbutazone as treatment – without proof of effectiveness in treating laminitis. Although longevity suggests effectiveness, until we have proof of our treatments, future generations may find them as quaint and misdirected as we find 'the skin of the weasel cut up in small pieces, together with butter, putrid egg, and vinegar' as the treatment recommended by Heresbach (1577)." Senior veterinary practitioners have personal experience of the confusion in the laminitis literature and a memoir by Donald Walsh relates the frustration of living through times of high expectation and bitter disappointment with what was delivered by laminitis researchers. It behooves laminitis researchers to listen to equine clinicians as they are still waiting for effective preventive and therapeutic strategies. Clinicians play an important role in laminitis research and retrospective analyses of their clinical records are urgently needed to shed light on what is truly making a difference in terms of prevention and treatment.

Responding to Nils Obel's 1948 statement that "a profound knowledge of the anatomical changes in the initial stages must be considered a prerequisite for the study of the patho-physiology of the disease," a revision entitled "The anatomy and physiology of the suspensory apparatus of the distal phalanx" is provided. The laminitis literature receives a comprehensive review and this is followed by articles with the latest information on the effect of laminitis induced by carbohydrate overload and black walnut extract. Current therapy is covered by 2 articles and a third reviews the preventive potential of distal limb hypothermia (cryotherapy). There are 2 articles on venography, 1 research based and the other clinical; these are to bring the reader up-to-date with the progress being made with this informative diagnostic technique. Chronic laminitis and its sequelae are reviewed from a clinician's viewpoint and then by a pathologist. Specific bone pathology of the distal phalanx following severe chronic laminitis has received little attention in the past and this article delivers important new information that segues appropriately into discussions on the destructive potential of the lamellar wedge and the indication for strategic hoof wall resection. For the first time in the veterinary literature, software that takes the information generated by the computed tomography scanner and renders it into a virtual three-dimensional model using MIMICS (Materialise, Belgium), is used to illustrate the lamellar wedge and its association with the pathologic lysis of the distal phalanx in severe chronic laminitis.

The final articles offer advice on supporting the chronically affected foot and how best to care for afflicted horses in their home environment. Of necessity, the topics of some articles reappear in Part II of this series as other experts are recruited to advance laminitis understanding.

ACKNOWLEDGMENTS

I am grateful to Dr Simon Turner and John Vassallo for the opportunity to serve as guest editor and author of the *Veterinary Clinics of North America: Equine Practice*.

The contributing authors are thanked for devoting the time to share their knowledge and experience with an audience that will learn much about laminitis within the pages of Parts I and II of *Advances in Laminitis*.

Christopher C. Pollitt, BVSc, PhD
School of Veterinary Science
The University of Queensland
St Lucia, Brisbane
Queensland 4072, Australia

The Laminitis Institute
University of Pennsylvania School of Veterinary Medicine
New Bolton Center
Kennett Square, PA, USA
E-mail address:
c.pollitt@uq.edu.au

REFERENCES

1. Hood DM. Laminitis in the horse. Vet Clin North Am Equine Pract 1999;15:287–94.
2. Obel N. Studies of the histopathology of acute laminitis: Almgvist and Wilcsells Bottrykeri Ab Uppsala (PhD thesis); Royal Veterinary College; Stockholm, Sweden; 1948.

A Historical Perspective of Laminitis

Henry W. Heymering, CJF, RMF

KEYWORDS

• Laminitis • History • Founder • Equine

What has been will be again, what has been done will be done again; there is nothing new under the sun. Is there anything of which one can say, "Look! This is something new"? It was here already, long ago; it was here before our time. There is no remembrance of men of old, and even those who are yet to come will not be remembered by those who follow.

–Ecclesiastes 1:9 to 11 New International Version.

History does not change; however, one's perspective of history changes as new research and discoveries emphasize previous ideas. Therefore, this article will have much in common with a previous work by Wagner and this author,[1] and another by this author alone.[2] I have separated the history into some generally recognized periods, adjusted slightly for seamless coverage. This article covers terms and treatments in the fields of veterinary (medications, surgery), farriery (trimming, shoeing), and management (diet, footing, exercise). Where possible, I have identified links from historical treatments to the postmodern period. Unless otherwise noted, for clarity I have mentioned only the earliest written record of each treatment that I could find.

ANCIENT HISTORY

In 3500 BC, the Sumerians were known to use most of the current methods of drug delivery (pills, poultices, infusions, ointments, troches, and other treatments),[3] and an ancient Sumerian script mentions cattle doctors.[4] The earliest known equine veterinary writings date to 2500 BC in China, 1900 BC in Egypt, and 1800 BC in India,[5] but the written record of laminitis is more recent.

Although attention to feeding and watering after exercise suggests the Hittites in 1350 BC were aware of laminitis,[6] Xenophon (380 BC) may have been the first to write about laminitis. Xenophon mentioned barley surfeit, without describing symptoms, and goes on to say, "diseases are easier to cure at the start than after they have become chronic and have been wrongly diagnosed."[7]

8621A Hunters Drive, Frederick, MD 21701, USA
E-mail address: horseu@earthlink.net

Vet Clin Equine 26 (2010) 1–11
doi:10.1016/j.cveq.2009.12.004 **vetequine.theclinics.com**
0749-0739/10/$ – see front matter

Aristotle (330 BC) also mentioned barley surfeit, but the signs of disease described ("evidence of the ailment is softening of the palate and hot breath"[8]) are not those of laminitis. Aristotle, however, described grass founder:

> *"Among horses, those at pasture are free of all ailments except foot-ill, but they suffer from this and sometimes cast the hooves. …the casting of the one hoof takes place simultaneously with the growing of the other hoof underneath. Evidence of the ailment: the right testicle twitches…."*[8]

Once again, the evidence described does not fit. Smith noted that Aristotle's writing (possibly the signs of disease?) may have been altered. "In Book VIII veterinary medicine is dealt with, and the translator warns us that this part bears evidence of an alien hand."[9]

ROMAN EMPIRE (27 BC TO 500 AD)

Columella (55 AD) described laminitis as blood descending to the feet. He noted that the feet were hot to the touch, and for treatment he recommended bleeding from the middle of the leg.[10] Bleeding is the first recorded treatment for laminitis. Bleeding for overeating (not necessarily laminitis) was described by Pliny (50 AD).[5]

Apsyrtus (early fourth century), the father of veterinary medicine, referred to acute laminitis as barley disease and treated it by dietary restriction and exercise in addition to bleeding. "Slowly and gradually the animal warmly clothed is driven up and down until sweating occurs; the body must then be dried."[11]

Chiron (fourth century), showed a clear understanding of laminitis, describing suffusion of the feet as the horse being unable to walk, with heat and blood in the hooves, and possible separation of the hoof wall from the laminae.[10] Chiron may have been a pseudonym for Hierocles,[4] a lawyer–veterinarian, who described laminitis as being caused by drinking quantities of cold water when heated.[11]

Publius Vegetius Renatus (480) made numerous references to the troubles from overfeeding of barley.[11] Vegetius in one part recognized laminitis as a suffusion in the feet caused by work and fatigue on a long journey. In another section, Vegetius dealt with laminitis under the heading of gout. For treatment, Vegetius recommended purges and febrifuge, in addition to moderate bleeding, diet, and exercise. Exercise is to be continued daily with a laxative diet of "green meat [fresh cut grass and other greens[12]] with nitre [potassium nitrate or saltpeter, used to reduce fever] sprinkled over it." If the animal did not respond to the treatments, then castration was recommended, "for gout seldom affects eunuchs."[11] Laminitis was confirmed to be more prevalent in stallions than geldings by Dorn (1975).[13]

DARK AGES (500 TO 900)

During the Dark Ages, the modern horse collar, the stirrup, and shoeing with iron shoes and nails were developed,[14] but there is no written record of their invention nor of any veterinary advances in laminitis during this period.

HIGH MIDDLE AGES (900 TO 1450)

Despite being very expensive, shoeing became so popular during the Crusades (1095 to 1291) that Guibert of Nogent wrote, "truly astonishing things were to be seen … poor people shoeing their oxen as though they were horses.[15] Jordanus Ruffus (1250), Senior Imperial Marshal (farrier),[16] was the first to mention the operation of unsoling (peeling back and removing the entire sole), which was used to treat laminitis for more than 600 years, until the practice was stopped by an Society for the Prevention of Cruelty to Animals lawsuit in the late nineteenth century.[11,17]

AGE OF DISCOVERY (1450 TO 1700)

Fitzherbert (1548)[18] was the first to recommend shoeing to treat morfounde or pomis, "... good paryng and shoynge as he ought to be will do good service." Presumably, this indicates that the heels were to be lowered and the toe dressed back, trimming away the unnatural growth, but specific directions did not appear until Russell (1878).[19]

Malbie[20] (1576) was the first to publish a book entirely on laminitis, guaranteeing a cure to acute laminitis largely by exercise. Snape (1683), serjeant-farrier[21] to Charles II, was the first to recommend vertical hoof grooving, which still is used today (**Fig. 1**).[22] Snape described one cause of what he called founder as standing in water after hard riding.[11]

MODERN ERA (1700 TO 1949)

Bridges (1751) recommended leaving the horse at liberty on a good bed,[23] which was proven effective by Hood and Stephans(1981).[24] Osmer[25] (1766) followed Snape in recommending vertical hoof grooving for founder, and directed when "a crisis of fever falls on the feet [laminitis] ... the proper method of acting is to cut them off round and short at the toe, till the blood appears...." Chest founder, as described by Osmer (1766) and then quoted by Freeman (1796), is navicular disease, not founder.[25,26]

Bourgelat (1771), founder of the veterinary school at Lyon, France, recommended an adjusted shoe, cradle-like in profile.[16] This style of shoe was used by Dollar (1898)[27] and Churchill (1912),[28] and a shoe with a similar profile of the ground surface was used by Roberge[29] (1894) to treat laminitis (**Fig. 2**). More recently, similar banana or rock n' roll shoes were recommended by Redden (2006),[30] and wooden or plastic clogs in similar profile have been recommended by Steward.[31,32]

Vial de Saint Bel (Sainbel, 1793), first head of the Veterinary College of London, coined the term laminae.[23] Mayo (1823) was the first to describe the secondary laminae.[33]

Youatt (1831)[34] noticed the digital pulse, saying, "the artery at the pastern will throb violently." Dadd (1866)[35] noted that, "this increased pulsation seems due to

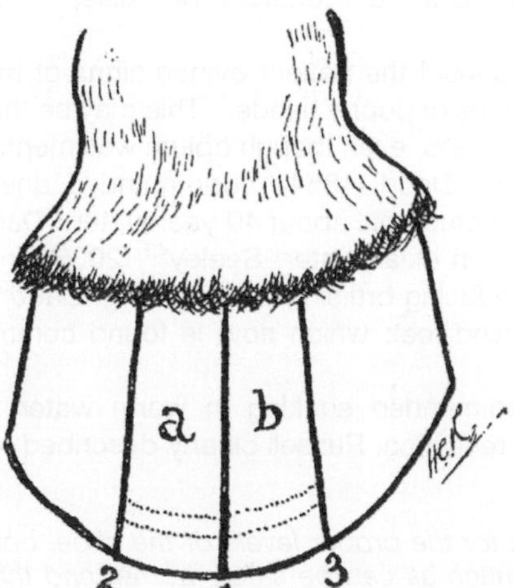

Fig. 1. Diagram of hoof showing the position of the three grooves made in the treatment of laminitis. (*From* Reeks HC. Diseases of the horse's foot. Chicago: Alex Eger; 1906. p. 278.)

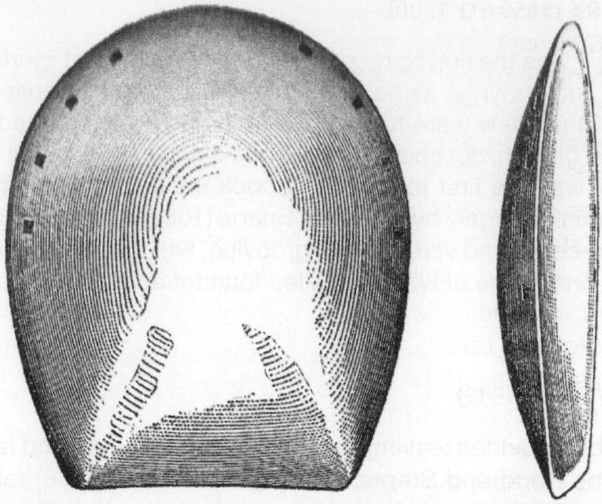

Fig. 2. A shoe made like a half ball, rocking in all directions, called a ball shoe or centerbearing shoe. (*From* Roberge D. The foot of the horse. New York: Wm R Jenkins; 1894. p. 39.)

obstruction in channels through which blood usually circulates with freedom, while the same or even an augmented force continues to impel it." Youatt[34] was the first to recommend pads to treat inflammation of the feet, but not for laminitis by name. Youatt[34] recommended wide-web barshoes, seated out to prevent direct sole pressure. Youatt[34] also recommended digitalis as a sedative. To relieve the pressure in the hoof, Youatt[34] recommended softening the hoof wall with poultices, removing the shoes, paring the sole as thin as possible, and rasping the outer hoof wall, especially at the quarters. Scheafer[36] (1863), in a book on homeopathic veterinary medicine, recommended homeopathic aconite, along with numerous other homeopathic medicines for laminitis. Holcombe (1890)[37] used aconite to treat laminitis, for the purpose of slowing the heartbeat. Homeopathic aconite currently is used as an early treatment for acute laminitis to help regulate the pulse,[38,39] and for reducing blood pressure.[40,41]

Dadd[35] (1866) said, "should the patient evince signs of much agony, give a few drenches of infusion of hops or poppy heads." This may be the first use of pain medication for treatment of laminitis, even though opium was mentioned as far back as the Ebers Papyrus (1550 BC).[5] Dadd (1854) recommended anesthesia for surgery on horses, but it was not adopted until about 40 years later.[5] Dadd[35] (1866) recommended arnica tincture given in clear water. Seeley[42] (2006) proved the usefulness of homeopathic arnica in reducing bruising and swelling. Dadd[35] (1866) reported laminitis affecting only the hind feet, which now is found commonly in cattle, but not horses.[43]

Russell[19] (1878) recommended soaking in warm water for the first 24 hours. Although not calling it a resection, Russell clearly described removing the wall at the toe, down to serum:

> *"In preparing the foot for the proper levels of the shoe, commence at the heel, lower both sides as much as can be safely borne, and this operation must be carried forward toward the quarters. ... The front part of the hoof must next be weakened, by rasping from coronet to ground surface, until serum is apparent, extending this operation back to the quarters," and a roller-motion shoe applied.*[19]

Resections were proven effective by Peremans and colleagues (1991).[44]

Zundel[45] (1886) described the laminar wedge and the sole being perforated by the tip of the coffin bone.[45] Zundel[45] spoke of laminitis of the opposite leg when one leg is unable to support weight, and also of laminitis from being kept in a sling. Zundel[45] implicated hot weather as a cause of laminitis, has and this also has been reported by Young (2004).[46] Zundel[45] mentioned hoof trauma, such as being crushed under a wagon wheel, as a cause of laminitis. Zundel[45] described chronic laminitis as, "a subinflammatory state of acute laminitis." Zundel[45] advises against taking off the shoes. Zundel[45] mentions treatment by forced recumbency. Zundel made no mention of medication to treat pain (only fever) from laminitis; however, he wrote about Bouley's use of neurotomy to treat laminitis. Still, Zundel[45] did not recommend it, because it often results in sloughing of the hoof. Zundel[45] described an operation by Gross of thinning the wall in a broad (4 cm) horizontal band near the coronet from heel to heel all around the hoof. Zundel[45] mentioned Silberman's use of a steel band, two fingers wide, similar to the currently marketed Nolan Hoof Plate (Mike Nolan's Farrier Service, Columbus, OH, USA).[47] Zundel[45] described an apparatus for the cooling of feet in laminitis, including the use of snow or crushed ice. This was proven effective in reducing laminitis in the developmental stage by van Eps and Pollitt (2004).[48]

Zundel recommended shoes and pads. "Between the shoe and the foot a piece of gutta percha [rubber], or felt or leather may be put on. Thus shod, a horse will still do long service, even in cities, and much more in the country."[45] In the late 1800s, numerous pads were developed to reduce concussion and slipping. Dollar[27] (1898) and Hunting[49] (1941) each devoted entire articles of their books to pads, but did not mention pads for treating laminitis.

Dollar (1898) recommended a full-rocker "cradling" eggbar shoe for dropped sole following laminitis. Dollar[27] illustrated a heartbar shoe but only recommended it for frog pressure, to widen the hoof, and he did not mention it for laminitis or founder. Chapman and Platt[50] promoted treating laminitis with heartbar shoes in the early 1980s.[51,52]

Axe[53] (1907) recommended stronger pain medication: "a full dose of morphia may be injected beneath the skin." While Zundel[45] mentioned "alkaline remedies ... to render the blood more fluid," Hodgins and Haskett[54] (1907) suggested the use of oral bicarbonate of soda (antacid) for laminitis. Histamine is only produced in the gut in quantity when the diet contains grain and the gut has become overly acidic.[55,56]

Martin[57] (1916)was the first to implicate microbes as a cause of laminitis. Martin spoke of injecting local anesthetic, but he found, "removal of pain in the feet, may cause the animal to place its entire weight for too long a time on its inflamed feet and thus cause a rapid descent of the pedal bones within the hoof, that might not otherwise have occurred."[57] For the same reason, George Platt (2006) said that giving phenylbutazone only makes laminitis worse by causing the coffin bone to sink.[58]

Merillat (1920) reviewed Straunard (1918), following his recommendations. Merillat said of bleeding, "jugular venesection is recommended. Six to 10 L of blood are withdrawn. This lowers the blood pressure for a definite time.... It may cure without delay."[41] Merillat said the following about exercise.

> *"Exercise is very beneficial in founder. The patient emerges from the stable with great difficulty and great apprehension, but after a few minutes walks easily. The pain noticeably diminishes and the blood pressure of the foot becomes lower. The pulsation of the metacarpals becomes more feeble, even after a few yards of walking. ... The walking should be continued for not less than a quarter of an hour. The longer the better."*[41]

In contrast, Backus[59] (1937) reported, "if the horse is forced to move, the evidence of pain partially subsides, but after the patient is allowed to rest, the pain is more severe than before."

Åkerblom (1934) successfully experimented with carbohydrate overload to induce laminitis.[6] Åkerblom was able to produce symptoms of laminitis by injecting repeated small doses of histamine intravenously and identified the bacterium responsible for the decarboxylation of histidine in the equine intestine as *Balantidium coli*.[60] Åkerblom also suggested that other toxic amines, particularly tyramine, may play a part.[60] Turner (1937) asserted, "the harmful effect (causing laminitis from overeating) is destroyed by cooking."[60]

Rodebaugh[61] (1938) recommended the addition of 0.75 inch heel caulks on the shoe to relax the deep digital flexor (DDF) tendon. Because caulks only act to raise the hoof angle on hard footing (footing that is contraindicated), effectively raising the hoof angle was not accomplished until Redden (1992).[62] Other writers on laminitis, such as Coffman and colleagues[40] (1970) Goetz[63] (1989), and Moore[64] (1916) insisted, "…elevating the heel increases the pain…." Research by McGuigan and colleagues[65] (2005) found that once 6° to 13° of rotation has taken place, the force pulling on the DDF tendon is zero for the first 40% of the stance phase.

Frank[66] (1944) recommended horizontal hoof wall grooving (0.25 inches wide instead of Gross' 1.5 inches wide) all the way around the hoof from heel to heel for treatment of some cases of chronic laminitis. Johnson[67] (1975) grooved just at the dorsal toe rather than from heel to heel, and Ritmeester and colleagues[68] (1998) proved its effectiveness. For acute laminitis, Frank injected 125 to 150 cc of autologous horse serum or whole blood, either subcutaneously or intramuscularly—also recommended by Thomas (1945),[69] Adams (1966),[70] and currently used to treat tendonitis in people.

Chavance[71] (1946) reported that injection with antihistamines was an effective treatment for laminitis. *Allisonella histaminiformans,* which produces histamine directly from histidine in grains, is found in the cecum of horses.[56] Histamine is involved with many of the different causes of laminitis. Nocek[72] (1997) noted, "histamine release can be caused by a variety of factors other than nutritional origin, such as environmental stress, concussion, trauma associated with concrete floors, overcrowding, and infectious diseases, causing tissue breakdown." Acute laminitis in cattle can be caused by subcutaneous injection with histamine, and bovine laminitis from overeating can be alleviated by antihistamine.[55]

Obel[73] (1948) gave veterinarians the familiar grading system for laminitis by his name. Obel[74] also found the separation in laminitis to take place in the "keratogenic" zone of cornification of the secondary epidermal laminae. Larsson and colleagues[75] (1956) then found, "methionine has been found to be incorporated to a much higher degree than cystine in those parts of the hoof matrix where the factors causing laminitis seem to strike primarily."

POSTMODERN (1949 TO PRESENT)

There was little progress in the postmodern period until the late 1980s, when there began an explosion of research and controversy, which continues today. Unfortunately, this has not yet resulted in a solid foundation of knowledge, but rather a sea of uncertainty.

There have been at least 25 books, monographs, or booklets (mostly for horse owners) written solely about laminitis. All but four of them were written in the postmodern period: Malbie (1576),[20] Jubin (1908),[76] Straunard (1918),[77] Obel (1948),[74]

Abdin-Bey (1984),[78] Chapman and Platt (1984),[50] Taylor (1988),[79] Eustace (1992),[80] Moore and Allen (1995),[81] Coumbe (1996),[82] Redden (1998),[83] Veterinary Clinics of North America (1999),[84] King and Mansmann (2000),[85] USDA (2000),[86] Jackson (2001),[87] Pollitt (2001),[88] Ramey (2003),[89] Strasser (2003),[90] Hamilton-Fletcher (2004),[91] Butler and Gravlee (2007),[92] Parker (2009),[93] American Farriers Journal (1997),[94] Buff (2000),[95] Buff (2005),[96] and Sillence and colleagues (2007).[97] Each of these publications has a different view, often diametrically opposed to others. Because there is so little solid evidence, these books are necessarily largely empiric and speculative.

Of the dozens of suspected causes of laminitis, only four have been shown to reliably create laminitis for the purposes of research: starch,[73] black walnut,[98] oligofructose,[99] and insulin.[100] Of the dozens of medicines and treatments recommended for laminitis, only seven (virginiamycin [only for pretreating for carbohydrate overload][101]; resection[44]; horizontal dorsal coronary wall grooving[68] deep, soft sand footing[24]; dimethyl sulphoxide[102]; 1,4-dihydropyridine 1000[103] [a calcium channel blocker given 4 hours after the initial insult]; and cryotherapy[48] [in the developmental stage]) have been proven by at least one controlled experiment to be effective.

For nearly 2000 years, bleeding has been used as treatment; there have been 1700 years of exercise as treatment, and more than 40 years of phenylbutazone as treatment, without proof of effectiveness in treating laminitis. Although longevity suggests effectiveness, until there is proof for these treatments, future generations may find them as quaint and misdirected as today's veterinarians find "the skin of the weasel cut up in small pieces, together with butter, rotten egg, and vinegar" as the treatment recommended by Heresbach (1586).[104]

REFERENCES

1. Wagner IP, Heymering H. Historical perspectives on laminitis. Vet Clin North Am Equine Pract 1999;5(2):295–309.
2. Heymering HW. A history of remedial shoeing. In: Curtis S, editor, Corrective farriery, vol. 2. Newmarket (UK): Newmarket Farriery Consultancy; 2006. p. 378–87.
3. Panati C. Extraordinary origins of everyday things. New York: Harper & Row; 1987. p. 245.
4. Dunlop RH, Williams DJ. Veterinary medicine: an illustrated history. St. Louis (MO): Mosby; 1996. p. 53.
5. Smithcors JF. Evolution of the veterinary art. Kansas City (MO): Veterinary Medicine Publishing; 1957. p. 11–27.
6. Rooney JR, Robertson JL. Equine pathology. Ames (IA): Iowa State U Press; 1996. p. 188.
7. Morgan HM. The art of horsemanship by Xenophon. London: J.A. Allen; 2004. p. 28.
8. Aristotle. History of animals books VII–X [edited and translated by D.M. Balme]. Cambridge (MA): Harvard University Press; 1927.
9. Smith F. The early history of veterinary literature. London: J.A. Allen; 1976.
10. Adams JN, Brill EJ. Pelagonius and Latin veterinary terminology in the Roman empire. Boston: Brill Academic Publishers; 1995.
11. Smith F. The early history of veterinary literature, vol. 1. London: J.A. Allen; 1976.
12. Stewart J. Stable economy: a treatise on the management of horses. 7th edition. London: William Blackwood and Sons; 1860.

13. Dorn RC, Garner HE, Coffman JR, et al. Castration and other factors affecting the risk of equine laminitis. Cornell Vet 1975;65:57–64.
14. White L Jr. Medieval religion and technology. Berkeley (CA): University of California Press; 1978.
15. Severin T. Retracing the first crusade. National geographic 1989;176(3):326–65.
16. Fleming G. Horse-shoes and horse-shoeing: their history, origin, uses, and abuses. London: Chapman and Hall; 1869.
17. Reeks HC. Diseases of the horse's foot. Chicago: Alex. Eger; 1906.
18. Fitzherbert A. Boke of husbandry. London: Thomas Berthelet; 1548.
19. Russell W. Scientific horseshoeing. Cincinnati: Robert Clarke & Company; 1879.
20. Malbie N. A plaine and easie way to remedy a horse that is foundered in his feete. London: T Purfoote; 1576.
21. Prince LB. The farrier and his craft. London: J.A. Allen; 1980.
22. Floyd AE. An approach to the treatment of the laminitic horse. In: Floyd AE, Mansmann RA, editors, Equine podiatry. St. Louis (MO): Saunders; 2007. p. 350.
23. Smith F. The early history of veterinary literature, vol. 2. London: J.A. Allen; 1976.
24. Hood DM, Stephens KA. Pathophysiology of equine laminitis. Compend Contin Educ Pract Vet 1981;3:S454.
25. Osmer W. A treatise on the diseases and lamness of horses. 3rd edition. London: T. Waller; 1766.
26. Freeman S. Observations on the mechanism of the horse's foot. London: W. Bulmer & Co; 1796.
27. Dollar JAW. Horseshoeing. New York: Wm R Jenkins; 1898.
28. Churchill FG. Practical and scientific horseshoeing. Kansas City (MO): Franklin Hudson; 1912.
29. Roberge D. The foot of the horse. New York: Wm R Jenkins; 1894. p. 188–90, illustration #42.
30. Redden RF. When and how to use the full rocker motion shoe. In: Proceedings Bain Fallon Memorial Conference. Coffs Harbour (AU), 2006. p. 36–42.
31. Steward ML. How to construct and apply atraumatic therapeutic shoes to treat acute or chronic laminitis in the horse. In: 15th Annual Bluegrass Laminitis Symposium. Louisville (KY), 2002. p. 31–3.
32. Steward ML. How to construct and apply atraumatic therapeutic shoes to treat acute or chronic laminitis in the horse. AAEP Proc 2003;49:337–46.
33. Smith F. The early history of veterinary literature, vol. 3. London: J.A. Allen; 1976.
34. Youatt W. The horse. London: Baldwin & Craddock; 1831.
35. Dadd GH. Modern horse doctor. New York: Orange Judd & Co; 1866. p. 351.
36. Scheafer JC. New manual of homeopathic veterinary medicine. New York: William Radde; 1863.
37. Holcombe AA. Diseases of the fetlock, ankle, and foot. In: Salmon DE, editor. Diseases of the horse. Washington, DC: Government Printing Office; 1890. p. 417.
38. Elliott M, Pinkus T. Horses and homeopathy. London: Ainsworths Homeopathic Pharmacy; 1994.
39. Macleod G. The treatment of horses by homeopathy. Saffron Walden (UK): C.W. Daniel Co; 1977.
40. Coffman JR, Johnson JH, Guffy MM, et al. Hoof circulation in equine laminitis. J Am Vet Med Assoc 1970;156:76–83.
41. Merillat LA. The treatment of acute laminitis. Am J Vet Med 1920;15:535–7.
42. Seeley BM, Denton AB, Ahn MS, et al. Effect of homeopathic arnica montana on bruising in face-lifts: results of a randomized, double-blind, placebo-controlled clinical trial. Arch Facial Plast Surg 2006;8(1):54–9.

43. Nilsson SA. Clinical morphological and experimental studies of laminitis in cattle. Acta Vet Scand 1963;4(Suppl 1):1–304.
44. Peremans K, Verschooten F, DeMoor A, et al. Laminitis in the pony: conservative treatment vs dorsal hoof wall resection. Equine Vet J 1991;23(4):243–6.
45. Zundel A. The horse's foot and its diseases. New York: Wm R Jenkins; 1886.
46. Jenkins D. Hot flash: laminitis. Am Farriers J 2004;30(4):86–9.
47. Casey R. The Nolan Hoof Plate informational DVD and TV shows 2007–2008. Presented at the AAEP 54th Annual Convention. LaFayette, Georgia.
48. van Eps AW, Pollitt CC. Equine laminitis: cryotherapy reduces the severity of the acute lesion. Equine Vet J 2004;36(3):255–60.
49. Hunting W. The art of horse-shoeing. Chicago: Alex Eger; 1898.
50. Chapman B, Platt GW. Laminitis and heart bar shoes. Brookfield (WI): American Farriers J; 2000.
51. Callcott MV, Chapman B. Convention preview: Chapman laminitis treatment. American Farriers J 1983;9(1):45–6.
52. Chapman B, Platt GW. Laminitis. Proc Annu Conv Am Assoc Equine Pract 1984;30:99–115.
53. Axe JW. The horse: its treatment in health and disease, vol. 6. London: Gresham; 1907.
54. Hodgins JE, Haskett TH. The veterinary science. London, Canada: The Voterinary Science Society; 1907.
55. Takahashi K, Young BA. Effects of grain overfeeding and histamine injection on physiological responses related to acute bovine laminitis. Jpn J Vet Sci 1981;43: 375–85.
56. Garner MR, Flint JF, Russell JB. *Allisonella histaminiformans* gen. nov., sp. nov. a novel bacterium that produces histamine, utilizes histidine as its sole energy source, and could play a role in bovine and equine laminitis. Syst Appl Microbiol 2002;25:498–506.
57. Martin WJ. Equine laminitis. Am J Vet Med 1916;11:297–302, 332–3.
58. Hall of fame vet says hold the bute! Am Farriers J 2006;32(6):23.
59. Backus ND. Lameness in the horse, with special reference to acute laminitis. J Am Vet Med Assoc 1937;91:64–72.
60. Turner AW. The etiology of laminitis. Aust Vet J 1937;13:254–6.
61. Rodebaugh HD. Surgical treatment of chronic laminitis. Vet Med 1938;33:288–9.
62. Redden RF. 18 degrees elevation of the heel as an aid to treating acute and chronic laminits in the equine. Proc Annu Conv Am Assoc Equine Pract 1992;375–9.
63. Goetz TE. The treatment of laminitis in horses. Vet Clin North Am Equine Pract 1989;5(1):73–108.
64. Moore RC. Equine laminitis or pododermatis. Am J Vet Med 1916;11:290.
65. McGuigan MP, Walsh TC, Pardoe CH, et al. Deep digital flexor tendon force and digital mechanics in normal ponies and ponies with rotation of the distal phalanx as a sequel to laminitis. Equine Vet J 2005;37:161–5.
66. Frank ER. Veterinary surgery notes. Minneapolis: Burgess Publishing Company; 1944.
67. Johnson JH. The foot in laminitis. Proc AAEP 1975;21:388–9.
68. Ritmeester AM, Blevins WE, Ferguson DW, et al. Digital perfusion, evaluated scintigraphically, and hoof wall growth in horses with chronic laminitis treated with egg bar-heart bar shoeing and coronary grooving. Equine Vet J Suppl 1998;26:111–8.
69. Thomas EF. Autogenous blood therapy in laminitis. North Am Vet 1945;26: 278–9.

70. Adams OR. Lameness in horses. 2nd edition. Philadelphia: Lea & Febiger; 1966.
71. Chevance J. Histamine theory and treatment of laminitis. Vet Med 1946;41: 199–201.
72. Nocek JE. Bovine acidosis: implications on laminitis. J Dairy Sci 1997;80:1018.
73. Garner HE, Coffman JR, Hahn AW, et al. Equine laminitis of alimentary origin: an experimental model. Am J Vet Res 1975;36:441–4.
74. Obel N. Studies on the histopathology of acute laminitis. Uppsala: Almqvist & Wiksells Boktryckeri AB; 1948.
75. Larsson B, Obel N, Aberg B. On the biochemistry of keratinization on the matrix of the horse's hoof in normal conditions and in laminitis. Nord Vet Med 1956;8: 761–76.
76. Jubin L. La fourbure du pied du cheval, these inaugurale. Lyon: A. Rey; 1908.
77. Straunard R. La fourbure du cheval. Paris: Jouve; 1918.
78. Abdin-Bey MR. Ätiologie und Pathogenese der Hufre beim Pferd—eine Literaturstudie [dissertation]. Hanover (Germany); 1984.
79. Taylor M. Treating founder without shoes. Hyannis (MA): Hoof Bond, Inc; 1988.
80. Eustace RA. Explaining laminitis and its prevention. Cherokee (AL): Life Data Labs; 1992.
81. Moore JN, Allen D. A guide to equine acute laminits. Trenton (NJ): Veterinary Learning Systems; 1995.
82. Coumbe K. All about laminitis. London: JA Allen; 1996.
83. Redden R. Understanding laminitis. Lexington (KY): Blood-Horse, Inc; 1998.
84. Hood DM, editor. The Veterinary Clinics of North America: Equine Practice, Laminitis. Philadelphia (PA): WB Saunders 1999;15(2).
85. King C, Mansmann RA. Preventing laminitis in horses. Cary (NC): Paper Horse; 2000.
86. USDA. Lameness and Laminitis in U.S. Horses. USDA: APHIS:VS, CEAH, National Animal Health Monitoring System. Fort Collins (CO). #N318.0400; 2000.
87. Jackson J. Founder prevention & cure the natural way. Harrison (AR): Star Ridge Publishing; 2001.
88. Pollitt C. Equine laminitis. Barton (Australia): RIRDC; 2001.
89. Ramey DW. Concise guide to laminitis. North Pomfret (VT): Trafalgar Square Publishing; 2003.
90. Strasser H. Who's afraid of founder? Qualicum Beach (Canada): Sabine Kells; 2003.
91. Hamilton-Fletcher R. Veterinary advice on laminitis. Dorking, Surrey (UK): Ringpress Books; 2004.
92. Butler KD, Gravlee F. Laminitis & founder: prevention and treatment for the greatest chance of success. Cherokee (AL): Life Data Labs, Incorporated; 2007.
93. Parker PM. Laminitis: Webster's timeline history 1887–2007. San Diego (CA): ICON Group, International; 2009.
94. American Farriers Journal, editors. 25 most frequently asked questions about laminitis, founder. Brookfield (WI): Lessiter Publications, Inc; 1997.
95. Buff E. How to successfully treat the foundered horse. Webster (NY): Esco Buff; 2000.
96. Buff E. The Founder Data Collection and Analysis — how to take, read and interpret radiographs for the prognosis and treatment of the foundered horse. Kearney (NE): Morris Publishing; 2005.
97. Sillence M, Asplin K, Pollitt C, et al. What causes equine laminitis? The role of impaired glucose uptake. Kingston (AU): Rural Industries Research and Development Corp; 2007.

98. Galey FD, Whiteley HE, Goetz TE, et al. Black walnut (*Juglans nigra*) toxicosis: a model for equine laminitis. J Comp Pathol 1991;104(3):313–26.
99. van Eps AW, Pollitt CC. Equine laminitis induced with oligofructose. Equine Vet J 2006;38(3):203–8.
100. Asplin KE, Sillence MN, Pollitt CC, et al. Induction of laminitis by prolonged hyperinsulinaemia in clinically normal ponies. Vet J 2007;174(3):530–5.
101. Rowe JB, Lees MJ, Pethick DW. Prevention of acidosis and laminitis associated with grain feeding in horses. J Nutr 1994;124:2742S–4S.
102. Said AH, Fahmy LS, Hegazy AA, et al. Dimethyl sulfoxide (DMSO) in the treatment of acute experimental laminitis in horses. Assiut Vet Med J 1992;27(53): 269–76.
103. Hood DM, Brumbaugh GW, Wagner IP. Effectiveness of a unique dihydropyridine (BAY TG 1000) for prevention of laminitis in horses. Am J Vet Res 2002; 63:443–7.
104. Heresbach C. Foure bookes of husbandrie. London: John Wright; 1586. p. 123–4.

80 Causes, Predispositions, and Pathways of Laminitis

Henry W. Heymering, CJF, RMF

KEYWORDS

• Laminitis • History • Founder • Equine

For most of history, the causes of laminitis have been based on observations. In the last 30 years or so, however, the number of theories has exploded, with only a few being confirmed by experiments. This article highlights these theories. **Box 1** lists these theories. Please note that included are simple theories, observations, disproved causes, and proved causes. Further information regarding these theories may be found elsewhere. The citations may speak for, or against, or both.

Of the dozens of suspected causes of laminitis, only five have been shown to reliably create laminitis for the purposes of research (starch,[52] black walnut,[37] oligofructose,[52] fructose,[53] and insulin[22]). Laminitis also has been caused experimentally by subcutaneous injection, or repeated intravenous injection, of histamine, and by lactic acid injected into the rumen of sheep.

8621A Hunters Drive, Frederick, MD 21701, USA
E-mail address: horseu@earthlink.net

Vet Clin Equine 26 (2010) 13–19
doi:10.1016/j.cveq.2009.12.003 vetequine.theclinics.com

Box 1
Possible causes of laminitis

Circulation

Theory only

- AVA shunts[1]
- Coagulopathy[2,3]
- Reperfusion[4,5]
- Starling forces—edema[6–8]
- Vasoconstriction[9]
- Vasodilation[8,10,11]

Observations

- Mechanical damage
  - Road founder[12,13]
  - Lack of circulation from inactivity, including supporting leg,[3] ship travel,[3] being kept in slings[13]
  - Trauma to the hoof—crushed under a wheel[13]
- Over-rehydration[6]

Endocrine

Theory only

- Equine Cushing disease[14]
- Equine metabolic syndrome[15]
- Estrogen (from plants[16] or pregnancy[17])
- Hyperadrenocorticism/cortisol[18]
- Insulin resistance[19]

Disproved causes

- Hypothyroidism[20,21]

Proved causes

- Insulin[22]

Observations

- Mares that do not come into heat[23]
- Mares that are in continual heat[23]
- Testosterone[24,25]

Enzymes

Theory only

- MMP2 & MMP9[8]

Hoof nutrients (lack)

Theory only

- Glucose[26]
- Methionine keratin synthesis blocked[27,28]

Inflammation/edema

Theory only

- Allergy[29]
- Iron excess[30,31]

Stress

Observations

- Colic[3]
- Cold snaps (John Arkley, Palmer AK, personal communication, June 2002)
- Draft/chill[13]
- Drinking cold water when hot[12]
- Heat[13,32]

Theory only

- Hypertension[33,34]
- Parturition[35]
- Standing in cold water after hard riding[12]
- Superpurgation[13]

Toxins

Theory only

- Avacado[36]
- Mercury[36]
- Rattlesnake venom[36]
- Red oak[36]
- Selenuim[36]

Observations

- Bee stings in great number (eg, 100 [Henry W. Heymering, CJF, RMF, personal observation, 1981])
- Endophytes[16,37]
- Endotoxins[38]
- Exotoxins[4,39]
- Histamine[29,40–42]
- Hoary alyssum (*Berteroa incana*)[43]
- Toxic amines[5,40]
- Infections
  - *Allisonella histiminiformans*[44]
  - *Balantidium coli*[40]
  - Bacterial lung infections[28]
  - Intestinal infections[36]
  - Lyme disease[45]
  - Potomac horse fever[46]
  - Retained placenta[21]
  - *Streptococcus equi*[36]
  - *Streptococcus bovis*[47]
  - Viral respiratory infections[23]

Proved causes
- Black walnut (*Juglans nigra*)[48]

Disproved causes
- Endotoxins[49]

Overeating
- Proved causes
  - Acidosis[41,50]
  - Carbohydrates (starch)[51]
  - Fructans[52]
- Observations
  - Beet tops[53]
  - Barley[12]
  - Grain[42]
  - Lactic acid[54,55]
  - Pasture[49]
- Theory
  - Protein[40,56]

Miscellaneous

Observations
- Abdominal surgery[57]
- Colic[6]
- Corticosteroid administration[58,59]
- Deworming/anthelmintics[53,58]
- Genetics[60]
- High nerving[43]
- Kidney disease (Burney Chapman, personal communication, 1992)
- Phenylbutazone[53]
- Strasser trim[61]
- Vaccinations[36,62]

Theory
- Fatty liver[63]
- Tumor necrosis factor[54]

REFERENCES

1. Robinson NE. Digital blood flow, arteriovenous anastomoses and laminitis. Equine Vet J 1990;22(6):381–3.
2. Hood DM, Gremmel SM, Amoss MS, et al. Equine laminitis III: coagulation dysfunction in the developmental and acute disease. J Equine Med Surg 1979; 39:355–60.

3. Rooney JR, Robinson JL. Laminitis. In: Rooney JR, Robinson JL, editors. Equine pathology. Ames (IA): Iowa State University Press; 1996. p. 188–93.
4. Hood DM, Grosenbaugh DA, Mostafa MB, et al. The role of vascular mechanisms in the development of acute equine laminitis. J Vet Intern Med 1993; 7(4):228–34.
5. Bailey SR. The pathogenesis of acute laminitis: fitting more pieces into the puzzle. Equine Vet J 2004;36:199–203.
6. West C. Bluegrass laminitis symposium: what we know about laminitis. Available at: http://www.thehorse.com/ViewArticle.aspx?ID=9247. Accessed December 20, 2009.
7. Butler KD, Gravlee F. Laminitis & founder: prevention and treatment for the greatest chance of success. Cherokee (AL): Life Data Labs, Incorporated; 2007.
8. Pollitt CC. Equine laminitis: a revised pathophysiology. AAEP Proceedings 1999; 45:188–92.
9. Coffman JR, Johnson JH, Guffy MM, et al. Hoof circulation in equine laminitis. J Am Vet Med Assoc 1970;156:76–83.
10. Trout DR, Horndoff WJ, Linford RL, et al. Scintigraphic evaluation of digital circulation during the developmental and acute phases of equine laminitis. Equine Vet J 1990;22:416–21.
11. Robinson NE, Scott JB, Dabney JM, et al. Digital vascular responses and permeability in equine alimentary laminitis. Am J Vet Res 1976;37:1171–4.
12. Smith F. The early history of veterinary literature. London: J.A. Allen; 1976. p. 27,48.
13. Zundel A. The horse's foot and its diseases. New York: Wm. R. Jenkins; 1886. p.172–3.
14. Donaldson MT. Equine Cushing's disease and laminitis. In: Proceedings of North American Veterinary Conference, vol. 18. Orlando (FL), January 17–21, 2004. p.118–20.
15. Johnson PJ. The equine metabolic syndrome (peripheral Cushing's syndrome). Vet Clin North Am Equine Pract 2002;18:271–93.
16. Rohrbach BW, Green EM, Oliver JW, et al. Aggregate risk study of exposure to endophyte-infected (Acremonium coenophialum) tall fescue as a risk factor for laminitis in horses. Am J Vet Res 1995;56(1):22–6.
17. Johnson PJ, Messer Iv NT, Ganjam SK, et al. Laminitis during pregnancy pathophysiological and practical considerations. In: Proceedings of the Fourth International Equine Conference on Laminitis and Diseases of the Foot. 2007. p. 1–11.
18. Johnson PJ, Messer NT, Wiedmeyer C, et al. Endocrinopathic laminitis in the horse. Clinical Techn Equine Pract 2004;3(1):45–56.
19. Coffman JR, Colles CM. Insulin tolerance in laminitic ponies. Can J Comp Med 1983;3:347–51.
20. Lowe JE, Baldwin BH, Foote RH, et al. Equine hypothyroidism: the long-term effects of thyroidectomy on metabolism and growth in mares and stallions. Cornell Vet 1974;64:276–95.
21. Stashak TS. Lameness. In: Stashak TS, editor. Adams' lameness in horses. 4th edition. Philadelphia: Lea & Febiger; 1987. p. 486–99.
22. Asplin KE, Sillence MN, Pollitt CC, et al. Induction of laminitis by prolonged hyperinsulinaemia in clinically normal ponies. Vet J 2007;174(3):530–5.
23. Stashak TS. Adam's lameness in horses. 4th edition. Philadelphia: Lea & Febiger; 1987. p. 487.
24. Dorn RC, Garner HE, Coffman JR, et al. Castration and other factors affecting the risk of equine laminitis. Cornell Vet 1975;65:57–64.

25. Amoss MS, Hood DM, Miller WG, et al. Equine laminitis: II. Elevation in serum testosterone associated with induced and naturally occurring laminitis. J Equine Med Surg 1979;3:171–5.
26. Pass MA, Pollitt S, Pollitt CC. Decreased glucose metabolism causes separation of hoof lamellae in vitro: a trigger for laminitis? Equine Vet J Suppl 1998;26:133–8.
27. Larsson B, Obel N, Aberg B. On the biochemistry of keratinization on the matrix of the horse's hoof in normal conditions and in laminitis. Nord Vet Med 1956;8: 761–76.
28. Adams OR. Lameness in horses. 3rd edition. Philadelphia: Lea & Febiger; 1974. p. 250.
29. Nilsson SA. Clinical morphological and experimental studies of laminitis in cattle. Acta Vet 1963;4(Suppl 1):1–304.
30. Pitzen D. Some laminitis problems in horses may be caused by excessive iron intake. Available at: http://74.125.93.132/search?q=cache:qztgQFipCN8J: www.naturalhorsetrim.com/Dan%2520Pitzen%2520on%2520excess%2520iron%2520and%2520laminitis.doc+Pitzen+iron&cd=4&hl=en&ct=clnk&gl=us&client=safari. Accessed December 21, 2009.
31. Pitzen D. The trouble with iron. Feed management 1993;44(6):9–10.
32. Jenkins D. Hot flash: laminitis. Am Farriers J 2004;30(4):86–9.
33. Merillat LA. The treatment of acute laminitis. Am J Vet Med 1920;15:535–7.
34. Hood DM. Current concepts of the physiopathology of laminitis. Proc Annu Conv Am Assoc Equine Pract 1980;25:13–20.
35. Martin WJ. Equine laminitis. Am J Vet Med 1916;11:297–302, 332–3.
36. Kellon E. Diseases leading to laminitis and the medical management of the laminitic horse. In: Floyd AE, Mansmann RA, editors. Equine podiatry. St. Louis (MO): Saunder Elsevier; 2007. p. 370–7.
37. Vanselow RU. Laminitis due to poisonous resistance factors in grass. The Farriers Journal 2009;137:6–10.
38. Hood DM, Stephens KA. Physiopathology of equine laminitis. Comp Cont Ed 1981;3(12):S455.
39. Mungall BA, Kyaw-Tanner M, Pollitt CC. In vitro evidence for a bacterial pathogenesis of equine laminitis. Vet Microbiol 2001;79:209–23.
40. Turner AW. The etiology of laminitis. Aust Vet J 1937;13:254–6.
41. Takahashi K, Young BA. Effects of grain overfeeding and histamine injection on physiological responses related to acute bovine laminitis. Jpn J Vet Sci 1981; 43:375–85.
42. Goetz TE. The treatment of laminitis in horses. Vet Clin North Am Equine Pract 1989;5(1):73–108.
43. Rooney JR, Roberston JL. Equine pathology. Ames (IA): Iowa University Press; 1996.
44. Garner MR, Flint JF, Russell JB. *Allisonella histaminiformans* gen. nov., sp. nov. a novel bacterium that produces histamine, utilizes histidine as its sole energy source, and could play a role in bovine and equine laminitis. Syst Appl Microbiol 2002;25:498–506.
45. Reilly F. Lyme disease laminitis—why it happens. Available at: http://equinemedsurg.com/Heiro%20article.html#lyme. Accessed December 21, 2009.
46. Mulville P. Equine monocytic ehrlichoisis (Potomac horse fever): a review. Equine Vet J 1991;23(6):400–4.
47. Rowe JB, Lees DW, Pethick DW, et al. Prevention of laminitis resulting from carbohydrate overload in horses. Australian Equine Vet 1994;12(1):29.

48. Galey FD, Whiteley HE, Goetz TE, et al. Black walnut (*Juglans nigra*) toxicosis: a model for equine laminitis. J Comp Pathol 1991;104(3):313–26.
49. Aristotle. History of animals books VII-X edited and translated by D.M. Balme. Cambridge (MA): Harvard University Press; 1927.
50. Butler D, Gravlee F. Laminitis and founder: prevention and treatment for the greatest chance of success. Cherokee (AL): Life Data Labs; 2007.
51. Garner HE, Coffman JR, Hahn AW, et al. Equine laminitis of alimentary origin: an experimental model. Am J Vet Res 1975;36:441–4.
52. van Eps AW, Pollitt CC. Equine laminitis induced with oligofructose. Equine Vet J 2006;38(3):203–9.
53. Adams OR. Lameness in horses. 2nd edition. Philadelphia: Lea & Febiger; 1966.
54. Hood DM, Brumbaugh GW, Wagner IP. Effectiveness of a unique dihydropyridine (BAY TG 1000) for prevention of laminitis in horses. Am J Vet Res 2002;63:443–7.
55. Morrow LL, Tumbleson ME, Kintner LD, et al. Laminitis in lambs injected with lactic acid. Am J Vet Res 1973;34:1305–7.
56. Frederick MF, Frederick S. Treating refractory laminitis: a field study of refractory laminitic cases that resolved on pergolide mesylate. In: 14th Annual Bluegrass Laminitis Symposium. Louisville (KY); 2001. p. 159–80.
57. Parsons CS, Orsini JA, Krafty R, et al. Risk factors for development of acute laminitis in horses during hospitalization: 73 cases (1997–2004). J Am Vet Med Assoc 2007;230(6):885–9.
58. Peremans K, Verschooten F, DeMoor A, et al. Laminitis in the pony: conservative treatment vs. dorsal hoof wall resection. Equine Vet J 1991;23(4):243.
59. Bailey SR, Elliott J. The corticosteroid laminitis story: 2. Science of if, when, and how. Equine Vet J 2007;39(1):7–11.
60. Hood DM, Beckham AS, Walker MA, et al. Genetic predisposition to chronic laminitis in horses. Proc Annu Conv Am Assoc Equine Pract 1994;40:45–6.
61. Heymering H. The Strasser method trim reconsidered. 2009, no.141 (December). p. 16–20.
62. Thomas EF. Autogenous blood therapy in laminitis. No Am Vet 1945;26:278–9.
63. Coffman JR. Chronic laminitis—fatty liver syndrome. Proc Annu Conv Am Assoc Equine Pract 1996;12:275–81.

Laminitis Treatment: A Personal Memoir

Donald M. Walsh, BS, DVM

KEYWORDS

• Equine • Laminitis • Farrier • Venogram

Memory is the selection of images, some elusive,
Others printed indelibly on the brain.
Each image is like a thread, each thread woven
Together to make a tapestry of intricate texture,
And the tapestry tells a story, and the story is our past.

"Eve's Bayou" Kasi Lemmons

This year I have completed 40 years as a veterinarian treating horses with laminitis. What follows is my recollection of the experience, of things that I have been told and ways I have tried to treat the disease. I consider myself one of the many veterinarians who have been humbled by laminitis while trying to treat its painful effects and intense suffering. So this is my story of treating laminitis.

In 1967, as a third year veterinary student, my first case in the University of Missouri Equine Clinic was a pony that belonged to a good friend. The pony had laminitis and was euthanized because of severe rotation of the distal phalanx. I asked my instructor what caused this to happen, dismayed that we could do nothing for my friend's pony. He said, "We don't know for sure but we think it is caused by histamine." "Can't we use antihistamine," I asked. "Yes," he said, "but antihistamines don't work very well in the horse, but corticosteroids do seem to help. There is also a new drug available now—phenylbutazone, but it's expensive. A 1-gram pill costs $1.00. You give 1 gram a day if the owner can afford it, but your friend's pony was too far gone for any drugs to help." There were no treatments available then, specifically for the feet, other than soaking; some people soaked the horse's feet in cold water and others used warm water.

In 1968, on my summer break between my third and fourth year of veterinary school, I worked in Paris, Kentucky with Dr Gordon Layton. A thoroughbred mare with a fever and diarrhea developed severe laminitis. She survived but was chronically lame after the episode. She was a valuable mare and was kept on phenylbutazone to keep her comfortable. However, she could barely walk from then on. We also saw a very fat pony with deformed feet and he could barely walk as well. We trimmed his ski-toed

Homestead Veterinary Hospital, 3615 Basset Road, Pacific, MO 63069, USA
E-mail address: walshvet@gmail.com

Vet Clin Equine 26 (2010) 21–28
doi:10.1016/j.cveq.2009.12.010 vetequine.theclinics.com
0749-0739/10/$ – see front matter

feet, put him on thyroid medication, and put him in a dry lot. He seemed to improve but still could not walk normally.

Colonel Sager, the long-time head veterinarian at Claiborne Farm, told us that in World War I the French and American horses often developed laminitis because the soldiers, when they arrived at a town, would overfeed them grain, trying to get some nutrition into the starving horses. Laminitis frequently occurred. The Americans rested their horses and tied them, standing in a creek if possible. The French troops forced theirs to keep moving during the laminitic attack. The Colonel said the French horses made better recoveries. Because the Colonel's word was "like God had spoken" in those days, I always held this information in high regard.

These 3 cases were the extent of my experience and knowledge about laminitis when I graduated from the University of Missouri Veterinary School in 1969 and went into private practice.

The first case of laminitis I attended in practice was a pony that broke into the grain room. I gave it mineral oil and dexamethasone for 5 days. The pony only showed minor Obel grade 1 symptoms for the first day. I had been successful with my first case and thought, "this isn't so difficult."

During the next few years Drs Harold Garner and James Coffman did a considerable amount of research at the University of Missouri showing that the starch overload model induced severe laminitis and caused considerable changes to the bacterial flora of the gut. Although it seemed that this model would enable improved treatment of laminitis, very little changed. We still used phenylbutazone and dexamethasone. There was talk that the horses were developing thrombosis in the vessels in the feet, and heparin was advocated with little or no success.

It was during this time in the mid-1970s that we started seeing horses develop laminitis, which were bedded on wood shavings. The typical call from a stable would be that they had 5 or 6 horses, all with acute laminitis. When the veterinarian arrived the horses were led out of the stalls. When these horses walked they had the typical posture of acute laminitis, but unlike typical laminitis all 4 legs were swollen, like stovepipes, up to the knees and hocks. If these horses were examined quickly and given a large dose of dexamethasone (20 mg) they would look normal the next day. However, if the treatment was delayed until the second day they would develop severe laminitis in all 4 feet, and many had to be put down.

Soon we discovered that the shavings had black walnut heartwood in them. The horses that normally ate new shavings were always the victims. For a while it was thought that something was being absorbed through the feet but my stable manager pointed out that the horses that regularly ate shavings, when their stalls were rebedded, were the ones showing signs.

It was about this time that we also recognized that corticosteroids administered to some horses could cause laminitis, and everyone stopped giving it to horses with laminitis. I continued to always use it on black walnut shavings cases. Eventually all the shavings suppliers were aware of the problem and avoided black walnut contamination of their supplies. By the early 1980s we rarely saw black walnut laminitis cases.

Now the laminitis group at Missouri included Dr Jim Moore, and they became convinced that endotoxin, released by the death of gram-negative bacteria, was causing the laminitis. A laminitis symposium was held at the University of Missouri and a great debate regarding the blood supply to the foot ensued. Was it increased or decreased during the start of laminitis? It is a question still debated today.

It was during this time that I began to question if phenylbutazone was really helping horses. I asked Dr Garner if the horses they induced to Obel grade 3 laminitis recovered. His reply was that most of them returned to normal after a month or so and a few stayed lame longer. I asked if he treated them and he replied that they were just turned out in paddocks. Soon after that I visited Dr David Hood at Texas A&M University and asked him the same question, because he was also inducing laminitis in horses. He told me that all of his horses got sore (Obel grade 3) and after the experiment they were given 4 g of phenylbutazone a day; however, most of them had to be euthanized because they were so severely foundered. Garner and Hood were inducing laminitis with a starch overload. At that time I was also wondering if we were overtreating horses with nonsteroidal anti-inflammatory drugs. Many veterinarians are now using phenylbutazone and flunixin (Banamine) in large doses on their laminitis cases. I never used both at the same time and from that time onward wondered about their benefit in treating laminitis. Is reducing the pain helpful or would it be better for the horse to seek relief by lying down and reducing the load on the laminae? My experience has proven the latter to be more helpful in recovery.

I remember telling Dr Garner in the mid-1980s that I thought there was a form of laminitis that was slow coming on, in overweight horses and ponies. It started with changes in the feet that gradually got worse and worse until the horses developed a full-blown attack of clinical laminitis. On my first visit to see them, their feet had chronic changes, dropped soles, and radiographs that showed stretching of the laminae causing an unparallel dorsal hoof wall relative to the distal phalanx. The owners claimed that the animal had never taken a lame step until that day. I doubted them because many of these cases were owned by backyard-horse people who kept them in a pasture. They were fat and seldom ridden.

But then a really good horseman presented one of these cases to me, and swore that the horse had never been lame and was used regularly. I then realized that this was a slow form of laminitis. I now realize that this was a separate form of laminitis, best recognized by farriers regularly observing the feet. I met with our local farriers' association and asked them to watch and see if I was correct. A year later they told me that I was correct and that, because many of these horses and ponies were trimmed infrequently, they just had not noticed the changes occurring.

Today good farriers often tell owners that their animal is developing changes in its feet and to call their veterinarian. All too frequently the veterinarian cannot see any obvious painful signs and tells the owner that the horse does not have laminitis. We now are beginning to understand the long-term adverse effects of high levels of insulin and other hormone changes in these overweight horses and ponies, and their tendency to show symptoms of laminitis after grass consumption.

It was about this time when more efforts were focused on treating the feet of the horse to prevent rotation. Hoof casts enjoyed some popularity for a short time, but often resulted in disaster, with the feet sloughing because of excess pressure. A farrier named Burney Chapman and a veterinarian named Dr George Platt started using a shoe that had been around for a long time, described in the US Cavalry Manual, known as a heartbar shoe. Chapman and Platt incorporated this shoe with a complete hoof wall resection of the dorsal hoof wall to allow the foot to regrow without any rotation. For the first time a farrier (Burney Chapman) gave a presentation at the American Association of Equine Practitioners convention.

Insurance companies became interested in this treatment and decided that it might save horses with severe laminitis, and therefore prevent having to pay claims for horses euthanized because of laminitis. The insurance industry held a big free meeting in Lexington, Kentucky in 1985, inviting speakers to promote this radical new procedure. This was the start of Dr Ric Redden's annual Bluegrass Laminitis Symposium. The problem with promoting this procedure among farriers and veterinarians was that it was designed for only the most severe cases, and resulted in ponies with mild laminitis being shod with heartbar shoes and having dorsal hoof wall resections. Other problems were that it really did not prevent a lamellar wedge from forming when the new hoof wall grew back down the foot, and that the resection of the dorsal wall sometimes destabilized the remaining medial and lateral hoof walls, and weakened the foot even more. There was never any controlled study to justify the procedure and although some horses made good recoveries, it lost favor over time and was discontinued.

During this period isoxsuprine, advocated as a treatment for navicular disease, was supposed to increase blood flow to the foot, hence people started using it to treat laminitis. This drug was used for years before any testing was done, and the tests showed that it had no effect on the blood flow to the foot.

The success of the heartbar shoe in helping horses led to the development of different types of frog support systems, such as Lily-Pads (Therapeutic Equine Products, Inc, Shelbyville, KY, USA), which are rubber pads that could be taped onto the horse's foot at the first signs of laminitis. Theraflex Pads (Thera-Flex, Inc, Lawrenceburg, KY, USA) had a frog support on the solar surface of a full pad. It was at this time that we started to recognize the value of moving the breakover of the foot back under the foot and unloading the dorsal laminae of the foot. The concept of the reverse shoe or the opened toe heartbar was a major help in relieving pain in the laminae. In my opinion this was the most significant improvement that occurred during my time in practice.

My frustration and confusion in treating laminitis drove me to look for other sources of information. In my practice area there lived a man who would best be described as a "lay practitioner." He had treated and rehabilitated horses with laminitis for many years. I recalled, as a boy, hearing about him and his renowned ability to treat laminitis. I remembered many cases over the years that were not improving or that shortly after diagnosis had disappeared, with the owner telling me that the horses had been taken to this man for treatment. Often the horses were gone for months, and I recall as a young veterinarian thinking that the man must have failed to improve a particularly refractory case that had been removed from my care. Then one day the horse reappeared and the owner said that it was good as new. I remember that the horse was standing in a paddock and, as I stared in disbelief, the horse turned away and galloped off with its tail over its back. The horse had been at the lay practitioner's place.

The man's name was Harry Bond. He was secretive about what he did to treat the horses because he had made his living doing this for years. Dr Coffman had once driven from the University of Missouri to Harry's home in Staunton, Illinois, to try to learn what he did to treat laminitis. The trip was a waste of his time; Harry revealed nothing. The nearest veterinarian to Harry was Dr Bill Brown, a well-known racetrack veterinarian, and I called him to find out what he knew about Harry and his treatment. To my surprise Dr Brown told me that he referred all his cases of laminitis to him because he hated treating them and Harry got good results. He knew more than most people about Harry's methods. He told me that Harry worked on the horse's feet daily; he put a substance on the sole of the foot and ignited it to cauterize the soles every day. He told me that he thought the cauterization somehow desensitized the sole pain and enabled the horse to walk, and he knew that part of the treatment involved ponying the horse with his old mare.

Dr Brown's testimonial convinced me that I needed to find out more about Harry's methods. By this time I had started the Animal Health Foundation, a nonprofit organization, to raise money to fund laminitis research. On my Board of Directors was a person who knew Harry well and had taken several horses with laminitis to him. He offered to introduce me, but I was skeptical that Harry would tell me anything.

I just happened to have at that time a large, part-draft mare that had severe unilateral laminitis in a rear foot. This was a case of supporting-limb laminitis that developed during the successful treatment of an injury and infection in the tendons of the opposite leg. The mare had broken open at the coronary band and the distal phalanx was penetrating the sole. We decided to take her over to Harry; this would give me a chance to meet him after having known of him for about 25 years. In brief, Harry and I became good friends. He was in his eighties then, and perhaps teaching me his methods allowed him to continue to see horses. I would drive over and pick him up and he would come with me to look at cases, then I would drive him home again. The driving time to do this was about 4 hours, hence it gave us a lot of time to talk about laminitis.

His treatment involved an examination to classify if the horse had infected, open, or closed feet. If there were any open areas of the soles or coronary band, then the feet were soaked in a weak solution of Lysol disinfectant. They were treated with iodoform ointment, which he made and placed on any open spots. Large cotton pads were then placed on the soles and the feet put inside denim boots that were made by cutting off worn-out blue jeans legs and sewing the bottoms shut. The horses were bedded in deep straw. As their feet healed and the soles closed, they were then treated like the horses with closed soles.

The feet of horses with intact soles were trimmed and Harry would cauterize the soles by igniting a solution made of turpentine, pine tar, iodine crystals, and mothballs. He would cauterize the feet every day and then put a strong white liniment on the coronary bands, then walk them, gradually increasing the exercise. Their diet was grass hay if they were fat, and if not fat, they received hay plus 0.9 kg of a mixture of 3-parts oats to 1-part bran. He removed all drugs except a handful of juniper berries morning and evening. When horses first arrived he often treated them with a mixture of 4 ounces of coffee, 4 ounces of sweet spirits of niter (ethyl nitrite), and 2 tablespoons ginger, 3 times a day. These medications usually produced a diuretic effect on the horse after administration. After President Ford introduced legislation that all alcohol-containing products be removed from over-the-counter sales, spirits of niter became no longer available; hence Harry substituted it with whiskey.

Ethyl nitrite is a powerful vasodilator, as is alcohol. Harry taught me that movement was good and an essential part of recovery, but at the right time. If exercise was done too early the horse would become worse. Harry's method appeared more of an art, but was actually based on sound medical principles.

The Animal Health Foundation received many donated horses during this time that owners could not afford to keep treating. These were horses that had failed to respond to conventional therapy and had true refractory laminitis; thus I was given the perfect situation to try Harry's method. Most of these horses arrived on high levels of phenylbutazone and to my surprise, when the phenylbutazone was stopped, they really looked to be in no severe pain. Many were thin with decubitus ulcers from lying on their sides all the time. The combination of Harry's treatment and foot care that moved the breakover back under the foot enabled many of these cases to make a good recovery. Today, some 25 years later, we are still using Harry's methods on laminitis cases at the Homestead Veterinary Hospital in Pacific, Missouri.

In 1990, Dr Redden started advocating raising the heels on laminitis cases, about 2 in, to remove the pull of the deep digital flexor tendon (DDFT). If initiated early in the disease, this was supposed to stop rotation of the distal phalanx. Dr Redden also was an advocate of cutting the deep flexor tendon to reduce the pull of the DDFT. At first, this was thought of as a salvage procedure for chronically rotated feet, but later it was advocated earlier in the disease, before rotation. If necessary the procedure was repeated, if the palmar angle of the distal phalanx started to increase.

This procedure is still used by practitioners who believe that the DDFT is the cause of rotation. It was also used in cases of chronic rotation when there was contracture of the DDFT; it gave relief to the animal and with careful hoof trimming allowed derotation of the distal phalanx. After initial success, after the tendon healed many horses slowly (more than a year or longer) returned to the same painful conformation, especially those that had suffered bone loss of the distal phalanx. However, some horses did remain in a state of reduced pain and became usable again. Controversy still surrounds this procedure, with mixed opinions regarding its usefulness.

Dr Redden has been one of the most innovative veterinary clinicians over the years. He has developed many shoes, such as the Redden Ultimate (heel elevation with improved breakover) and the Rocker Banana shoe. Many people are supporters of his theories and believe that his products have helped many horses. Dr Redden's annual Bluegrass Laminitis Symposium from 1986 to 2005 provided a wonderful forum to share information with people from around the world who were interested in the horse's foot.

A useful tool to gain more information about the circulation in the foot came about as the result of a video that was presented at Dr Redden's meeting in 1992 by Dr Chris Pollitt of Australia. It was entitled "Equine Foot Studies" and showed aspects of the circulation of the horse's foot using "state of the art" (for the 1990s) radiographic imaging techniques. Dr Pollitt injected radiopaque dye into the arterial blood supply of a cadaver foot and then loaded the foot with a hydraulic press. He demonstrated that the arterial blood flow was stopped during full weight bearing. He also showed that raising the heel allowed blood to enter the foot during weight bearing via a dorsal coronary branch. This gave more credence to raising the heel during laminitis, but did not definitely show that it worked.

This initial study led him to develop a method of injecting dye into the venous circulation with a tourniquet at the fetlock to outline the venous circulation. He called this technique a venogram. It was hoped that the information contained in a venogram would improve methods of treating feet. At first, it was used to show that some horses had no hope of recovery and so it would be better to euthanize them before a long, painful attempt to treat them. As time went on and more venograms were done, the technique became useful to indicate when more aggressive therapy could be initiated to treat laminitis. It has also come into use to monitor the progress of the recovery and response to different types of corrective shoeing and application of foot devices such as clogs. Over the last 15 years, venograms have been the only additional information, besides the standard radiograph, to evaluate the circulation of the foot of horses with laminitis. Today, with the availability of computed tomography and magnetic resonance imaging, much more information is becoming available to help evaluate circulation in feet, but it has had no significant effect on improving treatment as yet.

In the mid-1990s a farrier named Gene Ovnicek developed a shoe to treat laminitis that incorporated the use of rails on the medial and lateral side of the shoe. The rails were elevated more at the heel, and the toe of the shoe was rolled and the breakover occurred back under the foot. The rails seemed to reduce the torque on the laminae when the horse turned, and this made many horses more comfortable. This shoe gave rise to the Equine Digit Support System (Equine Digit Support System, Inc, CO, USA), which enabled farriers to alter the rail by having interchangeable rails and frog supports of different heights. These can be screwed into the shoe and if the horse does not seem comfortable, they can be replaced with a different size without removing the shoe.

Derotation is the process of reestablishing a more normal palmar angle to the distal phalanx by lowering the heel of the horse's foot. Derotation helps reestablish normal blood flow and repositions the hoof capsule relative to the distal phalanx. After this is done, the heel of the shoe is then elevated to make the horse walk heel-down first, and then toe. This is accomplished by increasing the heel height of the wedge rails until the horse walks heel-toe.

Coronary grooving is a technique that has been around for a long time, and has gained and lost favor; it is currently enjoying more use. A groove is cut into the dorsal hoof wall at the coronary band across the entire dorsal part of the hoof. This relieves the pinching at the coronary band and a venogram reveals that venous filling is reestablished. It is only necessary in the more severe cases of laminitis, but seems beneficial. The new hoof wall grows down with less deformity and at a more normal rate. It is difficult to know where this technique first started, but it can be found in the old literature.

In the last 5 years the acceptance and use of the Steward Clog has improved the lives of many chronic laminitic horses. Dr Mike Steward started applying wooden shoes on horses with laminitis and took note of the way the horse wore down the wood. He built wooden clogs that mimicked the wear pattern and tried applying them to horse's feet. He found that it offered them an improved range of movement in foot breakover at the toe and heel. It also increased sole support, which resulted in marked improvement in their comfort. These clogs are inexpensive and can be screwed and glued on the feet, avoiding the discomfort of hammering nails into the hoof.

With the exception of pergolide there have been no new drugs proven to be successful in treating laminitis. In the late-1990s low-dose pergolide was used successfully to treat pituitary adenoma, or as we now call it pituitary pars intermedia dysfunction, associated with equine Cushing disease. It was found to be successful in preventing repeated attacks of laminitis in these horses. Pituitary pars intermedia dysfunction, and the laminitis associated with it, had been driving practitioners crazy while trying to prevent recurrent attacks. At that time we had not sorted out the differences between equine Cushing horses and equine metabolic syndrome, therefore all of them were treated in the same way, with varying results. We now know that insulin resistance results in high circulating levels of insulin, and that hyperinsulinemia is associated with laminitis in Cushing disease and equine metabolic syndrome. Diet and exercise are the best treatment for insulin resistance, but equine Cushing horses need pergolide to control their insulin levels. Thyroid medication has also been used for years to treat the obesity in these animals with some success. If affected animals can lose weight, this seems to improve their insulin resistance and reduce the frequency of recrudescent bouts of laminitis. Many of these cases are given supplements containing magnesium and chromium, but no scientific study has proven them to be effective. These are the same horses that when exposed to high carbohydrate grass or hay develop clinical laminitis.

In recent years a better understanding of what factors play a role in developing high levels of carbohydrates in grass has enabled horse owners to prevent laminitis in their animals. Kathryn Watts' research, which showed that soaking hay in water before feeding significantly reduces carbohydrate levels in the hay, has been a great help in managing horses with difficult-to-control insulin resistance. This group of horses, that we call "easy keepers," may require a completely different nutritional management regimen to regular horses. Perhaps they are designed by nature to endure a period of dramatically reduced caloric intake in the winter, using their insulin-resistant state to live on their fat stores until spring arrives. It has always been difficult for me to understand why an animal eating its natural food would develop laminitis. Proper husbandry practices may eliminate this most commonly seen form of laminitis, once we completely understand the endocrinology and metabolic processes involved.

Today the only proven therapy that has been shown to prevent acute laminitis is the application of cold ice water from the knees and the hock down to the feet. This work, done by Drs Andrew van Eps and Chris Pollitt of Australia, scientifically proved that by icing the limbs, laminitis could be prevented in horses undergoing a carbohydrate induction of laminitis. The usefulness of icing after symptoms have started has not been proven in any trials to date. This treatment, along with encouraging the horse to lie down in a deep bed when not being iced, is listed in the US Calvary Manual for Stable Sergeants 1917 to treat laminitis in horses.

When we look back at the history of laminitis treatments we seem to recycle many types of treatment, and I think this is because we think that they are helping. Then because they do not work in all cases, we resort to trying other treatments. Laminitis is a difficult disease in which to compare the clinical results of treatments, because the degree of damage varies greatly from case to case and even from foot to foot. Perhaps this is evidence to support the concept that some cases will recover regardless of the treatment, and some cases are destined to fail no matter what we try to do for them.

Until we completely understand the pathophysiology of all the forms of laminitis, we will never know if we are treating them properly. Even then, because of the rapid severe damage that occurs so quickly, we will not always be successful. Nevertheless, if we had a true understanding of laminitis pathophysiology, we should be able to prevent many cases from occurring.

In closing, I would like to say that this article is not meant to be a complete review of the veterinary literature of laminitis for the last 40 years, but my personal recollection. I have greatly enjoyed practicing veterinary medicine for the last 4 decades. I am proud of the veterinary profession and of the many advancements that have been made in caring for animals. However, I must admit that I think the continued lack of a complete understanding of laminitis is an embarrassment to our profession. We need to free the horse of this disease and we need to do it now. Hopefully, one day I will get to write my final article on the treatment of laminitis, which will get to include that success story.

The Anatomy and Physiology of the Suspensory Apparatus of the Distal Phalanx

Christopher C. Pollitt, BVSc, PhD[a,b]

KEYWORDS

- Equine hoof wall • Secondary epidermal lamellae
- Suspensory apparatus • Distal phalanx
- Basement membrane • Hemidesmosome • Laminitis

Research into the structure and function of the suspensory apparatus of the distal phalanx (SADP) has proven fundamental to the understanding of how laminitis develops (**Fig. 1**). This review reports the results of recent studies on the normal structure and function of the equine hoof wall, its internal lamellar layer, the adjacent dermis and the parietal surface of the distal phalanx.

The hoof wall consists of 3 layers: the stratum externum, stratum medium, and stratum internum. The stratum medium is the thickest of the 3 layers and is characterized by its tubular and intertubular horn structure (**Fig. 2**). It is the main load support system of the equine foot[1] and serves, via the SADP, to transfer ground reaction forces to the appendicular skeleton.[2]

Members of the mammalian family Equidae represent the extreme result of unguligrade evolution. Single digits, encased in tough, keratinized hooves, on the end of lightweight limbs, have undoubtedly contributed to the speed and versatility of the soliped equids. This characteristic makes the horse (and the other Equidae) unique in the animal kingdom. The tough, hoof capsule protects the softer, more sensitive, structures within and allows the natural horse to gallop over dry, rocky terrain with apparent impunity. But at a price. Immobility and crippling result if the connection between hoof and bone, the SADP, fails.

Portions of this article previously appeared in Pollitt CC. Anatomy and physiology of the inner hoof wall. Clin Tech Equine Pract 2004;3:3–21.

[a] School of Veterinary Science, The University of Queensland, St Lucia, Brisbane, Queensland 4072, Australia

[b] The Laminitis Institute, University of Pennsylvania School of Veterinary Medicine, New Bolton Center, Kennett Square, PA, USA

E-mail address: c.pollitt@mailbox.uq.edu.au

Vet Clin Equine 26 (2010) 29–49
doi:10.1016/j.cveq.2010.01.005 **vetequine.theclinics.com**
0749-0739/10/$ – see front matter

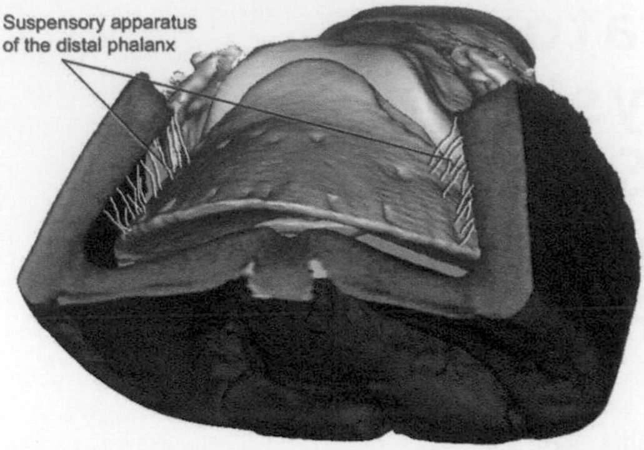

Fig. 1. The distal phalanx is suspended within the hoof capsule by the suspensory apparatus. The SADP (a small part of which is shown here diagrammatically) attaches the entire parietal surface of the distal phalanx to the lamellae of the inner hoof wall. Diagram created from computed tomography (CT) data using MIMICS software (Materialise, Leuven, Belgium).

HOOF WALL GROWTH

The hoof wall grows throughout the life of the horse to replace hoof lost to wear and tear at the ground surface. Continual regeneration of the hoof wall occurs at the coronet, where germinal cells (epidermal basal cells) produce populations of daughter cells (keratinocytes or keratin-producing cells) that mature and keratinize, continually

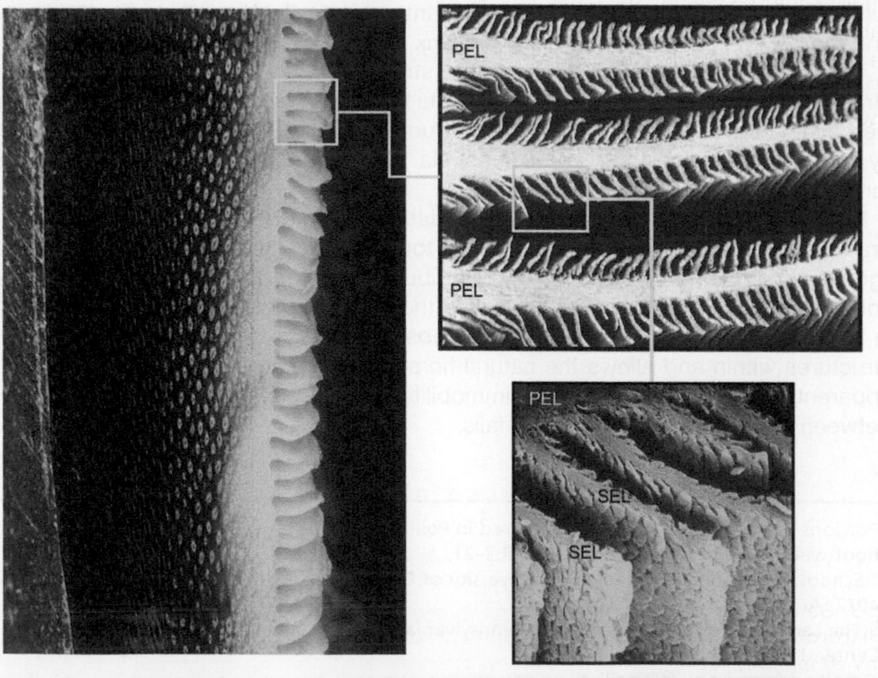

Fig. 2. The equine hoof wall and its inner lamellar layer. Secondary epidermal lamellae (SELs) increase the surface area of each leaflike primary epidermal lamella (PEL). Epidermal basal cells cover the surface of each SEL. (*From* Pollitt CC. Anatomy and physiology of the inner hoof wall. Clin Tech Equine Pract 2004;3:4; with permission.)

adding to the proximal hoof wall. Similarly, mitosis in the proximal hoof primary epidermal lamellae (PELs) also occurs.[3] Although mitotic figures among the basal cells of the proximal lamellar zone are easily observed, there is no convincing evidence that the more distal lamellae proliferate at all. The fundamental question is: how do the inner hoof wall lamellae remain attached to the connective tissue embedded on the surface of the stationary distal phalanx, while one moves over the other? Is it by continuous proliferation of the lamellar epidermis (laminar flow) or by some other remodeling process (which may somehow be involved in laminitis pathogenesis)? Cells in mitosis are rarely, if ever, found in normal lamellae below the proximal, proliferative zone. To determine precisely where in the hoof wall epidermal cell proliferation occurs, a proliferative index (PI) for basal cells of the coronet, lamellae and toe of the dorsal hoof wall of ponies has been calculated.[4] The thymidine analog (5-bromo-2′-deoxyuridine or BRdU), injected intravenously into living ponies, was incorporated into all cells undergoing mitosis, during a 1-hour study period. Histologic sections of hoof tissue were stained immunohistochemically, using monoclonal antibodies against BRdU. As expected the highest PI values (mean ± standard error) were in the coronet: 12.04% ± 1.59 and proximal lamellae (7.13% ± 1.92) (**Fig. 3**).

These are the growth zones of the proximal hoof wall (**Fig. 4**). Distal to this the PI values of more distal lamellae were lower. They ranged from 0.11% ± 0.04 to 0.97% ± 0.29; significantly lower ($P<.05$) than the proximal lamellar growth zone. Evidence for a constant supply of new cells in the lamellar region, generating a downward laminar flow, was not provided by this study. The few proliferating cells detected in the main lamellar region had a patchy distribution and were located at the PEL tips, not in cap-horn arcades. A 20-fold PI decrease between proximal and more distal lamellae suggests that most of the normal lamellae are nonproliferative and their main function is to suspend the distal phalanx within the hoof capsule. However, the most distal lamellae and the tubular hoof of the white line and dorsal sole had a PI approaching the proximal hoof, as expected in a zone in which considerable new hoof production occurs to create the white line and sole (**Fig. 5**).

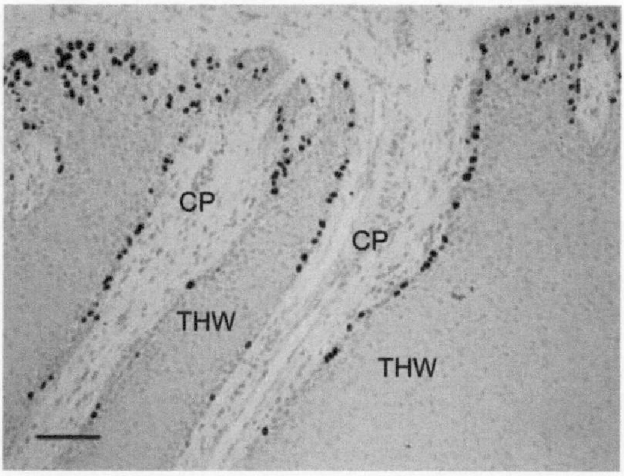

Fig. 3. Basal cell proliferation in the coronary band. Longitudinal section of proximal hoof wall (coronary band) immunostained for BRdU that was injected intravenously into a normal pony 60 minutes previously. The positive, brown staining, cells are basal cells that incorporated BRdU as they underwent mitosis during the previous 60 minutes. The tubular and intertubular hoof show a high rate of basal cell mitosis. CP, coronary papilla; THW, tubular hoof wall; bar = 100 μm. (*From* Pollitt CC. Anatomy and physiology of the inner hoof wall. Clin Tech Equine Pract 2004;3:6; with permission.)

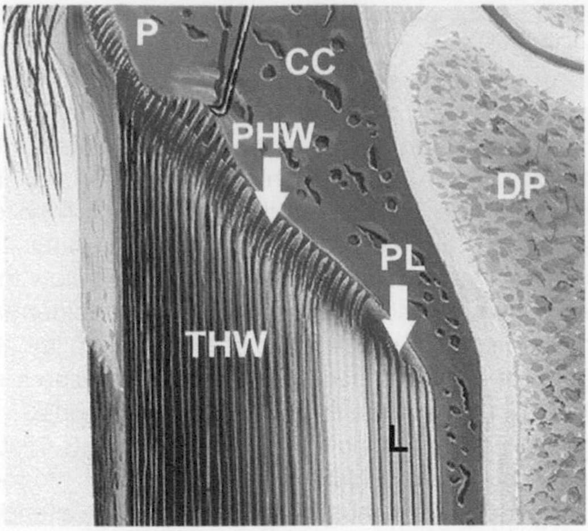

Fig. 4. The growth zones of the hoof (highlighted in red) are confined to the top or proximal region of the wall. Basal cells of the tubular hoof wall and periople proliferate nonstop throughout the life of the horse. The proximal lamellae also proliferate at a rate similar to the hoof wall proper, but the rate is near zero in the lamellar regions below this. CC, coronary corium; DP, distal phalanx; P, periople; PHW, proximal hoof wall; PL, proximal lamellae; THW, tubular hoof wall; L, lamellae. (*From* Pollitt CC. Anatomy and physiology of the inner hoof wall. Clin Tech Equine Pract 2004;3:7; with permission.)

Remodeling within the hoof wall epidermal lamellae, which must occur as the hoof wall moves past the stationary distal phalanx, seems to be a process not requiring epidermal cell proliferation. Remodeling of epidermis and the extracellular matrix (ECM) to which it is attached probably involves the controlled release of activated matrix metalloproteinases (MMPs) and their subsequent inhibition by tissue inhibitors

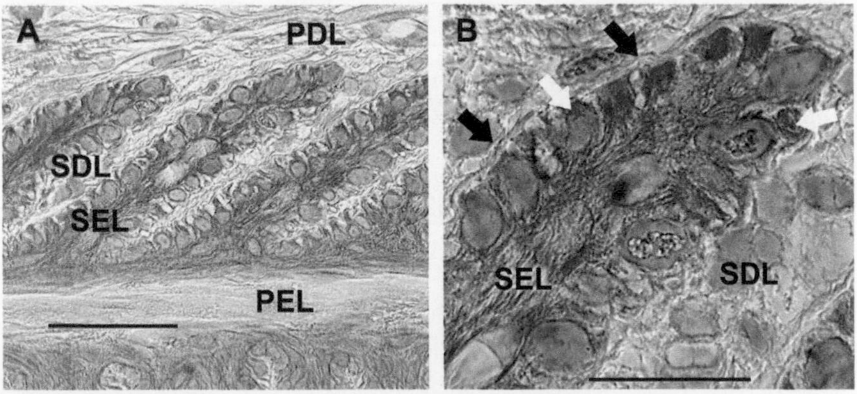

Fig. 5. Immunostaining of normal hoof SEL with anti-MMP-2. Dark brown, positive cytoplasmic staining was located mainly in lamellar basal and parabasal cells (*A*). PEL and primary dermal lamellae (PDL) did not stain. Basal cell MMP-2 of SELs (*B*) was located in cytoplasm (*solid white arrows*) adjacent to the BM (*solid black arrows*). Nuclei of epidermal cells and fibroblasts stained blue by the hematoxylin counterstain. (*A*) Bar = 50 μm; bar; (*B*) bar = 20 μm. (*From* Pollitt CC. Equine laminitis: current concepts. Rural Industrial Research and Development Corporation, 2008. Publication no. 08/062. Kingston, Australia; with permission.)

of metalloproteinases (TIMPs).[5] MMPs have been shown to exist in lamellar hoof (**Fig. 6**)[6] and their uncontrolled activation has been proposed as a mechanism for the pathogenesis of laminitis.[6,7]

The molecular components of desmosomes, hemidesmosomes (HDs), and basement membranes (BMs) are substrates for MMP activity,[5] so the mechanistic concept[8] of formation and destruction of desmosomes in a staggered ratchetlike manner now has a well-referenced, biologic explanation. Lamellar epidermal cells and their adjacent BM are constantly responding to the stresses and strains of growth and locomotion by releasing MMPs and TIMPs to accomplish whatever cellular reorganization is required. Because this involves enzymes capable of destroying key components of the attachment apparatus between distal phalanx and inner hoof wall, triggering this loaded gun has dire consequences for the future health of the foot. Inadvertent or uncontrolled lamellar MMP activation makes horses, with their evolutionary reliance on a single digit per limb, uniquely susceptible to the destructive effects of laminitis.

HOOF WALL TUBULES

Examination of the hoof capsule, with its contents removed, shows thousands of small, circular holes pocking the surface of the concave, coronary groove (**Fig. 7**). A sagittal section of the proximal hoof wall shows that the holes continue distally into the body of the wall for 4 to 5 mm, gradually tapering to a point. A layer of confluent epidermal basal cells covers the surface of the holes and the surface of the coronary groove between the holes.

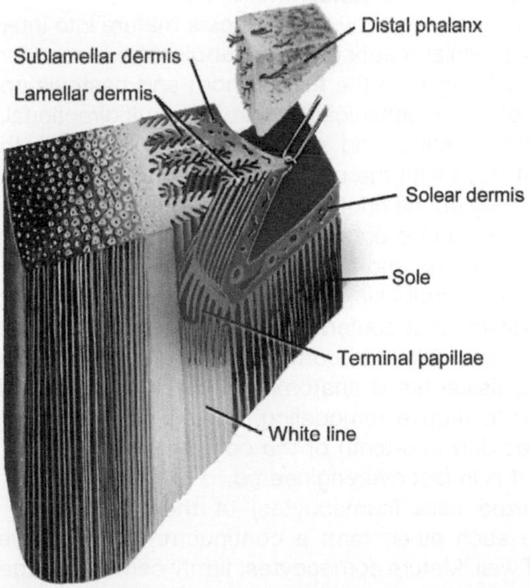

Fig. 6. The growth zones of the distal hoof (highlighted in red). Epidermal basal cells of the distal lamellae, white line and sole tubules, similar to the proximal hoof, also proliferate non-stop throughout the life of the horse. (*From* Pollitt CC. Equine laminitis: current concepts. Rural Industrial Research and Development Corporation, 2008. Publication no. 08/062. Kingston, Australia; with permission.)

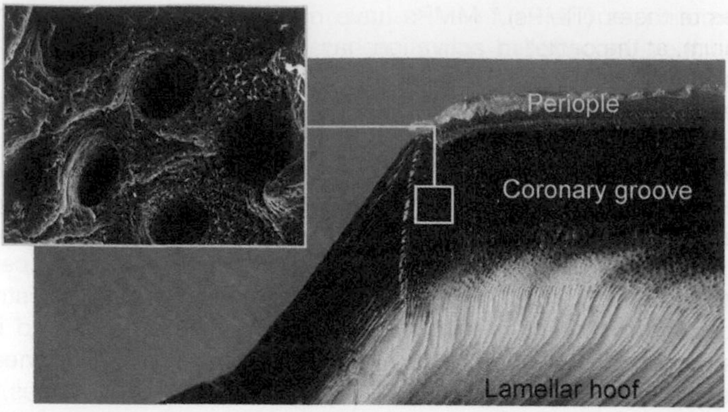

Fig. 7. The hoof capsule, with its contents removed, shows thousands of small, circular, holes pocking the surface of the concave, coronary groove. Germinative epidermal basal cells cover the surface of the holes and the surface of the coronary groove between the holes (*inset*). (*From* Pollitt CC. Anatomy and physiology of the inner hoof wall. Clin Tech Equine Pract 2004;3:8; with permission.)

As described earlier, coronet basal cells undergo mitosis throughout the life of the horse, producing stratum medium daughter cells that mature and keratinize, undertaking a journey, up to 8 months in duration, in the direction of the ground surface. Maturing keratinocytes, arising from basal cells lining the holes, become organized into thin, elongated cylinders or tubules approximately 0.2 mm in diameter.[2] In cross section the keratinocytes of individual hoof wall tubules are arranged around a central hollow medulla in nonpigmented concentric layers.

The keratinocytes generated between the holes mature into intertubular hoof, thus forming a keratinized cellular matrix in which tubules are embedded. The intertubular horn is formed at right angles to the tubular horn and bestows on the hoof wall the unique property of a mechanically stable, multidirectional, fiber-reinforced composite.[9] Hoof wall is stiffer and stronger at right angles to the direction of the tubules, a finding at odds with the usual assumption that the ground reaction force is transmitted proximally up the hoof wall parallel to the tubules. The hoof wall seems to be reinforced by the tubules but the intertubular material accounts for most of its mechanical strength stiffness and fracture toughness. The tubules are 3 times more likely to fracture than intertubular horn.[8,10] The stratum medium is considered to have an anatomic design that confers strength in all directions. Unlike bone, which is a living tissue and remodels to become stronger along lines of stress, the stratum medium is nonliving tissue but is anatomically constructed to resist stress in every direction and never to require remodeling. During normal locomotion the stratum medium experiences only one-tenth of the compressive force required to cause its structural failure.[11] It is in fact overengineered.

The fully keratinized cells (corneocytes) of the tubular and intertubular hoof, cemented firmly to each other, form a continuum: the tough yet flexible stratum medium of the hoof wall. Mature corneocytes, firmly cemented together, form a tough protective barrier, preventing the passage of water and water-soluble substances inwards and the loss of body fluids, imparted by the highly vascular dermis, outwards. In addition to acting as a permeability barrier, hoof wall corneocytes, arranged in their specialized tubular and intertubular configuration, have the crucial job of ultimately supporting the entire weight of the horse.[12]

The tubules of the equine hoof wall are not arranged randomly. The tubules of the stratum medium, at the center of the toe, are arranged into recognizable zones based on the density of tubules in the intertubular horn.[13,14] The zone of highest tubule density is the outermost layer and the density declines stepwise toward the internal lamellar layer. Because the force of impact with the ground (the ground reaction force) is transmitted proximally up the wall[11] the tubule density gradient across the wall seems to be a mechanism for smooth energy transfer, from the rigid (high tubule density) outer wall to the more plastic (low tubule density) inner wall, and ultimately, via the SADP to the distal phalanx. The gradient in tubule density mirrors the gradient in water content across the hoof wall and together these factors represent an optimum design for equine hoof wall. The hoof wall also has a powerful dampening function on vibrations generated when the hoof wall makes contact with the ground during locomotion. It is able to reduce the frequency and maximal amplitude of the vibrations.[15] By the time the shock of impact with the ground reaches the first phalanx, around 90% of the energy has been dissipated, mainly at the lamellar interface.

THE CORIUM

The highly vascular corium or dermis underlies the hoof wall and consists of a dense matrix of tough connective tissue containing a network of arteries, veins, capillaries, and sensory and vasomotor nerves. All parts of the corium, except for the lamellar corium, have papillae that fit tightly into the holes in the adjacent hoof. The lamellar

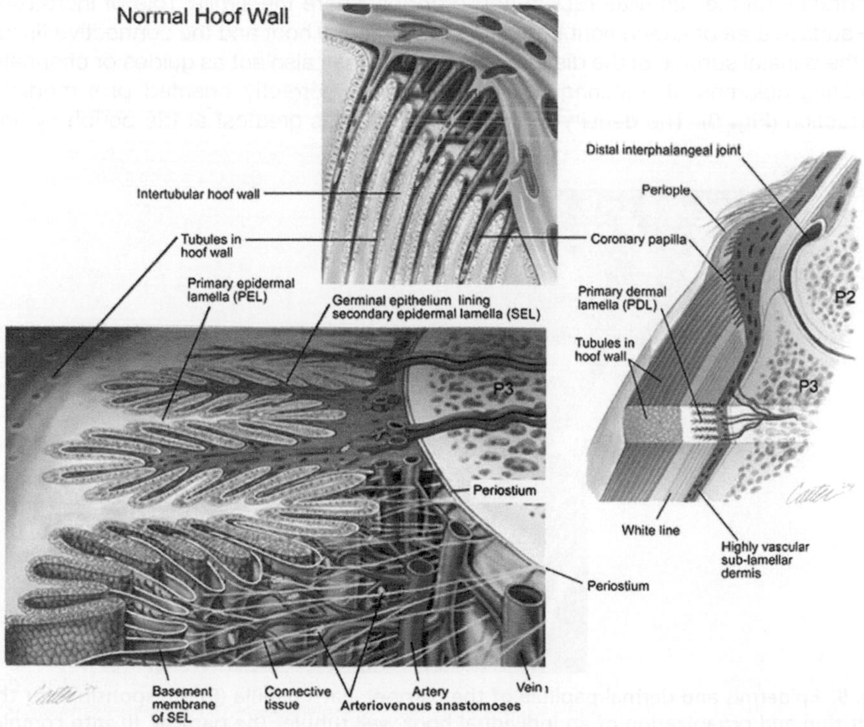

Fig. 8. The dermal papillae of the coronet and interdigitating lamellae of the inner hoof wall. (*From* Pollitt CC. Anatomy and physiology of the inner hoof wall. Clin Tech Equine Pract 2004;3:10; with permission.)

corium has dermal lamellae that interlock with the epidermal lamellae of the inner hoof wall and bars (**Fig. 8**). The vascular system of the corium provides the hoof with nourishment. The dense matrix of corium connective tissue connects the BM of the dermal-epidermal junction to the periosteal, parietal surface of the distal phalanx and thus suspends the distal phalanx from the inner wall of the hoof capsule.

THE CORONET CORIUM

The coronet corium fills the coronary groove and blends distally with the lamellar corium. Its inner surface is attached to the extensor tendon and the ungual cartilages of the distal phalanx by the subcutaneous tissue of the coronary cushion. Collectively, the coronary corium and the germinal epidermal cells that rest on its BM are known as the coronet or coronary band. A feature of the coronet corium is the large numbers of hairlike papillae projecting from its surface. Each tapering papilla fits into 1 of the holes on the surface of the epidermal coronary groove and is responsible for nurturing an individual hoof wall tubule.

The BM surface of the hoof wall corium was examined with the scanning electron microscope after treatment of hoof tissue blocks with a detergent enzyme mixture.[16] A clean separation could be made between dermal and epidermal tissues, enabling the surface of the dermal BM to be examined in detail. The BM of the coronary and terminal papillae was folded into numerous ridges parallel with the long axis of the papilla. These longitudinal ridges on the surface of the papillae are analogous to the secondary dermal lamellae (SDLs) and probably share the similar role of increasing the surface area of attachment between the epidermal hoof and the connective tissue on the parietal surface of the distal phalanx. They may also act as guides or channels, directing columns of maturing keratinocytes in a correctly oriented proximodistal correction (**Fig. 9**). The density of coronary papillae is greatest at the periphery and

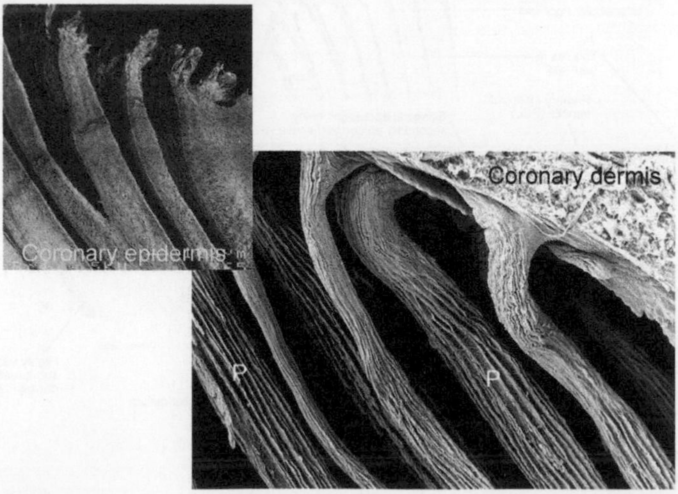

Fig. 9. Epidermis and dermal papillae of the coronet. Each papilla (P) is responsible for the nutrition and organization of an individual hoof wall tubule. The papillae fit into complementary sockets in the coronary groove of the epidermal hoof wall (*upper inset*). (*From* Pollitt CC. Anatomy and physiology of the inner hoof wall. Clin Tech Equine Pract 2004;3:11; with permission.)

least adjacent to the lamellae, mirroring the arrangement of the hoof wall tubules of the stratum medium in zones based on tubule size and density.[14]

THE SOLE CORIUM

As in the coronet each dermal papilla of the sole corium fits into a socket in the epidermal sole. At the distal end of each dermal lamella is a set of papillae known as the terminal papillae (**Fig. 10**). The epidermis surrounding the terminal papillae is nonpigmented and forms the inner part of the white zone (white line). The white zone is soft and flexible and effectively seals the sole to the hoof wall. It is sometimes subject to degeneration and infection, usually described as seedy toe or white line disease.

THE BLOOD SUPPLY OF THE FOOT

Digital Arteries

The medial and lateral digital arteries arise by division of the medial palmar artery (common digital artery) between the suspensory ligament and the deep digital flexor tendon and enter the digit on the abaxial surfaces of the proximal sesamoid bones of the fetlock (**Fig. 11**).

At the level of the proximal interphalangeal joint, the digital arteries send major branches to the heels, which supply the digital cushion, frog, lamellar corium of the heels and bars, and the palmar perioplic and coronary coria. Opposite the middle of the second phalanx, each digital artery again branches and forms an artery that runs deep to the cartilages and the extensor tendon, and connects with the artery of the opposite side, to form an arterial circle around the second phalanx and coronary band. This coronary circumflex artery supplies the digital extensor tendon and distal interphalangeal joint and supplies numerous branches to the coronary corium and proximal lamellae of the toe and dorsal quarters.

Proximal to the navicular bone each digital artery gives off a dorsal branch that passes through the notch or foramen in the palmar process of the distal phalanx and, running in the parietal groove on the dorsal surface of the distal phalanx, supplies

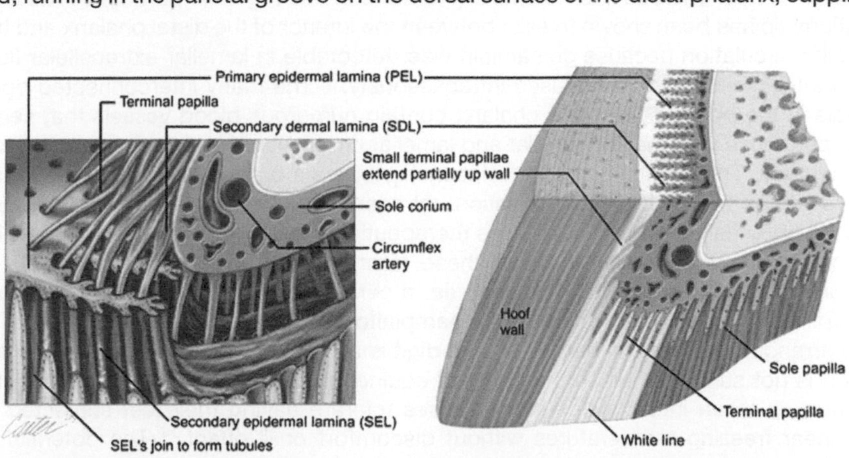

Fig. 10. On the distal end of all dermal lamellae are numerous terminal papillae. Germinal epidermis lining the terminal papillae are responsible for generating keratinized epidermal cells that fill the space between the PELs as they grow toward the ground surface. (*From* Pollitt CC. Anatomy and physiology of the inner hoof wall. Clin Tech Equine Pract 2004;3:11; with permission.)

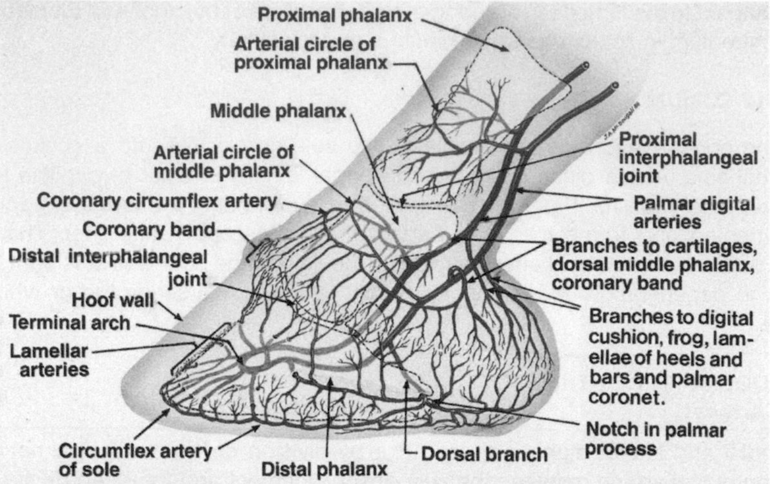

Fig. 11. The arteries of the equine foot. Design C.C. Pollitt, artwork J. McDougall. (*From* Pollitt CC. Anatomy and physiology of the inner hoof wall. Clin Tech Equine Pract 2004;3:12; with permission.)

the lamellar coria of the quarters and heels and forms anastomoses with the palmar part of the circumflex artery of the sole.

The terminal medial and lateral branches of the digital artery enter the solar canal of the distal phalanx via foramina and unite with the artery of the opposite side to form the terminal arch deep within the bone. Branches of the terminal arch (4–5 middorsally and 8–10 distally, near the solar border) radiate outwards through foramina in the dorsal surface of the distal phalanx and supply the lamellar corium and, after forming the circumflex artery, the corium of the sole.

In addition to the 12 to 15 main foramina, the dorsal surface of the distal phalanx is perforated by numerous finer foramina (the bone in this region is porous). A vascular relationship has been shown to exist between the interior of the distal phalanx and the lamellar circulation because gentamicin was detectable in lamellar extracellular fluid soon after gentamicin was infused intraosseously.[17] The many interconnected bony canals in the body of the distal phalanx contain numerous blood vessels that seem to anastomose with the sublamellar and lamellar circulation, forming an interconnecting network. This unique anatomic relationship offers a practical way to access, and deliver drugs to, the lamellar circulation. Intraosseous infusion of the distal phalanx has the potential to deliver antilaminitis therapeutic agents directly to the hoof lamellar region. Many of the vessels within these foramina are arranged anatomically to perform countercurrent heat exchange (ie, a central artery surrounded by a sheath of capillaries and venules, similar to the pampiniform plexus of the mammalian testis). This arrangement implies that the equine digit is an efficient thermoregulatory organ, which is not surprising when the range of equine habitats, from the subarctic to the equator, is taken into consideration. Horses tolerate having their feet subjected to low, near freezing temperatures without discomfort or ill effect.[18] The potential of long-term cryotherapy has been validated by keeping the distal limbs of horses in an ice-water slurry for 48 h while the remaining feet were at room temperature[18] or keeping all 4 limbs in very cold circulating water for 3 days.[19] The horses seemed oblivious to the wide disparity (30 vs 5°C) of foot temperatures they were experiencing. This evolutionary adaptation can be exploited therapeutically. Two to three days of continuous distal limb cryotherapy prevents the onset of acute, experimentally induced laminitis.[19–21]

The lamellar corium derives most of its blood supply from the branches of the terminal arch that perforate the parietal surface of the distal phalanx. Numerous anastomoses form an arterial lattice between the epidermal lamellae and blood can flow proximally to the coronary circumflex artery and distally to the solar circumflex artery (**Fig. 12**).

The circumflex artery of the sole is an anastomosis of all the distal branches of the terminal arch and the dorsal arteries of the distal phalanx and forms a complete arterial loop, supplying the corium at the junction of the distal lamellae and peripheral sole close to the sharp solar margin of the bone. All of the arterial blood supply of the sole (except for the angle between the bars and the heels) comes from axially directed arteries branching inwards from the circumflex artery (**Fig. 13**).

There are no vascular foramina perforating the solar surface of the distal phalanx (except over the palmar processes), which means that almost the entire corium of the sole depends on a blood supply that arises first on the dorsal surface of the distal phalanx and then curls under the margin of the distal phalanx. The solar corium is sandwiched between the epidermal sole and the unyielding solar surface of the distal phalanx and is therefore prone to damage from compressive forces. If a horse is deliberately forced to stand or walk on the soles of its feet (by overzealous trimming of the ground surface wall) the sharp distal rim of the distal phalanx effectively cuts off the blood circulation to the central solar corium and results in severe lameness and, in some cases, necrosis of the sole. Laminitis-induced descent of the distal phalanx into the hoof capsule also causes dorsal sole necrosis by a similar mechanism.

Digital Veins

There are 3 interconnected valveless venous plexuses in the foot (**Fig. 14**).

The dorsal venous plexus lies in the deep part of the lamellar corium. The palmar/plantar venous plexus lies in the deep part of the sole corium and on the inner axial

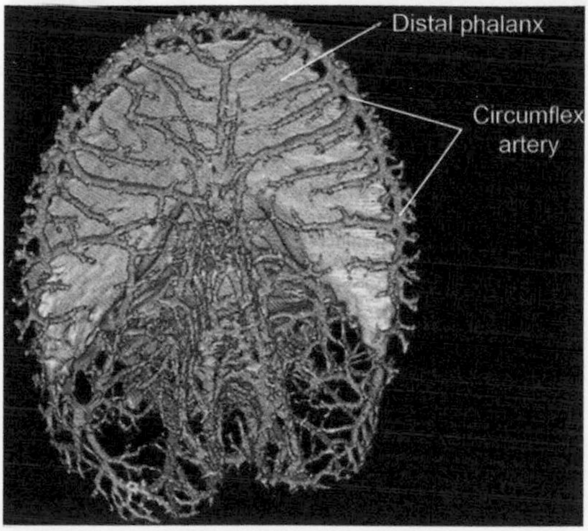

Fig. 12. Three-dimensional reconstruction of a CT scanned horse's foot with the arterial circulation injected with contrast material. Note how arteries exit through foraminae in the dorsal surface of the distal phalanx and anastomose proximally with vessels of the coronet and distally to form the circumflex artery.

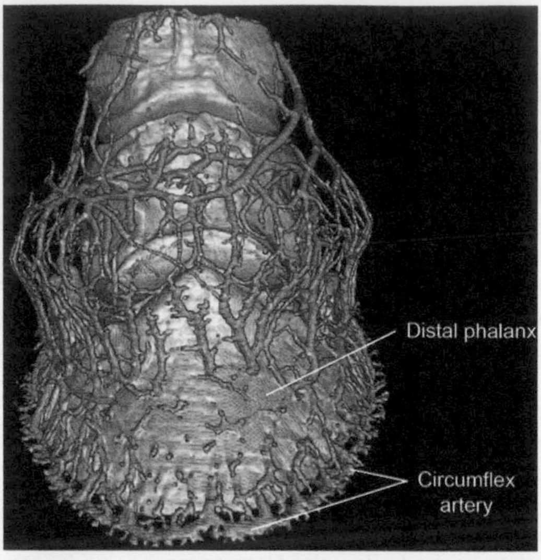

Fig. 13. Three-dimensional reconstruction of a CT scanned horse's foot with the arterial circulation injected with contrast material. Note how axially directed branches of the circumflex artery supply the sole. (*Modified from* Pollitt CC. Anatomy and physiology of the inner hoof wall. Clin Tech Equine Pract 2004;3:12; with permission.)

surfaces of the cartilages of the distal phalanx. The coronary venous plexus lies in the coronary cushion, covering the digital extensor tendon and the outer abaxial surfaces of the cartilages of the distal phalanx. It anastomoses with the palmar/plantar venous plexus via foramina in the cartilages (both sides of the cartilages are covered by plexuses of veins). The 3 plexuses are drained by the medial and lateral digital veins. The

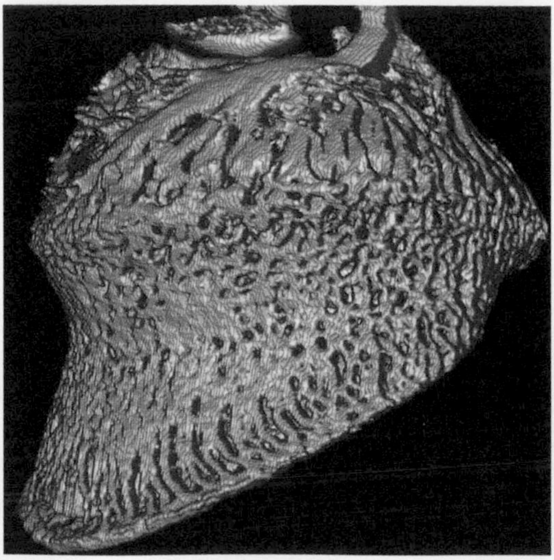

Fig. 14. Three-dimensional reconstruction of a CT scanned horse's foot with the venous circulation injected with contrast material. Note the extensive degree of anastomosis among the valveless venous plexuses. (*From* Pollitt CC. Anatomy and physiology of the inner hoof wall. Clin Tech Equine Pract 2004;3:14; with permission.)

deep veins within the foot are valveless, although valves occur in the more superficial coronary, subcoronary, and heel veins.

Reactions of the Venous Blood in the Foot When Loading

The hoof is subjected to a range of weight-bearing and locomotor forces. These forces are believed to cause expansion of the frog and to deform all the soft tissue of the hoof, including the digital cushion, the cartilages, and the vascular systems. Because the soft tissues of the hoof are encased by the hard keratinized wall, which cannot expand substantially,[22] the internal deformation of the hoof forces evacuation of the venous blood from the hoof quickly. The multiple routes of drainage of the wall and sole venous plexuses, the absence of valves in most veins of the hoof, the presence of valves in the proper digital veins and caudal hoof veins, and the presence of a double layer of venous plexuses on either side of the flexible cartilages are all mechanisms to evacuate the venous blood quickly and to distribute pressure evenly. The absence of valves would help evacuation by allowing venous blood to take any convenient path. The presence of the valves in the caudal hoof veins and proper digital veins prevents retrograde blood flow to the hoof and thereby ensures the efficient venous return of blood to the heart.[23,24]

THE INNER HOOF WALL

In common with all epidermal structures the lamellae of the inner hoof wall are avascular and depend on capillaries in the microcirculation of the adjacent dermis for gaseous exchange and nutrients. The epidermal cells closest to the dermis form the basal cell layer (germinal cell layer or stratum germinativum).

THE DERMAL MICROCIRCULATION

Numerous (500/cm^2) arteriovenous anastomoses (AVAs) connect the axial arteries and veins of the dermal lamellae.[25] AVAs are present throughout the dermal lamellae but are larger and more numerous around the axial vessels close to their bases (**Fig. 15**). Studies with the transmission electron microscope (TEM) show that AVAs are richly innervated by autonomic vasomotor nerves and their associated peptidergic nerves, and have thick walls of smooth muscle and a specialized, characteristically tall, endothelium.[26]

Their normal role is in relation to thermoregulation and pressure modulation. Dilated AVAs bring hot arterial blood to the inner hoof wall and can cause rapid and large temperature fluctuations of the hoof wall. AVAs are equally numerous around the bases of the papillae of the coronary corium and the lamellar terminal papillae. The vascular architecture of a dermal papilla is basically the same whatever its source and the blood vessels of the papillary dermis of the periople, coronary band, terminal papillae, sole, and frog regions share a common structural organization.

SECONDARY EPIDERMAL LAMELLAE

The innermost layer (stratum internum) of the hoof wall and bars of horses and ponies bears the stratum lamellatum (layer of leaves), named after the 550 to 600 epidermal lamellae (PELs) that project from its surface in parallel rows. Examination of the hoof capsule, with its contents removed, shows that the lamellae of the dorsal hoof wall are shaped like long thin rectangles approximately 7 mm wide and 50 mm long. One long edge of the rectangle is incorporated into the tough, heavily keratinized hoof wall proper (stratum medium) and the other long edge is free, facing the outer surface of

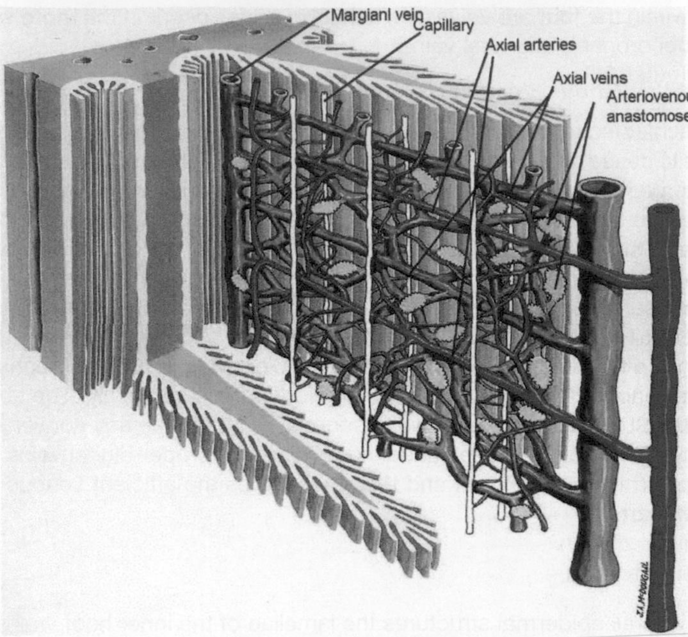

Fig. 15. The dermal microcirculation. AVAs (short yellow vessels) are numerous and more concentrated near the bases of primary dermal lamellae. SDL capillaries (white) are shown reduced in number for diagrammatic reasons. (*From* Pollitt CC. Anatomy and physiology of the inner hoof wall. Clin Tech Equine Pract 2004;3:15; with permission.)

the distal phalanx (**Fig. 16**). The proximal short edge is curved and forms the inner shoulder of the coronary groove. The distal short edge merges with the sole and becomes part of the white zone visible at the ground surface of the hoof.

If the role of the epidermal lamellae is indeed suspensory, then an anatomic specialization increasing the surface area for the attachment of the multitude of collagenous fibers emanating from the parietal surface of the distal phalanx would be expected. The secondary epidermal lamellae (SELs) are just such a specialization. During the

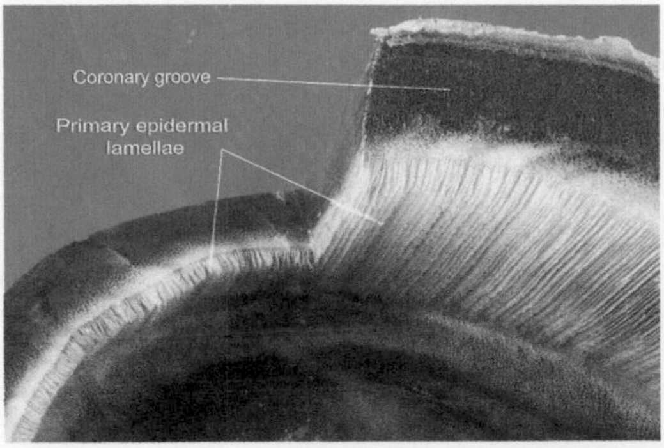

Fig. 16. Hoof with contents removed showing the lamellae of the inner hoof wall. (*Modified from* Pollitt CC. Anatomy and physiology of the inner hoof wall. Clin Tech Equine Pract 2004;3:15; with permission.)

formation of an epidermal lamella, on the shoulders of the inner coronary groove, the basal cell layer proliferates, causing folds (secondary lamellae) to form along the lamellar perimeter. The basal cell proliferation index is high on the shoulders of the coronary groove in the region of secondary lamella formation.[4] The folds elongate to form 150 to 200 secondary lamellae along the length of each of the 550 to 600 primary lamella. Normal SELs have a constant histologic appearance (**Fig. 17**), which only laminitis alters. A description of hoof lamellar anatomy forms the basis of the histologic grading system of laminitis histopathology.[27]

Special stains such as periodic acid Schiff (PAS) are required to highlight the BM and locate the glycoprotein constituents of the BM, for example laminin. PAS staining of normal hoof lamellae show the BM of each SEL as a dark magenta line closely adherent to the SEL basal cells. There are no polymorphonucleocytes (PMNs) either in capillaries or in the dermis. The BM of normal lamellae penetrates deeply into the crypt between pairs of SELs and clearly outlines the tapered tip of each SDL. The proximity of the SDL tip to the keratinized axis of the PEL is, therefore, readily appreciated; it is always a distance equivalent to the length of 1 or 2 epidermal basal cells. The club-shaped tips of the SELs, as outlined by the BM, are always rounded and never tapered or pointed. The tips of the lamellae (primary and secondary) all orientate toward the distal phalanx, thus indicating the lines of tension to which the lamellar suspensory apparatus are subjected.

The surface area of the equine inner hoof wall has been calculated to average 0.8 m^2[28] (about the size of the surface area of the skin of a small adult human) (a considerable increase over the inner surface area of bovine hooves, which lack secondary lamellae). This large surface area for suspension of the distal phalanx and the great compliance of the interdigitating lamellar architecture help reduce stress and ensure even energy transfer during peak loading of the equine foot. The hoof distal phalangeal suspensory apparatus is strong; during peak loading the hoof wall and the distal phalanx move in concert and separate only when laminitis interferes with lamellar anatomy.

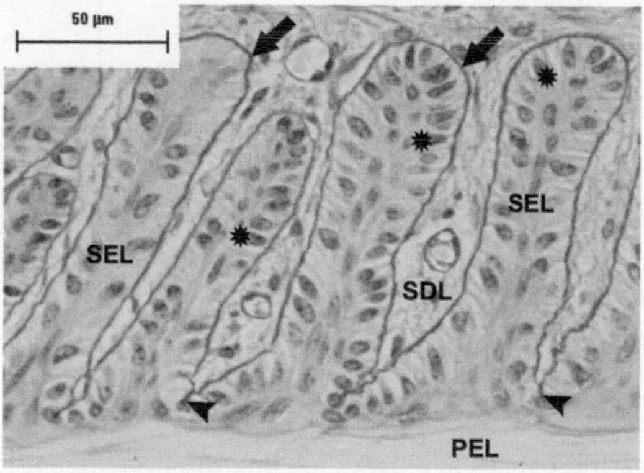

Fig. 17. Micrograph of normal hoof lamellae stained to highlight the BM. The BM (*arrowed*) of each SEL shows as a dark magenta line closely adherent to the SEL basal cells. Between the bases of each SEL the BM penetrates deeply (*arrowheads*) and is close to the anuclear, keratinized PEL. The SEL tips are rounded (club-shaped). The basal cell nuclei are oval (*stars*) and positioned away from the BM at the apex of each cell. The long axis of each basal cell nucleus is at right angles to the long axis of the SEL. The SDLs are filled with connective tissue right to their tips, between the SEL bases. These parameters of hoof lamellar anatomy form the basis of the histologic grading system of laminitis histopathology. PAS stain; bar = 10 µm. (*From* Pollitt CC. Anatomy and physiology of the inner hoof wall. Clin Tech Equine Pract 2004;3:16; with permission.)

THE BM

At the interface of the epidermal and the dermal lamellae is a tough, unbroken sheet of ECM called the lamellar BM. This key structure partitions lamellar epidermal cells from the lamellar dermis. On 1 side of the BM epidermal basal cells are firmly attached, whereas on the other, (dermal) side, tendonlike connective tissue, emanating from the parietal surface of the distal phalanx, is tightly woven into the matlike structure of the BM. The signature lesion of laminitis, failure of the attachment between lamellar dermis and epidermis, occurs at the lamellar dermoepidermal junction and involves the lamellar BM. The ultrastructure of the equine hoof BM is essentially the same as in other animals but with some important specializations. It is a sheetlike three-dimensional latticework of fine interconnecting cords. The axial skeleton of the cord network consists of filaments of collagen IV. The collagen IV filaments are ensheathed with glycoproteins, in particular laminin-1, nidogen, perlecan, fibronectin, and heparin,[29] which together form the electron dense lamina densa (**Fig. 18**). Innumerable extensions of the lamina densa and banded anchoring fibrils (consisting of collagen VII) in the shape of recurved hooks intermesh with the type I collagen fibrils of the connective tissue of the lamellar corium, forming an important part of the attachment mechanism

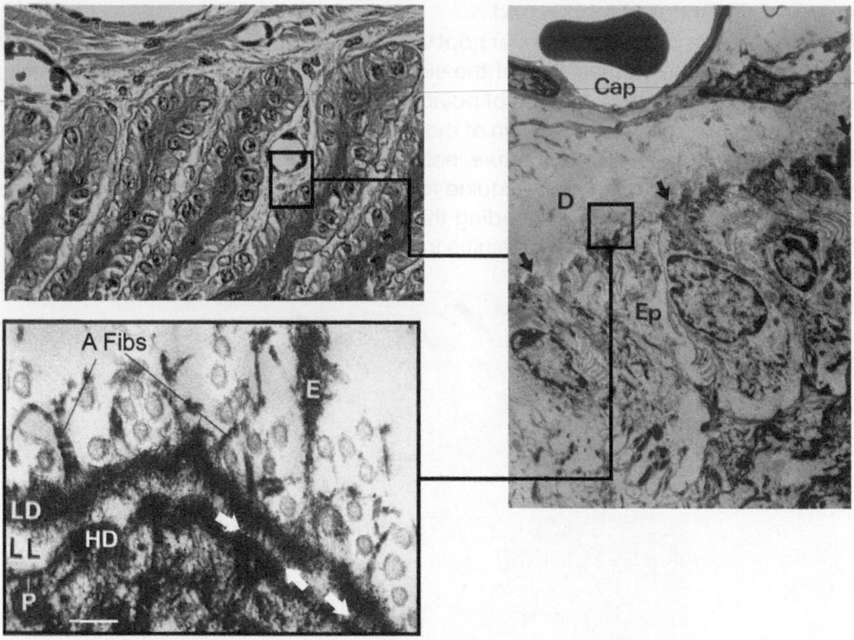

Fig. 18. The BM of each SEL stains as a dark blue line closely adherent to the SEL basal cells in light microscopic sections stained by Masson's trichrome. In low magnification TEMs the BM is just visible (*arrows*) and follows the contours of the SEL basal cells (Ep). High magnification TEMs show the lamina densa (LD) of the BM separated from the plasmalemma (P) of the basal cell by a gap; the lamina lucida (LL). Inserted in the basal cell plasmalemma are numerous attachment plaques called HDs. Extensions of the lamina densa (E) and banded anchoring fibrils (AFibs) intermesh with collagen fibrils of the connective tissue of the lamellar dermis (D). Bridging the gap between HDs and the lamina densa are numerous fine anchoring filaments (*white arrows*). Cap = capillary; bar = 10 nm. (*From* Pollitt CC. Anatomy and physiology of the inner hoof wall. Clin Tech Equine Pract 2004;3:17; with permission.)

between dermis and epidermis. The equine lamellar BM has a high density of lamina densa extensions and anchoring fibrils around the tips of the SELs, a feature perhaps not surprising in a large ungulate, weight bearing on single digits.[16]

Laminin-1, 1 of the key proteins of the BM, forms receptor sites and ligands for a complex array of growth factors, cytokines, adhesion molecules, and integrins. Without an intact, functional BM, the epidermis, to which it is attached, falls into disarray. Disintegration and separation of the lamellar BM are features of acute laminitis. Laminin-1 and collagen IV disappear from the BM, which progressively loses its close attachment to the basal cells and strips away from the epidermal lamellae.[30]

HDS

When viewed with the TEM the BM is dominated by the electron dense lamina densa, which appears as a dark line following the contours of the epidermal basal cells (see **Fig. 18**). The plasma membrane (plasmalemma) at the base of each basal cell is attached to the BM by numerous electron dense adhesion plaques or HDs. The various proteins of each HD occur on both sides of the basal cell plasmalemma, thus forming a bridge linking the interior of the basal cell to the exterior connective tissue (**Fig. 19**). The intracytoplasmic HD proteins that attach basal cells to the BM are named plectin, BP230, BP180, and integrin $\alpha_6\beta_4$.

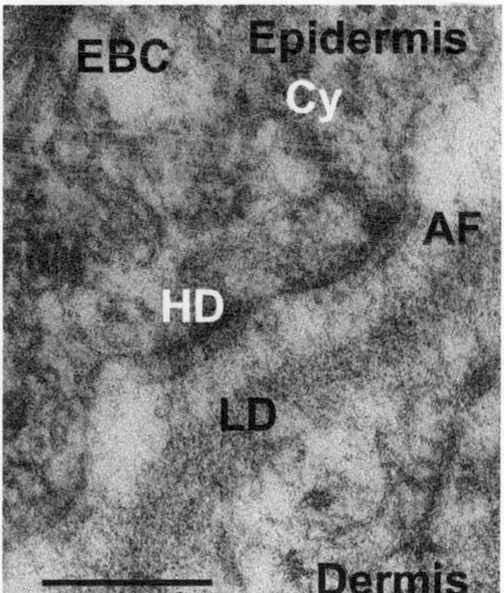

Fig. 19. HDs at the dermoepidermal junction. The electron dense lamina densa (LD) is the major structural component of the BM. HDs are attachment plaques that serve to keep the lamina densa of the BM firmly adherent to all lamellar epidermal basal cells (EBC). Each HD is constructed of several proteins that stain darkly when viewed by TEM. The internal skeleton or cytoskeleton (Cy) of the basal cell is constructed of fine keratin filaments that attach to the intracytoplasmic dense plaque of HDs and interconnect to desmosomes and the nucleus. Bridging the gap between the dense plaque of the HD (H) and the lamina densa are numerous submicroscopic anchoring filaments (AF). Bar = 10 nm. (*From* Pollitt CC. Anatomy and physiology of the inner hoof wall. Clin Tech Equine Pract 2004;3:18; with permission.)

HDs are maintained and assembled by glucose-consuming phosphorylation reactions. Integrin $\alpha_6\beta_4$ and BP180 have domains on both sides of the plasmalemma and form part of the extracytoplasmic, subbasal dense plaque of the HD. The protein that bridges the gap between the HD and the lamina densa is laminin-5.[31,32] TEM resolves laminin-5 as innumerable fine anchoring filaments spanning the lamina lucida, the space between the basal cell and the lamina densa (**Fig. 20**). The essential nature of hoof lamellar HDs and anchoring filaments is illustrated by horses that inherit mutations in the genes expressing HD proteins.

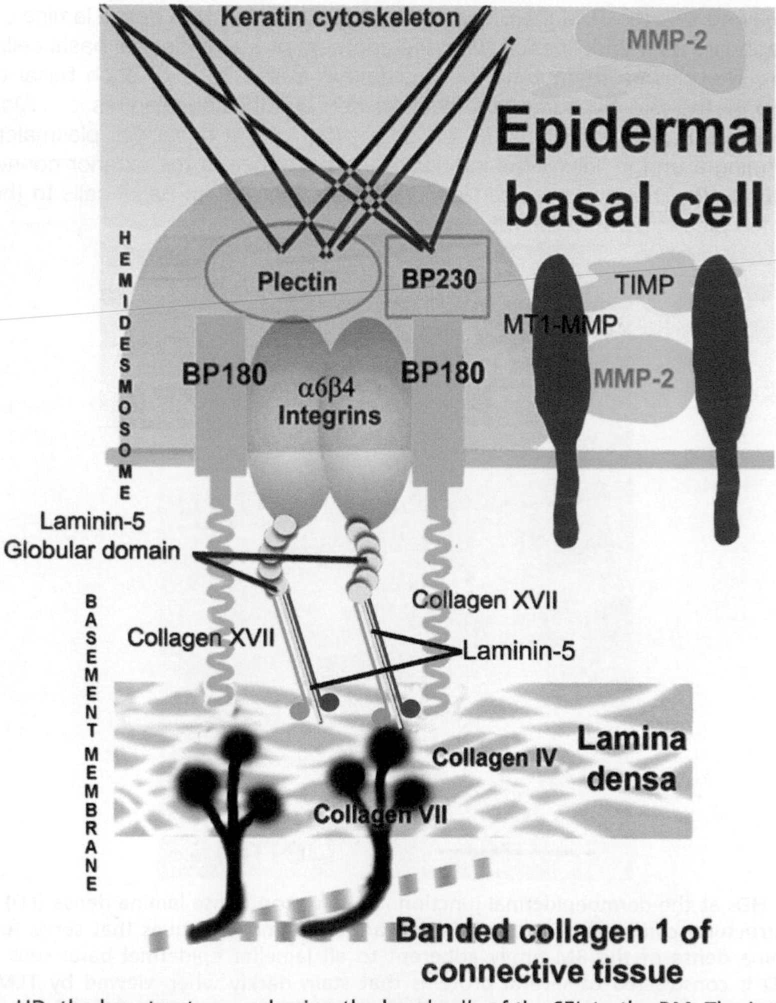

Fig. 20. HD, the key structure anchoring the basal cells of the SEL to the BM. The intracytoplasmic plaque consists of the proteins plectin, BP180, and integrin $\alpha_6\beta_4$. Keratin intermediate filaments of the cell cytoskeleton connect to plectin, which in turn communicates with laminin-5 anchoring filaments via integrin $\alpha_6\beta_4$. Integrin $\alpha_6\beta_4$ and BP180 have domains on both sides of the plasmalemma and form part of the extracytoplasmic, subbasal dense plaque of the HD. The anchoring filaments are incorporated into the matrix of the BM.

Within the Belgian horse population, an autosomal, recessive mutation within the gene encoding the $\gamma 2$ chain of laminin-5 has been identified. The mutation causes a premature termination codon and consequently the expression of the laminin-5, anchoring filament protein is absent,[32] resulting in widespread dermoepidermal separation in skin and hoof lamellae. Belgian foals afflicted with this hereditary, junctional epidermolysis bullosa suffer hoof exunguilation and generalized skin lesions at pressure points and mucocutaneous junctions and die or are killed within a few days of birth.[33] Loss of plectin from the HD adhesion complex of a Quarterhorse foal is a second example of congenital, lamellar dysadhesion.[34] The foal had fragile skin and hooves that indicated acute and chronic laminitis. The distal phalanx had sunk into the hoof capsule and had perforated the sole. Although the loss of plectin was ubiquitous in hooves and skin, only the forefeet showed lesions; the anatomy and histology of the hind feet were normal, thus illustrating how closely the lesions of laminitis follow foot load distribution. If clinicians could do more to lessen the effect of weight bearing during the developmental stage, the destructiveness of laminitis pathology in adult horses could be diminished.

A firm attachment between epidermal basal cells and the dermis is essential in weight-bearing hoof lamellae. This attachment is ensured by the ordered array of molecules linking the epidermal basal cell cytoskeleton to HDs, anchoring filaments and the BM. Any defect that weakens a link in this chain also weakens epidermal-dermal adhesion.

LAMELLAR REMODELING ENZYMES

Connective tissue and keratinocytes are now known to remodel and continually upgrade their spatial organization by the tightly controlled production of a specific class of enzymes known as MMPs. MMPs are a group of zinc-dependent enzymes that, when activated, degrade ECM and BM components, and the activity of MMPs (particularly the gelatinases MMP-2 and MMP-9) correlates strongly with BM destruction and the associated degree of malignancy and invasiveness of tumors.[35,36] Two members of the MMP family (MMP-2 and MMP-9) can be isolated from homogenized normal hoof wall lamellae and from normal lamellar explants cultured in tissue culture medium.[37] Secreted as inactive proenzymes and, when activated, promptly inhibited by locally produced inhibitors (TIMPs), MMP activity is likely responsible for the remodeling of the various classes of epidermal cells between the BM, SELs, and PELs.

The protein constituents of the BM (type IV collagen, type VII collagen and laminin-1) are known substrates of MMP-2 and MMP-9.[38,39] In addition, laminin-5, the anchoring filament molecule bridging the lamellar basal cell to its underlying BM, loses its firm attachment to integrin $\alpha_6\beta_4$ activity during laminitis development.[40] The disorganization of the epidermal cells of the SELs, the wholesale separation of basal cells from the BM, and lysis of BM that occurs early in the pathology of laminitis[27] are now believed to be caused by the triggering of activation of uncontrolled, excessive MMP production.[6] MMPs, present in the cells of the SELs, presumably for normal remodeling purposes, seem to be important players in laminitis pathogenesis.

REFERENCES

1. Bowker RM. The growth and adaptive capabilities of the hoof wall and sole: functional changes in response to stress. In: Proceeding of the 49th Annual Convention of the American Association of Equine Practitioners. New Orleans, November 21–25, 2003. p. 146–68.

2. Kasapi MA, Gosline JM. Exploring the possible functions of the equine hoof wall. Equine Vet J Suppl 1998;26:10–4.
3. Leach DH. The structure and function of the equine hoof wall. [PhD thesis], Department of Veterinary Anatomy, Western College of Veterinary Medicine, University of Saskatchewan; 1980.
4. Daradka M, Pollitt CC. Epidermal cell proliferation in the equine hoof wall. Equine Vet J 2004;36:210–6.
5. Woessner FJ. Matrix metalloproteinases and their inhibitors in connective tissue remodeling. FASEB J 1991;5:2145–54.
6. Kyaw-Tanner M, Pollitt CC. Equine laminitis: increased transcription of matrix metalloproteinase-2 (MMP-2) occurs during the developmental phase. Equine Vet J 2004;36:221–5.
7. Kyaw-Tanner MT, Wattle O, van Eps AW, et al. Equine laminitis: membrane type matrix metalloproteinase-1 (MMP-14) is involved in acute phase onset. Equine Vet J 2008;40:482–7.
8. Leach DH, Oliphant LW. Ultrastructure of the equine hoof wall secondary epidermal lamellae. Am J Vet Res 1983;44:1561–70.
9. Bertram JEA, Gosline JM. Functional design of horse hoof keratin: the modulation of mechanical properties through hydration effects. J Exp Biol 1987;130: 121–36.
10. Bertram JEA, Gosline JM. Fracture toughness design in horse hoof keratin. J Exp Biol 1986;125:29–47.
11. Thomason JJ, Biewener AA, Bertram JEA. Surface strain on the equine hoof wall in vivo: implications for the material design and functional morphology of the wall. J Exp Biol 1992;166:145–65.
12. Pollitt CC. The anatomy and physiology of the hoof wall. Equine Vet Educ 1998; 10:318–25.
13. Reilly JD, Cottrell DF, Martin RJ, et al. Tubule density in equine hoof horn. Biomimetics 1996;4:23–36.
14. Reilly JD, Collins SN, Cope BC, et al. Tubule density of the stratum medium of horse hoof. Equine Vet J Suppl 1998;26:4–9.
15. Dyhre-Poulsen P, Smedegaard HH, Roed J, et al. Equine hoof function investigated by pressure transducers inside the hoof and accelerometers mounted on the first phalanx. Equine Vet J 1994;26:362–6.
16. Pollitt CC. The basement membrane at the equine hoof dermal epidermal junction. Equine Vet J 1994;26:399–407.
17. Nourian AR, Mills PC, Pollitt CC. Development of an intraosseous infusion method to access the lamellar circulation in the standing, conscious horse. Vet J 2009; 183:272–7.
18. Pollitt CC, van Eps AW. Prolonged, continuous distal limb cryotherapy in the horse. Equine Vet J 2004;36:216–20.
19. Van Eps AW, Pollitt CC. Equine laminitis model: cryotherapy reduces the severity of lesions evaluated 7 days after experimental induction with oligofructose. Equine Vet J 2009;41:741–6.
20. van Eps AW, Pollitt CC. Equine laminitis: cryotherapy prevents development of the acute lesion. Equine Vet J 2004;36:255–60.
21. van Eps AW, Pollitt CC. Equine laminitis model: lamellar histopathology seven days after induction with oligofructose. Equine Vet J 2009;41:735–40.
22. Fischerleitner TE. Rontgenographische untersuchungen uber den einfluss der lagever-anderungen des hufserahlund kronbeines auf die mechanic der homkapsel des pferdes imbelsastungsgerac. Inaugural dissertation. Vienna; 1974.

23. Mishra PC, Leach DH. Extrinsic and intrinsic veins of the equine hoof wall. J Anat 1983;136:543–60.
24. Mishra PC, Leach DH. Electron microscopic study of the veins of the dermal lamella of the equine hoof wall. Equine Vet J 1983;15:14–21.
25. Pollitt CC, Molyneux GS. A scanning electron microscopical study of the dermal microcirculation of the equine foot. Equine Vet J 1990;22:79–87.
26. Molyneux GS, Haller CJ, Mogg KC, et al. The structure, innervation and location of arteriovenous anastomoses in the equine foot. Equine Vet J 1994;26:305–12.
27. Pollitt CC. Basement membrane pathology: a feature of acute equine laminitis. Equine Vet J 1996;28:38–46.
28. Daradka M. The equine foot: growth, repair and dimensions. Lamellar surface area. Brisbane (Australia): The University of Queensland; 2000. 99–134.
29. McMillan JR, Akiyama M, Shimizu H. Ultrastructural orientation of laminin 5 in the epidermal basement membrane: an updated model for basement membrane organization. J Histochem Cytochem 2003;51:1299–306.
30. Pollitt CC, Daradka M. Equine laminitis basement membrane pathology: loss of type IV collagen, type VII collagen and laminin immunostaining. Equine Vet J Suppl 1998;26:139–44.
31. French KR, Pollitt CC. Equine laminitis: cleavage of key hemidesmosome proteins associated with basement membrane dysadhesion. Equine Vet J 2004;36:242–7.
32. Spirito F, Charlesworth A, Linder K, et al. Animal models for skin blistering conditions: absence of laminin 5 causes hereditary junctional mechanobullous disease in the Belgian horse. J Invest Dermatol 2002;119:684–91.
33. Shapiro J, McEwen B. Mechanobullous disease in a Belgian foal in eastern Ontario. Can Vet J 1995;36:572.
34. French KR, Pollitt CC. Equine laminitis: congenital, hemidesmosomal plectin deficiency in a Quarterhorse foal. Equine Vet J 2004;36:299–303.
35. Giannelli G, Falk-Marzillier J, Schiraldi O, et al. Induction of cell migration by matrix metalloprotease-2 cleavage of laminin-5. Science 1997;277:225–8.
36. Stetler-Stevenson WG. Type-IV collagenases in tumour invasion and metastasis. Cancer Metastasis Rev 1990;8:289–303.
37. Pollitt CC, Pass MA, Pollitt S. Batimastat (BB-94) inhibits matrix metalloproteinases of equine laminitis. Equine Vet J Suppl 1998;26:119–24.
38. Salamonsen LA. Matrix metalloproteinases and endometrial remodelling. Cell Biol Int 1994;18:1139–44.
39. Birkedal-Hansen H. Proteolytic remodeling of extracellular matrix. Curr Opin Cell Biol 1995;7:728–35.
40. Goldfarb RH, Liotta LA. Proteolytic enzymes in cancer invasion and metastasis. Semin Thromb Hemost 1986;12:294–307.

Overview of Current Laminitis Research

Susan C. Eades, DVM, PhD

KEYWORDS

- Laminitis • Inflammatory response syndrome
- Lamellae • Cytokine

All cases of laminitis are characterized by failure of the attachment of the epidermal cells of the epidermal laminae to the underlying basement membrane of the dermal laminae despite the diversity of diseases that underlie the syndrome. Disease states associated with laminitis include sepsis and systemic inflammation (eg, gastrointestinal disease, pneumonia, septic metritis, black walnut extract laminitis, and carbohydrate overload), equine metabolic syndrome, and mechanical overload (supporting limb laminitis). The understanding of the pathophysiology and progression of the disease is incomplete, and this limits efforts to prevent and treat this devastating disease successfully. However, scientific investigations are occurring at a phenomenal rate and shedding light on the pathophysiologic events involved with laminitis.

Development of acute laminitis often follows diverse primary diseases; therefore the mechanisms involved in the pathogenesis of laminitis are also numerous but interrelated. In a retrospective case-control study of hospitalized horses, development of laminitis was marginally associated with the lowest and highest fibrinogen concentrations, the highest packed cell volume, and the lowest total solids concentration and significantly associated with pneumonia, endotoxemia, diarrhea, abdominal surgery for colic, and vascular abnormalities.[1] Endotoxemia emerged from this study as a critical risk factor and the common clinical finding in hospitalized horses that developed laminitis. The systemic inflammatory response syndrome is an important part of the disease in these patients. In addition, pasture-associated laminitis accounts for 54% of cases of equine laminitis.[2] Increased serum insulin concentrations, associated with an equine metabolic syndrome, have also been characterized.[3] Based on this clinical information and discussions from the 2007 Havemeyer Meeting, inflammation and extracellular matrix degradation, metabolic disease, and endothelial and vascular dysfunction are currently considered as pivotal events in the development of laminitis.[4]

A modified version of this article originally appeared in: Eades SC. Overview of What We Know About the Pathophysiology of Laminitis. Journal of Equine Veterinary Science 2010;30(2):83–6.
Department of Veterinary Clinical Sciences, Equine Health Studies Program, Louisiana State University, Baton Rouge, LA 70803, USA
E-mail address: seades1@lsu.edu

Vet Clin Equine 26 (2010) 51–63
doi:10.1016/j.cveq.2010.01.001 vetequine.theclinics.com
0749-0739/10/$ – see front matter

CHARACTERIZATION OF LESIONS

Characterization of laminitis began with the evaluation of the histologic changes during alimentary carbohydrate overload models. Histology provides a snapshot of the laminar changes occurring at the time of euthanasia; so knowledge of the continuum of laminar events during the disease is lacking. Secondary epidermal laminar (SEL) swelling and edema, endothelial cell swelling and deformation, red blood cell accumulation in capillaries, perivascular leukocyte infiltration, and migration of leukocytes to the epithelial layer were documented as vascular events occurring 32 to 72 hours after cornstarch overload (4–24 hours after lameness).[5] Evaluation of the epithelium in this same model documented thinning and lengthening of the laminar structures with flattening and displacement of epithelial cells, redirection of the base of the SELs toward the distal phalanx, redirection of the tip of the SELs toward the hoof wall, epithelial cell swelling, vacuolization, and pyknosis with leukocyte infiltration. In this model, epidermal cell vacuolization and pyknosis, with dissolution of basal cells in the presence of an intact basement membrane, suggested that epidermal cell damage precedes basement membrane dissolution.[5]

Pollitt[6] characterized histologic changes in greater detail, creating a grading system for the evaluation of laminar pathology (**Table 1**). These lesions were identified in tissues taken 48 hours after administration of wheat starch. Distinct abnormalities were identified in the secondary dermal lamellae, the secondary epidermal lamellae, the basement membrane, and the epidermal cells. These results suggested that the extracellular matrix damage precedes and exceeds the changes in the epidermal cells, resulting in significant structural alteration before epidermal dissolution. Perivascular leukocyte infiltration was only observed in grade 3 lesions. The change in position in the epidermal cell nuclei may also result from damage to the cytoskeleton as a result of changes in enzyme activity. These alterations in the extracellular matrix and cytoskeleton were further evaluated ultrastructurally in a fructan model of

Table 1
Summary of scoring system for laminitis lesions induced by administration of wheat starch

Grade Score	Secondary Dermal Lamellae (SDL)	Secondary Epidermal Lamellae (SEL)	Basement Membrane	Epidermal Cells
Normal	Close to the primary epidermal lamellae (PEL)	Club-shaped tip	Can be identified with silver methylamine stain	Nucleus opposite basement membrane
Grade 1	Close to PEL	Narrow, elongated, pointed	Absent in some areas	Some nuclei centrally located
Grade 2	Separated from PEL	Narrow, elongated, pointed	More extensive loss and separation apparent at base of SEL	More extensive centralization
Grade 3	Extensive separation from PEL	Extremely elongated	Only apparent at SEL tip, separation extensive	More extensive centralization

Data from Pollitt CC. Basement membrane pathology: a feature of acute equine laminitis. Equine Vet J 1996;28:38–46.

laminitis.[7] Separation of the basement membrane from the SELs was characterized by loss of anchoring filaments and separation of the lamina densa from the epidermal plasmalemma. The lamina densa detached in many areas where hemidesmosomes were reduced in number. The severity of lamina densa separation correlated with the increased dose of fructan.

INFLAMMATION

Systemic sequelae of inflammation (systemic inflammatory response syndrome) commonly plague equine patients undergoing treatment for numerous conditions, including pleuropneumonia, colitis, enteritis, peritonitis, endometritis, and hepatitis. The pathogenesis of laminar failure is similar to that of organ failure in human sepsis.[8] Data from several laboratories have documented laminar changes similar to those in organs at risk of failure in human sepsis in which organ injury and dysfunction can occur even though energy and substrate delivery are adequate. Subsequently, cellular necrosis amplifies the inflammatory response. Although end-organ damage from the systemic inflammatory response can include damage to numerous body tissues, there is no complication more common and devastating during equine inflammatory disease than acute laminitis. Although researchers once questioned whether the disease should be called "laminar degeneration" because of the minimal neutrophil infiltration present histologically, application of more sensitive research tools has produced abundant evidence of inflammatory changes during laminitis.

Evidence of Laminar Cytokine Activation

Fontaine and colleagues[9] provided the earliest evidence of inflammatory changes during equine laminitis by documenting interleukin (IL)-1β messenger RNA (mRNA) expression in perivascular and interstitial cells of small laminar venules and capillaries at 3 hours after induction of black walnut heartwood extract (BWHE) laminitis. Subsequent studies using these earliest stages of BWHE laminitis revealed significant upregulation of cyclooxygenase (COX) 2 without changes in the expression of COX-1.[10] Differential display revealed regulation of a gene related to cytokine production, molecule possessing ankyrin-repeats induced by lipopolysaccharide (MAIL), accompanied by a 4-fold increase in MAIL mRNA expression, with increased expression of cytokines related to this gene (IL-6 160 fold and IL-1β 30 fold).[10] A summary of these early findings along with more recent studies of prodromal BWHE (3 hours), onset of lameness in BWHE laminitis, and onset of lameness using oligofructose documents inflammation in both BWHE and carbohydrate overload laminitis (**Table 2**).[9–13] Laminitis induced by BWHE results in a very early inflammatory response that precedes the onset of lameness and laminar damage.[13] This early response is characterized by an increase in gene expression of IL-8, which may be associated with neutrophil infiltration into the laminar tissue.[13] Dramatic increase in the expression of IL-1β and IL-6 is accompanied by a decrease in the antiinflammatory cytokine IL-10. Later in the disease, at the onset of lameness, expression of other cytokines typical of a mixed adaptive immune response increases.[13] Similarly, the onset of lameness induced by administration of oligofructose is accompanied by a mixed innate and helper T cell (T_H) 1 adaptive immune response (IL-2, IL-6, IL-8, and interferon) that is characteristic of the response to systemic inflammation induced by *Escherichia coli*.[13] The IL-1β response in the developmental stages of oligofructose-induced laminitis has not been studied; however, a significant early inflammatory response typical of innate immunity has been documented in plasma

Table 2
Laminar cytokine mRNA expression in horses with black walnut heartwood extract (BWHE)–induced and oligofructose (OF)–induced laminitis with values expressed as fold increase or no significant change (NS)

mRNA Expression	Laminae BWHE 3 h	Laminae BWHE at Onset of Lameness	OF at Onset of Lameness	Liver BWHE 1.5 h	Liver BWHE 3 h	Lung BWHE 3 h
IL-1β	↑30×	↑8.7×	NS	NS	NS	↑15.8×
IL-2	NS	NS	↑13	ND	ND	ND
IL-4	NS	↑2.7×	ND	NS	NS	NS
IL-6	↑160×	↑1351×	↑201×	↑4.6×	↑11.3×	↑83×
IL-8	↑20×	↑9.9×	↑8×	↑2.5×	↑2.4×	↑4.8×
IL-10	↓8.2×	NS	NS	↓2.9×	NS	NS
IL-12	NS	↑2.3×	NS	ND	ND	ND
IL-18	NS	NS	NS	ND	ND	ND
IFN-γ	NS	NS	↑4.3×	ND	ND	ND
TNF-α	NS	NS	NS	↑1.9×	↑4.7×	↑2.4×

Abbreviations: NS, significant change not seen; ND, values not determined.

Data from Stewart AJ, Pettigrew A, Cochran AM, et al. Indices of inflammation in the lung and liver in the early stages of the black walnut extract model of equine laminitis. Vet Immunol Immunopathol 2009;129(3–4):254–60; Belknap JK, Giguère S, Pettigrew A, et al. Lamellar proinflammatory cytokine expression patterns in laminitis at the developmental stage and at the onset of lameness: innate vs. adaptive immune response. Equine Vet J 2007;39(1):42–7.

12 hours after administration of oligofructose.[14] These early increases in tumor necrosis factor α (TNF-α) were accompanied by signs of endotoxemia.

Systemic Inflammatory Response During Laminitis

Pivotal to our understanding of the systemic inflammatory response syndrome during equine laminitis is the recent discovery of increased expression of pulmonary and hepatic inflammatory mediators in horses that are administered BWHE.[12] The pattern of proinflammatory cytokine expression in the lung and liver in the BWHE model (see **Table 2**) was similar to that reported in other sepsis models, with increases in the expression of TNF-α, IL-6, IL-8, and IL-1β within 1.5 hours after administration of BWHE. However, the increases in IL-1β, IL-6, and IL-8 in the lung and liver were all much smaller in magnitude than those occurring in the laminae at the same time in the BWHE model.[13,15] The reason for the heightened laminar inflammatory response is not known. An increase in TNF-α was seen in lung and liver[12] but not in laminae[13] possibly because of the monocyte-lineage cells that are in contact with the circulation in these former organs. Unlike what has been shown to occur in human sepsis models, the expression of antiinflammatory cytokines IL-10 and IL-4 did not increase after BWHE administration in lung, liver, or laminae.[12,13] Furthermore, neutrophil infiltration (as adjudged by CD13 immunohistochemistry) in liver and lung was a very early event (within 3 hours) after BWHE administration.[12]

In addition to this intense laminar cytokine response, there is evidence for a diverse laminar inflammatory reaction. Noschka and colleagues[16] used an equine-specific cDNA microarray to screen gene expression in laminar tissues collected at 1.5, 3, and 12 hours after BWHE administration. As early as 1.5 hours after BWHE administration, genes associated with leukocyte activation and emigration were upregulated.

Other genes involved in inflammatory processes, antioxidant processes, and antimicrobial processes were upregulated at the onset of Obel grade 1 laminitis. Immunohistochemical analysis has revealed that COX-2 is markedly increased in the basal epithelial cells during the first few hours after BWHE administration coincident with leukopenia.[17]

Oxidants

Oxidant injury plays an important role in the end-organ insult resulting from the systemic inflammatory response syndrome. Loftus and colleagues[15] evaluated laminar tissues for the presence of xanthine oxidase (XO)–dependent production of superoxide anion after administration of BWHE. Tissues from liver, lung, and skin from control and BWHE-treated horses contained superoxide dismutase (SOD).[15] Laminar samples from both groups of horses were devoid of SOD. Tissues from liver, lung, skin, and laminae from control and BWHE-treated horses all had endogenous XO and catalase. The levels of XO and catalase were similar in the extracts of laminae from control and BWHE-treated horses. The absence of increased XO activity suggests against the involvement of this reactive oxygen intermediate generating system in the development of laminar pathology in BWHE-treated horses. However, the absence of SOD suggests that the equine digital laminae are highly susceptible to damage by superoxide anion.[15] Yin and colleagues[18] evaluated 4-hydroxy-2-nonenal (4-HNE), a lipid aldehyde that forms as a result of lipid peroxidation, and demonstrated evidence of oxidant stress in laminar, lung, liver, and intestinal tissues of horses with BWHE laminitis. The laminar concentrations of 4-HNE increased significantly in horses with laminitis; however, it remained normal in lung, liver, and intestinal tract. It is possible that antioxidant systems prevent lipid peroxidation in these tissues, whereas damage occurs in the unprotected laminae.

Evidence of Laminar Cellular Infiltration

In laminitis, neutrophils were found aggregated to platelets in the early prodromal stage and at the onset of lameness.[19–21] Carbohydrate overload laminitis (cornstarch) was prevented in 8 ponies by pretreatment with an antagonist of platelet aggregation (platelet fibrinogen receptor antagonist peptide).[20] Using immunoperoxidase and CD13 monoclonal antibodies, Black and colleagues[22] documented emigration of neutrophils to perivascular tissues of the skin and laminae during prodromal stages (3–4 hours) and at the onset of lameness after administration of BWHE. Neutrophil emigration from the circulation is accompanied by a reduction in numbers of circulating neutrophils and monocytes.[23] Neutrophil and/or monocyte activation in skin, plasma, and laminae 3 and 12 hours after BWHE administration confirmed the activation of peripheral white blood cells (WBCs) and the initiation of the systemic inflammatory response syndrome.[24] These activated neutrophils produce increased quantities of reactive oxygen species.[23] Furthermore, it was determined that neutrophil activation and emigration, as measured by CD13 immunohistochemical staining of tissues, occurred concurrently with peaks in matrix metalloproteinase (MMP) 9 activity.[25]

In addition, laminar immunohistochemical staining of calprotectin, a marker of remote tissue inflammation and damage during the systemic inflammatory response syndrome in people, is increased at 12 hours after the onset of black walnut–induced laminitis in horses.[26] Immunohistochemical staining of calprotectin was perivascular, near the epithelial basement membrane, and mostly associated with neutrophil emigration. Furthermore, calprotectin signaling of epithelial damage occurred 12 hours after administration of BWHE, which is 9 hours after the initial onset of neutrophil emigration, suggesting that WBC emigration is a primary event that is not initiated by epithelial damage. In human keratinocyte preparations, inflammatory cytokines induce production of calprotectin and calprotectin causes further induction of cytokines. Calprotectin can induce cellular apoptosis, a documented event in equine laminitis.[27] Taken together, these results confirm that WBC activation is a significant early event in acute laminitis and that WBCs may be a significant source of damage to the extracellular matrix and epithelium.

ENZYMATIC DYSREGULATION

The separation of the dermal and epidermal laminae results from damage to the attachments of epidermal basal cells to the basement membrane.[28] Acceleration of enzymatic activity increases MMP-2 and MMP-9 concentrations and degrades laminin and type IV and type VII collagen.[28–33] Laminar damage (histology scores) and lameness in horses with oligofructose-induced laminitis were significantly reduced in 1 forelimb subjected to continuous cryotherapy (ice water slurry continuously below 5°C for 48 hours) compared with the opposite untreated limb. Cryotherapy significantly reduced lameness scores and expression of MMP-2. It also reduced laminar damage by reduced enzymatic activity, thereby underscoring the importance of enzymatic dysregulation in the pathogenesis of laminitis.[34]

The extracellular matrix is a diverse structure formed of structural proteins, proteoglycans, regulatory proteins, proteases, and protease inhibitors that are responsible for the maintenance of structural support, movement, growth, remodeling, and healing along with the modulation of cytokines, inflammation, healing, and cell migration.[35] Protease enzyme dysfunction during laminitis can result from alteration in gene transcription producing latent pro-MMP zymogens, activation of pro forms of MMPs, and changes in production of tissue inhibitors of metalloproteinases (TIMPs).[36] Numerous events associated with laminitis development result in MMP activation.[36] First, laminar degradation may be linked with an inflammatory response that upregulates MMP-9 to facilitate the destructive process. Examination of laminar samples (gelatin zymography for MMP-9 and MMP-2, myeloperoxidase enzyme-linked immunosorbent assay and real time–polymerase chain reation (RT-PCR) for pro–MMP-2 processing genes) from horses with naturally occurring laminitis and those administered starch gruel revealed that MMP-9 concentrations correlate directly with the activation of neutrophils, suggesting production or induction by inflammatory leukocytes.[37] Increased laminar concentrations of IL-8 during the developmental states of laminitis may attract neutrophils that can release MMP on activation.[13] In contrast, MMP-2 regulation occurred independent of myeloperoxidase concentration, suggesting that dysregulation of MMP-2 is independent of inflammatory processes.[37] Increased laminar expression of other cytokines, such as IL-1β, may directly upregulate MMPs.[13]

In addition, direct activation of MMPs may occur via toxins absorbed from the intestinal lumen. Pro–MMP-2 and pro–MMP-9 were activated in vitro in laminar explants by a bacterial exotoxin (thermolysin) and streptococcal exotoxin B, and this process was blocked by an MMP inhibitor.[38,39] This in vitro activation of pro–MMP-2 and pro–MMP-9 correlated with the weakening of laminar attachments. Although an intestinal trigger has not been identified, significant intestinal alterations have been documented. For example, the population of intestinal bacteria changes within 8 hours after administration of oligofructose.[40] Significant increases in intestinal permeability may increase absorption of intestinal triggers.[41] The concentration of amines increases significantly in the cecal contents of horses grazing spring and summer pastures.[42,43] Similar changes in amine concentration can be induced in vitro by increasing the concentration of cornstarch or fructan in cecal contents incubated anaerobically.[42,43] *Lactobacillus* spp and *Streptococcus bovis* are among the amine-producing bacteria.[42,43]

Recent studies have more specifically characterized enzyme changes in laminar tissue during laminitis. Expression of genes coding for proteins containing a disintegrin and metalloproteinase (ADAM) domain and genes encoding the natural inhibitors of these enzymes (TIMP) in horses with carbohydrate overload, BWHE, and naturally occurring laminitis were studied.[44] *ADAMTS-4* gene expression was strongly upregulated in nearly all horses with experimentally induced and naturally acquired laminitis.[44] The expression of MMPs (MMP-9) and *ADAMTS-5* was also increased, and expression of TIMP-2 was decreased in horses with the most severe form of the disease.[44] From these results, it was proposed that milder cases are primed by the degradation of aggrecan exposing the basement membrane, thereby allowing progression of the disease when MMP-9 expression is increased and TIMP-2 is decreased.[44] RT-PCR documented increased tissue expression of MMP-14 concurrent with decreased amounts of TIMPs in horses with laminitis induced by administration of oligofructose.[45] Activation of MMP-14 releases MMP-2 from TIMP-2 inhibition and is capable of degrading components of the extracellular matrix from its membrane-bound position. There is evidence in both BWHE and oligofructose-induced laminitis that destruction of laminar attachments is in part contributed by MMP activity escaping inhibition by TIMP.[44,45]

METABOLIC SYNDROME

Endocrinopathic laminitis is a term that has been used to describe laminitis that occurs in horses with obesity, insulin resistance, or pituitary dysfunction or occurs after glucocorticoid administration.[3] Insulin resistance is commonly diagnosed in a large number of these horses. Although the relationship among insulin resistance, glucotoxicity, lipotoxicity, and endothelial dysfunction that results in organ failure is well characterized in the human metabolic syndrome,[45] we are in the early stages of understanding these relationships in horses.

Of importance to the understanding of the pathophysiology of laminitis in the metabolic syndrome is the characterization of the metabolic profile of cases that develop laminitis. Characterization of risk factors in human metabolic syndromes of diabetes mellitus and coronary artery disease has increased the understanding of pathophysiology and has enabled preventative strategies for "at-risk" individuals. Small-scale studies have initiated efforts toward these goals in horses. One study differentiated metabolic data of 54 laminitic ponies from those of 106 nonlaminitic ponies.[46] Body condition score, serum triglyceride concentration, and serum insulin concentration were significantly greater in ponies that had history of laminitis when compared with a cohort of nonlaminitic ponies.[46] Proxy measures of insulin resistance, serum insulin concentration, and measures of body condition score (coined as the "prelaminitic profile") predicted development of laminitis in 11 of 13 ponies.[46] Furthermore, serum insulin concentrations were significantly higher in ponies that recurrently develop laminitis on pasture than those that do not.[47] In addition, Carter and colleagues[48] documented that serum leptin concentrations and neck measurements have predictive value. However, it still remains true that there is an overlap in the serum insulin, leptin and triglyceride concentrations and measure of generalized and regional adiposity in laminitic and nonlaminitic horses, making prediction of disease and prognosis difficult (**Table 3**).

Although a causal relationship of these risk factors with laminitis in horses with metabolic disease has not been demonstrated, veterinarians often attribute laminitis

Table 3
Comparison of values for serum insulin, triglycerides, leptin, mean blood pressure, mean body condition score, neck crest height, and neck circumference from 3 publications evaluating ponies with the metabolic syndrome that never had laminitis, those that were previously laminitic, and those with active clinical laminitis

	Never Laminitic	Previously Laminitic	Clinically Laminitic
Insulin	12.0 ± 1.1 μU/L[46] 21.5 ± 3.5 μU/mL[47] 8.8 mU/L median[48]	21.5 ± 3.2 μU/L[46] 69.5 ± 19.8 μU/mL[47] 20.5 mU/L median[48]	103.7 ± 24.0 μU/L[46] 59.5 median[48]
Triglycerides	40.1 ± 2.1 mg/dL[46] 34 ± 2.7 mg/dL[47] 39 mg/dL median[48]	42.3 ± 4.2 mg/dL[46] 49 ± 3.6 mg/dL[47] 53 mg/dL median[48]	62.6 ± 5.3 mg/dL[46] 47 mg/dL median[48]
Leptin	4.9 ng/mL median[48]	5.1 ng/mL median[48]	11.4 ng/mL median[48]
Mean blood pressure	76.8 mm Hg median[47] 84 mm Hg median[48]	89.6 mm Hg median[47] 81 mm Hg median[48]	74 mm Hg median[48]
Body condition score	5.8 ± 0.1[46] 5.78 ± 0.29[47] 6.5 median[48]	6.4 ± 0.1[46] 5.51 ± 0.26[47] 7 median[48]	7.5 median[48]
Neck crest height	6.12 ± 0.49 cm[47]	7.05 ± 0.60 cm[47]	
Neck circumference	81.20 ± 2.22 cm[47]	80.67 ± 1.82 cm[47]	

to hyperinsulinemia, dyslipidemia, and altered glucose metabolism by extrapolating from the human metabolic syndrome. Obesity with high body condition score and neck measurements are common findings in laminitic horses with the metabolic syndrome. Adipose tissue may play an important role in immune, vascular, and metabolic functions via production of adiponectin, leptin, TNF-α, and cytokines.[49] Increased plasma concentrations of leptin documented in laminitic animals with the metabolic syndrome are capable of proinflammatory effects.[50] Horses with metabolic syndrome are rarely hyperglycemic, making glucotoxicity an unlikely pathophysiologic factor. However, a pivotal discovery that has advanced the understanding of the pathogenesis of laminitis revealed that intravenous infusion of insulin via a euglycemic hyperinsulinemic clamp technique for 48 or 72 hours induced Obel grade 2 laminitis with a mean serum insulin concentration around 1000 μU/mL in healthy ponies and Standardbred horses compared with control horses.[51,52] Although these serum insulin values exceed those in most horses with naturally occurring laminitis and the metabolic syndrome, these results confirm that hyperinsulinemia has the ability to play a key role in triggering laminitis.[51]

Mediators of inflammation and oxidant damage may induce laminar injury, thus increasing the risk for laminitis in obese or insulin resistant ponies. Treiber and colleagues[53] evaluated markers of inflammation and redox status in pastured ponies with a history of laminitis and determined that there were no differences between markers of antioxidant function and oxidant pressure in ponies with laminitis and those without laminitis. However, laminitic ponies had higher serum concentrations of TNF than nonlaminitic ponies.

ALTERATION OF ENDOTHELIAL AND VENOUS FUNCTION

Many of the vascular events during equine laminitis were recently summarized by Robertson and colleagues.[54] Laminar edema caused by venous constriction was among the earliest vascular events identified in the early stages of BWHE-induced and carbohydrate-induced laminitis.[55,56] This increased venous resistance is concurrent with increased concentrations of endothelin 1 and can be prevented by administration of an antagonist of endothelin 1.[21,57] Endothelin 1 causes intense vasoconstriction of laminar veins, an effect that is enhanced 4 fold by L-N^G-Nitroarginine methyl ester.[58] Weiss and colleagues[19] demonstrated platelet activation and platelet-neutrophil activation in carbohydrate overload laminitis.[20] Localized platelet activation causes vasoconstriction via release of thromboxane and serotonin, which causes greater laminar vein constriction than laminar arteriolar constriction. Furthermore, vasoactive amines are formed by bacteria in the gastrointestinal tract and may enter the circulation, thus contributing to the pathogenesis of laminitis. Insulin resistance alters endothelial function that can create a proinflammatory condition, leading to platelet and leukocyte activation, increased endothelin production, and production of mediators of inflammation and oxidant stress.[49] The earliest laminar events in BWHE-induced laminitis include the activation of endothelial adhesion molecules and leukocyte emigration.[59]

Garner and colleagues[60] first introduced, in 1975, the hypothesis that the predominant cause of laminitis after carbohydrate overload is a disturbance in the digital blood flow. Contrast radiography was used to demonstrate reduced perfusion in the terminal vasculature of the foot.[61] Tracing radioactive albumin particles through the foot during the development of laminitis demonstrated a reduction in laminar capillary perfusion and shunting of blood at the level of the coronary band.[62] Pollitt and Davies[63] demonstrated increases in hoof temperature, suggesting an increase in blood flow to the tissues encased within the hoof capsule. Conversely, Hood and colleagues[62] demonstrated a decrease in hoof temperature after carbohydrate overload. These documented reductions in digital perfusion are transient and inconsistent, thus reducing the likelihood of substantial ischemia during laminitis.[64] In fact, Loftus and colleagues[15] did not observe a significant increase in XO generation in BWHE-induced laminitis, an event that would have occurred had ischemia/hypoxia been present.

Although changes in digital blood flow and altered concentrations of vasoactive substances may not have an important effect on regional blood flow, these alterations do signal alteration in vascular and endothelial function.[21] The end result of altered endothelial function during laminitis may be the creation of a proinflammatory state with increased oxidant stress rather than oxygen deprivation.

SUMMARY

The preponderance of evidence supports roles for inflammation, metabolic derangement, endothelial and venous dysfunction, and matrix degradation as causes of laminitis. Inflammation, oxidant stress, and matrix degradation may be factors common to each of these mechanisms that lead to the laminar damage of laminitis.

REFERENCES

1. Parsons TS, Orsini JA, Krafty R, et al. Risk factors for development of acute laminitis in horses during hospitalization: 73 cases (1997–2004). J Am Vet Med Assoc 2007;230:885–9.
2. USDA. Lameness and laminitis in U.S. horses. #N318.0400. Fort Collins (CO): USDA, APHIS, VA, CEAH, National Animal Health Monitoring System; 2000.
3. Johnson PJ. The equine metabolic syndrome peripheral Cushing's syndrome. Vet Clin North Am Equine Pract 2002;18:271–93.
4. Belknap JK, Moore JN, editors. Special issue: inflammatory aspects of equine laminitis. Vet Immunol Immunopathol 2009;(T3–4):149–262.

5. Hood DM, Grosenbaugh DA, Mostafa MB, et al. The role of vascular mechanisms in the development of acute equine laminitis. J Vet Intern Med 1993;7:228–34.
6. Pollitt CC. Basement membrane pathology: a feature of acute equine laminitis. Equine Vet J 1996;28:38–46.
7. French KR, Pollitt CC. Equine laminitis: loss of hemidesmosomes in hoof secondary epidermal lamellae correlates to dose in an oligofructose induction model: an ultrastructural study. Equine Vet J 2004;36(3):230–5.
8. Belknap JK, Moore JN, Crouser EC. Sepsis—from human organ failure to laminar failure. Vet Immunol Immunopathol 2009;129:155–7.
9. Fontaine GL, Belknap JK, Allen D, et al. Expression of interleukin-1beta in the digital laminae of horses in the prodromal stage of experimentally induced laminitis. Am J Vet Res 2001;62(5):714–20.
10. Waguespack RW, Kemppainen RJ, Cochran A, et al. Increased expression of MAIL, a cytokine-associated nuclear protein, in the prodromal stage of black walnut-induced laminitis. Equine Vet J 2004;36:285–91.
11. Waguespack RW, Cochran A, Belknap JK. Expression of the cyclooxygenase isoforms in the prodromal stage of black walnut-induced laminitis in horses. Am J Vet Res 2004;65:1724–9.
12. Stewart AJ, Pettigrew A, Cochran AM, et al. Indices of inflammation in the lung and liver in the early stages of the black walnut extract model of equine laminitis. Vet Immunol Immunopathol 2009;129(3–4):254–60.
13. Belknap JK, Giguère S, Pettigrew A, et al. Lamellar proinflammatory cytokine expression patterns in laminitis at the developmental stage and at the onset of lameness: innate vs. adaptive immune response. Equine Vet J 2007;39(1):42–7.
14. Bailey SR, Adair HS, Reinemeyer CR, et al. Plasma concentrations of endotoxin and platelet activation in the developmental stage of oligofructose-induced laminitis. Vet Immunol Immunopathol 2009;129:167–73.
15. Loftus JP, Belknap JK, Stankiewicz KM, et al. Laminar xanthine oxidase, superoxide dismutase and catalase activities in the prodromal stage of black-walnut induced equine laminitis. Equine Vet J 2007;39(1):48–53.
16. Noschka E, Vandenplas ML, Hurley DJ, et al. Temporal aspects of laminar gene expression during the developmental stages of equine laminitis. Vet Immunol Immunopathol 2009;129(3–4):242–53.
17. Blikslager AT, Yin C, Cochran AM, et al. Cyclooxygenase expression in the early stages of equine laminitis: a cytologic study. J Vet Intern Med 2006;20(5):1191–6.
18. Yin C, Pettigrew A, Loftus JP, et al. Tissue concentrations of 4-HNE in the black walnut extract model of laminitis: indication of oxidant stress in affected laminae. Vet Immunol Immunopathol 2009;129(3–4):211–5.
19. Weiss DJ, Evanson OA, McClenahan D, et al. Evaluation of platelet activation and platelet-neutrophil aggregates in ponies with alimentary laminitis. Am J Vet Res 1997;58(12):1376–80.
20. Weiss DJ, Evanson OA, McClenahan D, et al. Effect of a competitive inhibitor of platelet aggregation on experimentally induced laminitis in ponies. Am J Vet Res 1998;59(7):814–7.
21. Eades SC, Stokes AM, Johnson PJ, et al. Serial alterations in digital hemodynamics and endothelin-1 immunoreactivity, platelet-neutrophil aggregation, and concentrations of nitric oxide, insulin, and glucose in blood obtained from horses following carbohydrate overload. Am J Vet Res 2007;68(1):87–94.
22. Black SJ, Lunn DP, Yin C, et al. Leukocyte emigration in the early stages of laminitis. Vet Immunol Immunopathol 2006;109(13–4):161–6.

23. Hurley DJ, Parks RJ, Reber AJ, et al. Dynamic changes in circulating leukocytes during the induction of equine laminitis with black walnut extract. Vet Immunol Immunopathol 2006;110(3–4):195–206.
24. Riggs LM, Franck T, Moore JN, et al. Neutrophil myeloperoxidase measurements in plasma, laminar tissue, and skin of horses given black walnut extract. Am J Vet Res 2007;68(1):81–6.
25. Loftus JP, Belknap JK, Black SJ. Matrix metalloproteinase-9 in laminae of black walnut extract treated horses correlates with neutrophil abundance. Vet Immunol Immunopathol 2006;113(3–4):267–76.
26. Faleiros RR, Nuovo GJ, Belknap JK. Calprotectin in myeloid and epithelial cells of laminae from horses with black walnut extract-induced laminitis. J Vet Intern Med 2009;23(1):174–81.
27. Faleiros RR, Stokes AM, Eades SC, et al. Assessment of apoptosis in epidermal lamellar cells in clinically normal horses and those with laminitis. Am J Vet Res 2004;65:578–85.
28. French KR, Pollitt CC. Equine laminitis: cleavage of laminin 5 associated with basement membrane dysadhesion. Equine Vet J 2004;36:242–7.
29. Kyaw-Tanner M, Pollitt CC. Equine laminitis: increased transcription of matrix metalloproteinase-2 (MMP-2) occurs during the developmental phase. Equine Vet J 2004;36:221–5.
30. Mungall BA, Pollitt CC. Zymographic analysis of equine laminitis. Histochem Cell Biol 1999;112(6):467–72.
31. Pollitt CC, Daradka M. Equine laminitis basement membrane pathology: loss of type IV collagen, type VII collagen and laminin immunostaining. Equine Vet J Suppl 1998;26:139–44.
32. Johnson PJ, Kreegor JM, Keeler M, et al. Serum markers of lamellar basement membrane degradation and lamellar histopathological changes in horses affected with laminitis. Equine Vet J 2000;32(6):462–8.
33. Pollitt CC. Equine laminitis: a revised pathophysiology. Proc Am Assoc Equine Pract 1999;45:188–92.
34. Van Eps AW, Pollitt CC. Equine laminitis: cryotherapy reduces the severity of the acute lesion. Equine Vet J 2004;36:255–60.
35. Black SJ. Extracellular matrix, leukocyte migration and laminitis. Vet Immunol Immunopathol 2009;129:161–3.
36. Clutterbuck AL, Harris P, Allaway D, et al. Matrix metalloproteinases in inflammatory pathologies of the horse. Vet J 2008. DOI:10.1016/j.tvjl.2008.09.022.
37. Loftus JP, Johnson PJ, Belknap JK, et al. Leukocyte-derived and endogenous matrix metalloproteinases in the lamellae of horses with naturally acquired and experimentally induced laminitis. Vet Immunol Immunopathol 2009;129(3–4):221–30.
38. Mungall BA, Pollitt CC. Thermolysin activates equine lamellar hoof matrix metalloproteinases. J Comp Pathol 2002;126:9–16.
39. Mungall BA, Kyaw-Tanner M, Pollitt CC. In vitro evidence for a bacterial pathogenesis of equine laminitis. Vet Microbiol 2001;79:209–23.
40. Millinovich GJ, Trott DJ, Burrell PC, et al. Changes in equine hindgut bacterial populations during oligofructose-induced laminitis. Environ Microbiol 2006;8:885–98.
41. Bailey SR, Marr CM, Elliott J. Identification and quantification of amines in the equine caecum. Res Vet Sci 2003;74:113–8.
42. Bailey SR, Rycroft A, Elliott J. Production of amines in equine cecal contents in an in vitro model of carbohydrate overload. J Anim Sci 2002;80:2656–62.

43. Coyne MJ, Cousin H, Loftus JP, et al. Cloning and expression of ADAM-related metalloproteases in equine laminitis. Vet Immunol Immunopathol 2009;129(3–4): 231–41.
44. Kyaw-Tanner MT, Wattle O, et al. Equine laminitis: membrane type matrix metalloproteinase-1 (MMP-14) is involved in acute phase onset. Equine Vet J 2008;40:482–7.
45. Kim J, Montagnani M, Kwang KK, et al. Reciprocal relationships between insulin resistance and endothelial dysfunction: molecular and pathophysiological mechanisms. Circulation 2006;113:1888–904.
46. Treiber KH, Kronfeld DS, Hess TM, et al. Evaluation of genetic and metabolic predispositions and nutritional risk factors for pasture-associated laminitis in ponies. J Am Vet Med Assoc 2006;228:1538–45.
47. Bailey SR, Habershon-Butcher JL, Ransom KJ, et al. Hypertension and insulin resistance in a mixed breed population of ponies predisposed to laminitis. Am J Vet Res 2008;69(1):122–9.
48. Carter RA, Treiber KH, Geor RJ, et al. Prediction of incipient pasture-associated laminitis from hyperinsulinaemia, hyperleptinaemia and generalised and localised obesity in a cohort of ponies. Equine Vet J 2009;41(2):171–8.
49. Geor R, Frank N. Metabolic syndrome-From human organ disease to laminar failure in equids. Vet Immunol Immunopathol 2009;129(3–4):151–4.
50. Radin MJ, Sharkey LC, Holycross BJ. Adipokines: a review of biological and analytical principles and an update in dogs, cats, and horses. Vet Clin Pathol 2009;38(2):136–56.
51. Asplin KE, Sillence MN, Pollitt CC, et al. Induction of laminitis by prolonged hyperinsulinaemia in clinically normal ponies. Vet J 2007;174:530–5.
52. De Laat MA, McGowan CM, Sillence MN, et al. Equine laminitis: Induced by 48, h hyperinsulinaemia in Standardbred horses. Equine Vet J 2009;41. DOI: 10.2746/042516409X475779.
53. Treiber K, Carter R, Gay L, et al. Inflammatory and redox status of ponies with a history of pasture-associated laminitis. Vet Immunol Immunopathol 2009; 129(3–4):216–20.
54. Robertson TP, Bailey SR, Peroni JF. Equine laminitis: a journey to the dark side of venous. Vet Immunol Immunopathol 2009;129(3–4):164–6.
55. Allen D, Clark ES, Moore JN, et al. Evaluation of equine digital Starling forces and hemodynamics during early laminitis. Am J Vet Res 1990;51(12):1930–4.
56. Eaton SA, Allen D, Eades SC, et al. Digital Starling forces and hemodynamics during early laminitis induced by an aqueous extract of black walnut (*Juglans nigra*) in horses. Am J Vet Res 1995;56:1338–44.
57. Eades SC, Stokes AM, Moore RM. Effects of an endothelin receptor antagonist and nitroglycerin on digital vascular function in horses during the prodromal stages of carbohydrate overload-induced laminitis. Am J Vet Res 2006;67: 1204–11.
58. Keen JA, Hillier C, McGorum BC, et al. Endothelin mediated contraction of equine laminar veins. Equine Vet J 2008;40:488–92.
59. Loftus JP, Black SJ, Pettigrew A, et al. Early laminar events involving endothelial activation in horses with black walnut-induced laminitis. Am J Vet Res 2007;68: 1205–11.
60. Garner HE, Coffman JR, Hahn WE, et al. Equine laminitis associated with hypertension: a review. J Am Vet Med Assoc 1975;166:56–7.
61. Ackerman N, Garner HE, Coffman JR, et al. Angiographic appearance of the normal equine foot and alterations in chronic laminitis. J Am Vet Med Assoc 1975;166:58–62.

62. Hood DM, Wager IP, Brumbaugh GW. Evaluation of hoof wall surface temperature as an index of digital vascular perfusion during the prodromal and acute phases of carbohydrate-induced laminitis in horses. Am J Vet Res 2001;62:1167–72.
63. Pollitt CC, Davies CT. Equine laminitis its development coincides with increase sublamellar blood flow. Equine Vet J Suppl 1998;27:125.
64. Adair HS, Goble DO, Schmidhammer JL. Laminar microvascular flow, measured by means of laser Doppler flowmetry, during the prodromal stages of black walnut-induced laminitis in horses. Am J Vet Res 2000;61:862–8.

Carbohydrate Alimentary Overload Laminitis

Christopher C. Pollitt, BVSc, PhD[a,b,*], Michelle B. Visser, PhD[c]

KEYWORDS

- Equine laminitis • Carbohydrate overload
- Oligofructose • Basement membrane

Although not the first to describe the microscopic appearance of equine laminitis associated with alimentary overload with carbohydrate, Nils Obel in 1948 produced the first detailed descriptions. He expressed astonishment that this had not been done before considering the devastating nature of laminitis. He also stated "a profound knowledge of the anatomic changes in the initial stages must be considered a prerequisite for the study of the pathophysiology of the disease."[1]

Obel always doubted a vascular basis to laminitis pointing out that, clinically, many ill horses have subcutaneous edema in the distal limbs that is not accompanied by laminitis and conversely, in 50 cases of postparturient laminitis, distal limb edema was by no means a consistent finding. It seemed logical to him that if there was serious injury of lamellar vessels then this would be manifest throughout the organism, which is not the case. Describing the histopathology of laminitis induced by carbohydrate overload, Obel noted many of the changes that have been described in more recent studies. Consistently there was mitosis among epidermal basal cells, leukocytic infiltration, and attenuation of secondary epidermal lamellae.

He described the absence of secondary dermal lamellae between adjacent secondary epidermal lamellae (SELs) and how SELs, thus separated from their dermis, "were in direct contact with each other."[1] Obel seemed unaware of basement membrane (BM) pathology and although his published figures clearly show separation of dermis from epidermis along the BM lamellar interface, and spectacular dislocation between these 2 compartments, the connection to basement membrane pathology was not made. Making the BM connection to laminitis pathology and observing BM

[a] School of Veterinary Science, The University of Queensland, St Lucia, Brisbane, Queensland 4072, Australia
[b] The Laminitis Institute, University of Pennsylvania School of Veterinary Medicine, New Bolton Center, Kennett Square, PA, USA
[c] School of Veterinary Science, Faculty of Natural Resources, Agriculture and Veterinary Science, The University of Queensland, Queensland 4072, Australia
* Corresponding author.
E-mail address: c.pollitt@uq.edu.au

Vet Clin Equine 26 (2010) 65–78
doi:10.1016/j.cveq.2010.01.006 vetequine.theclinics.com

dislocation early in the course of laminitis development[2] encouraged mechanistic thinking and asked the question "how can epidermis and dermis separate from each other at the microscopic and the ultrastructural level and lead eventually to gross dislocation of hoof wall from distal phalanx?" Answering this question led to the inflammatory/enzymatic theory of laminitis pathophysiology that at least partially explains why the suspensory apparatus of the distal phalanx (SADP) fails.

The prefix of the word laminitis correctly identifies the laminae, or more correctly, lamellae, of the inner hoof wall as the focus of laminitis pathology. The suffix -itis implies a role for inflammation. The hoof wall lamellae are certainly inflamed in the acute phase. Tissue damage has occurred; there is pain, redness, and swelling beneath the hoof wall. The mystery is why?

In acute laminitis, the tissue suspending the distal phalanx from the inner hoof wall fails, specifically at the junction between the connective tissue of the dermis or corium (the bone side) and the basal cell layer of the epidermal lamellae (the hoof side). This junction, the BM zone or lamellar interface, seems to be the weak link in an otherwise robust and reliable structure. In acute laminitis there is wholesale epidermal cell detachment from, and lysis of, the lamellar BM and this leads to failure of the lamellar anatomy and, ultimately, failure of the suspensory attachment between hoof and distal phalanx. There is a good correlation between the grade of severity, as seen with the microscope (histopathology), and the degree of lameness (using the Obel grading system) shown by the horse.[2] Thus, when the horse first starts to show the foot pain of laminitis, it means that the anatomy of the hoof wall lamellae is being destroyed. The worse the lameness, the worse the damage. Any activity that places stress on an already weakened lamellar attachment apparatus (such as forced exercise) will cause further damage and is contraindicated. The use of nerve blocks and potent analgesic drugs to eliminate pain will encourage locomotion and potentially precipitate more damage.

ALIMENTARY CARBOHYDRATE OVERLOAD MODEL

Much of what is known about laminitis and the metabolic events surrounding it has been derived from studies on horses that have been experimentally dosed with excess soluble carbohydrate (the alimentary carbohydrate overload model). The diet of horses in their natural state is grass- and legume-based and consists mainly of complex structural carbohydrates, in the form of cellulose, hemicellulose, and lignin, as well as non-structural carbohydrates (NSC) in the form of sugars, fructans, or starch. The structural carbohydrates and fructans are indigestible to mammals without the aid of active microbial hindgut fermentation and a large portion of the equine abdomen is occupied by the cecum and colon where complex carbohydrates and fructans are fermented to absorbable end products.

Domestic horses and ponies sometimes encounter excessive quantities of starch and fructan in their diet when they consume cereal grain or the sward of certain cultivated pastures. Pony breeds, having evolved metabolic adaptations for survival in harsh, low nutrient environments, are particularly prone to laminitis if given unrestricted access to cultivated pasture. Most of the consequences of carbohydrate overload occur after the arrival of the carbohydrate in the hindgut and relate to the rapid proliferation of hindgut bacteria flourishing in the presence of excess substrate.

On mixing with the normally neutral cecal contents, excess starch or fructan undergoes rapid fermentation to lactic acid. With the arrival of more and more substrate, fermentation favors the rapid proliferation of hindgut gram-positive bacteria *Streptococcus bovis* and *Streptococcus equinus* (now *Streptococcus lutetiensis*).[3–5]

This results in very acidic conditions in the hindgut with pH as low as 4. Two isomers of lactic acid, D- and L-lactate, are produced in almost equal proportions by bacterial fermentation in the equine hindgut. However, only L-lactate is produced by the metabolic activities of mammals, so the concentration of D-lactate in venous blood can be used as an accurate indicator of bacterial lactic fermentation in the hindgut.[6] Plasma D-lactate concentration peaks around 20 hours after dosing and then declines as does fecal pH.

Low pH in the large intestine initiates a series of secondary events that often, but not always, culminate in laminitis. One of the most important consequences is the death and lysis of large numbers of bacteria and the release of the toxic components of their cell walls (endotoxins, exotoxins) and genetic material (microbial DNA). Toxins absorbed from the gut into the bloodstream during developmental laminitis and toxemia following alimentary carbohydrate overload creates a severe illness for the horse. Low concentrations of endotoxin, detectable in the plasma of horses dosed with oligofructose (OF) to induce laminitis, peak 8 hours after dosing and decline at 12 hours.[7] This correlates with the finding of Milinovich and colleagues[3] (see article by Milinovich and colleagues elsewhere in this issue for further exploration of this topic) who found that *Escherichia coli*, presumably the source of lipopolysaccharide endotoxin, disappears from the cecal microflora as oligofructose-fermenting hindgut streptococci rapidly flourish and bloom. The endotoxin peak also coincides with pyrexia onset and a decline in lymphocytes and an increase in polymorphs circulating in the blood.[6]

Experimental administration of endotoxin itself has never been able to cause laminitis. In addition, endotoxemia can be effectively controlled by a range of drugs (eg, polymyxin B,[8–10] flunixin meglumine[11]) and laminitis develops regardless of their use. It remains difficult to directly associate genuine endotoxemia with laminitis onset. Many ill horses appear endotoxic, but this is usually inferred from clinical signs rather than confirmed by endotoxin assay. During the development of OF-induced laminitis low concentrations of endotoxin are detected and may be sufficient to activate platelets, which in turn could activate leukocytes and thus contribute to lamellar inflammatory pathways.[7]

In field cases, grain founder occurs following the consumption of excessive amounts of grain, either from accidental access by the horse or by a misguided, intentional, dietary increase by its keeper. Although the amount of grain required to induce laminitis varies between individuals, the consumption of 5 to 8 kg of wheat grain by the average 400 to 450 kg horse causes fecal acidity (pH 4–5 instead of the normal 6.8–7.5), lactic acidemia, profuse watery diarrhea and fever, all of which are associated with laminitis. The likelihood of laminitis following grain consumption correlates directly with the starch content of the grain, the amount that passes undigested to the hindgut, and the rate at which the undigested carbohydrate is fermented. The type of grain and the manner in which it is processed in the stomach and small intestine are also important in determining the amount of starch that passes undigested to the hindgut. Grains such as wheat, sorghum, corn, and barley are considered to be most dangerous with respect to the risk of laminitis. The feeding of oats is relatively safe. Gorging on bread can result in significant amounts of readily fermentable carbohydrate passing to the hindgut and is also a recorded cause of laminitis.

As early as 24 hours after carbohydrate overload, the epithelial cells lining the cecum show degenerative changes and the bowel becomes leaky.[12] There is widespread desquamation and sloughing of cecal epithelial cells,[13] sufficient to allow passage of lactic acid, toxins, and laminitis trigger factors into the circulation (**Fig. 1**). The consequences can be catastrophic. About 10% to 15% of horses die

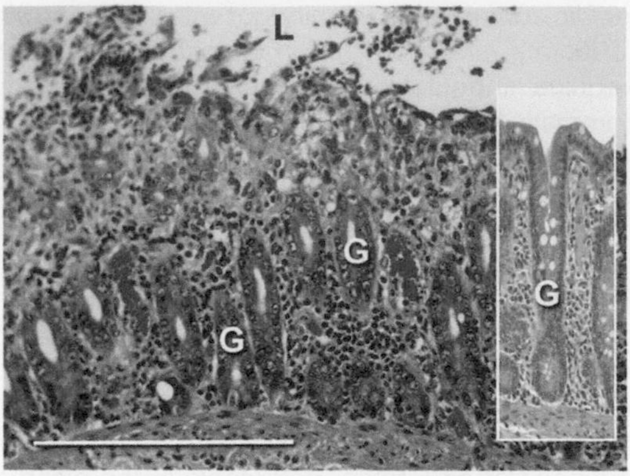

Fig. 1. The leaking hindgut of a horse developing carbohydrate overload laminitis. The hindgut lumen normally has an intact layer (the mucosal barrier) of tightly joined epithelial cells covering its surface (*inset*). This prevents harmful bacteria and their toxins from being absorbed into the circulation. The hindgut wall is glandular and the cells of the mucosal barrier line the glands (G) and the lumen (L) of the bowel. During carbohydrate-induced colitis the mucosal barrier is damaged providing a possible pathway for laminitis trigger factors to enter the circulation. The submucosa is heavily infiltrated with leukocytes and seems to be a site of intense inflammatory activity. Hematoxylin and eosin (H&E) stain. Bar = 100 μm.

from cardiovascular shock after the accidental consumption of excess grain. High heart rates, rapid breathing, fever, sweating, colic, diarrhea, and depression are the signs of horses suffering grain overload. Just when the horse turns the corner and responds to treatment and the severity of the clinical signs decreases, the signs of foot pain appear; laminitis has arrived on the scene.

The gram-positive bacteria responsible for the lactic acid production resulting from carbohydrate overload are sensitive to a range of antibiotics. The laminitis induction following carbohydrate overload does not occur if the activities of the bacteria are controlled. Virginiamycin, in the patented formulation Founderguard (Virbac, Australia), administered at 5 g/kg body weight, 4 days before wheat grain starch overload, prevented laminitis and D-lactic acid production in all cases.[2] The correct formulation of virginiamycin is important for the active ingredient to enter and mix properly with the cecal and colonic digesta. Unfortunately, virginiamycin has to be present in the cecum before the arrival of carbohydrate for laminitis prevention to occur. When virginiamycin was administered 6 to 8 hours after dosing with carbohydrate, laminitis did occur. For this reason, Founderguard is considered a useful laminitis prophylactic for horses and ponies with a high carbohydrate intake, but has little value therapeutically. The efficacy of Founderguard against the oligofructose laminitis induction model has not been tested.

LAMINITIS HISTOPATHOOGY

Many descriptions of laminitis histopathology derive from laminitis induced experimentally with a single large dose of carbohydrate of either grain starch or oligofructose.[1,6] The sequences of microscopic events that lead to clinical laminitis follow a consistent temporal pattern,[14] and the stages of histologic laminitis can be identified by the degree of severity of these changes. Lamellar biopsies taken from horses developing OF-induced laminitis at 12, 18, 24, 30, 36 and 48 hours after dosing have been used to develop a timeline of events that characterize lesion development.[14,15]

Multiple serial lamellar biopsy has been validated in normal horses and shown to neither inflame adjacent tissues nor be particularly painful for the horse.[16] Making the lamellar BM clearly visible is important and requires staining lamellar tissues with periodic acid Schiff (PAS) stain or with immunohistochemical methods using basement membrane–specific antibody.[17]

Normal lamellar anatomic characteristics, assessed before allocating a laminitis grade to a section of lamellar hoof tissue, are as follows (see the article by Pollitt in this issue):

- The tips of the SELs are always rounded (club-shaped) and never tapered or pointed.
- The basal cell nucleus is oval, with the long axis of the oval at a right angle to the long axis of the SEL. These parameters can be satisfactorily assessed using routine hematoxylin and eosin (H&E) staining of sections.
- The BM penetrates deeply into the crypts between the SELs and outlines the wafer-thin, but connective tissue–filled, secondary dermal lamellae.
- The BM tightly adheres to the basal cells of each SEL. The PAS or immunohistochemical stains show this best.[2]

GRADE 1 LAMINITIS HISTOPATHOLOGY

The earliest change attributable to laminitis is loss of shape and normal arrangement of the lamellar basal and parabasal cells. The basal cell nuclei become rounded instead of oval and take an abnormal position in the cytoplasm of the cell. The SELs become stretched, long, and thin, with tapering instead of club-shaped tips. These changes were present at 12 hours in serial lamellar biopsies taken after oligofructose dosing (**Fig. 2**).[14]

First noticeable at the tips of the SELs are teat-shaped bubbles of loose BM form (**Fig. 3**).

Examination of laminitis tissues with the electron microscope confirms lysis and separation of the lamellar BM.[18] The greater magnification shows widespread loss of basal cell adhesion plaques (hemidesmosomes) and contraction of the basal cell

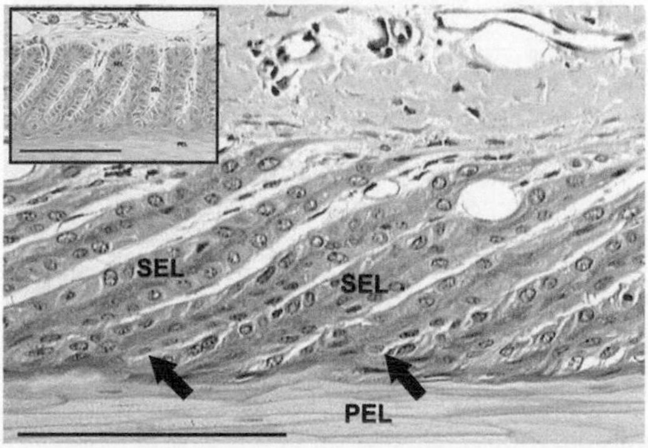

Fig. 2. Grade 1 histologic laminitis (H&E stain). The SELs are longer and thinner than normal and the SELs have pointed instead of the normal rounded tips. The basal cell nuclei are no longer oval in shape and have become round and situated abnormally close to the BM. The tips of the secondary dermal lamellae (*arrowed*) are still situated close to the primary epidermal lamella (PEL), which is normal. Inset shows normal lamellae. H&E stain. Bar = 10 μm.

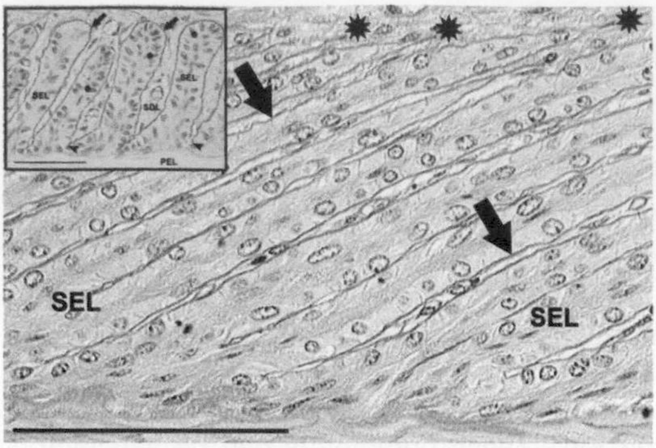

Fig. 3. Grade 1 histologic laminitis (PAS stain). Micrograph showing hoof lamellar tissues stained to highlight the BM. The BM (*arrowed*) is stained dark magenta. At the now tapered tips of the secondary epidermal lamellae (SEL) the BM has lifted away (stars) from the underlying basal cells. Between the SEL bases, the BM is in its normal position, close to the primary epidermal lamella (PEL). Inset shows normal lamellae. PAS stain. Bar = 10 μm.

cytoskeleton away from the inner cell surface. Electron microscopy shows why the BM separates from the feet of the basal cells. The filaments that anchor hemidesmosomes to the lamina densa of the BM no longer bridge the dermal/epidermal interface (Fig. 4).[19]

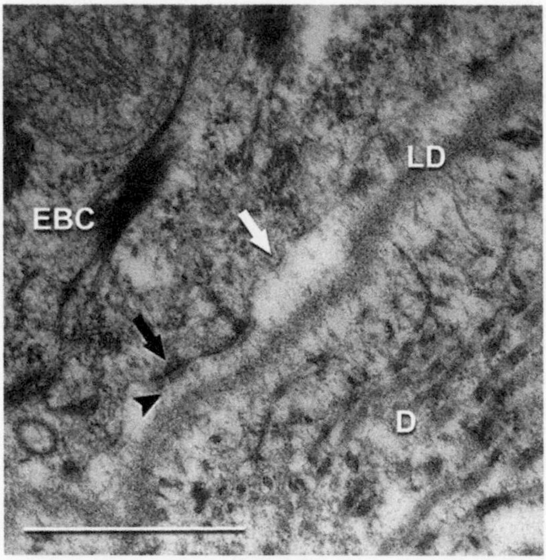

Fig. 4. Electron micrograph of hoof lamellar tip developing laminitis. The lamina densa (LD) of the BM has separated from the plasmalemma of the lamellar epidermal basal cell (EBC). Some hemidesmosomes (*black arrow*) appear undamaged but others (*white arrow*) have faded and have lost their anchoring filament attachment to the EBC plasmalemma. Normally, anchoring filaments (*arrowhead*) bridge the lamina densa firmly to the EBC but when functional hemidesmosomes are lost (*white arrow*) the LD separates from the EBC. Bar = 200 nm. D, dermis.

GRADE 2 LAMINITIS HISTOPATHOLOGY

Because the BM is no longer completely tethered to the basal cells, it slips farther away with each cycle of weight bearing by the horse. Portions of the lamellar BM are lysed initially between the bases of the SELs (**Fig. 5**). The BM retracts from the tips of SELs taking with it the dermal connective tissue. The lamellar epidermal cells, now free of their BM, seem not to be undergoing necrosis, at least initially, and clump together to form amorphous, basement membrane–free masses on either side of the lamellar axis.[2]

Electron microscopy of the attenuated lamellar tips of grade 2 histologic laminitis confirm BM separation from the plasmalemma of the lamellar epidermal basal cell (**Fig. 6**).[19] Usually the adjacent dermis seems unaffected by the laminitis process.

GRADE 3 LAMINITIS HISTOPATHOLOGY

In laminitis the worst-case scenario is a rapid and near-total BM separation from all the epidermal lamellae of the hoof toe, quarters, heels, and bars. Sheets of BM peel away to form aggregations of loose, isolated basement membrane in the connective tissue adjoining the lamellae. The epidermal lamellar cells are left as isolated columns on either side of the keratinized axis of the primary epidermal lamella, with little viable connection to the dermal connective tissue still attached to the distal phalanx (**Fig. 7**). Similar lesions were described by Obel in 1948.[1] The hoof lamellar tips slide away from the BM connective tissue attachments, at first microscopically, but as the degree of separation increases, the distance between hoof and distal phalanx becomes measurable in millimeters (**Fig. 8**) and can be detected radiographically.[20] This manifests clinically as the sinker. Because the BM is the key structure bridging the epidermis of the hoof to the connective tissue of the distal phalanx, wholesale loss and disorganization of the lamellar basement membrane follows and inexorably leads to the pathology of hoof and bone that characterizes the chronic stage of laminitis.[20]

The laminitis process also affects the lamellar capillaries. As the BM and the connective tissue between the SELs disappear, so do the capillaries. They become obliterated, compressed against the edges of the primary dermal lamellae. Without

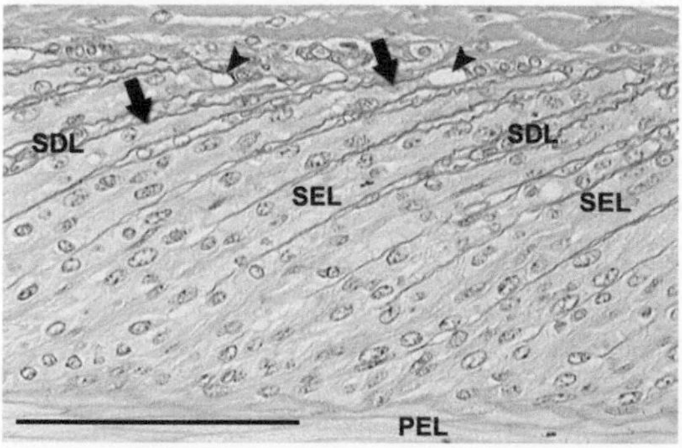

Fig. 5. Grade 2 histologic laminitis (PAS stain). The BM is stained dark magenta. At the tips of the now pointed secondary epidermal lamellae (SEL) the basement membrane (*arrowed*) has continued to lift from the underlying basal cells to form empty, BM-enclosed, teat-shaped caps (*arrowheads*). The BM has disappeared at the tips of secondary dermal lamellae (SDL), between SEL bases. The lamellar BM is no longer close to the primary epidermal lamella (PEL). There is a reduced amount of connective tissue between SELs. Bar = 10 μm.

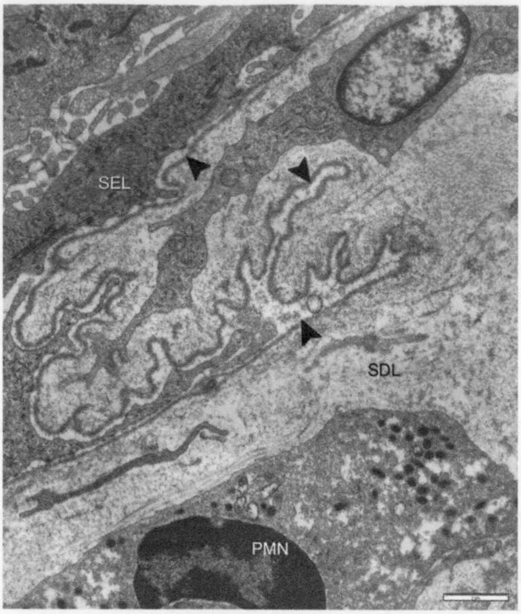

Fig. 6. Transmission electron micrograph of SEL tip affected by grade 2 histologic laminitis. Much of the lamellar basement membrane (*arrowheads*) is no longer attached to the plasmalemma of SEL basal cells. A polymorphonuclear leukocyte (PMN) is in the dermis of the secondary dermal lamella (SDL). Bar = 2 μm.

a full compliment of capillaries in the lamellar circulation, blood probably bypasses the capillary bed through dilated arteriovenous shunts[21] changing the nature of the foot circulation. A bounding pulse becomes detectable by finger palpation of the digital arteries. Furthermore, epidermal cell necrosis, intravascular coagulation, and edema

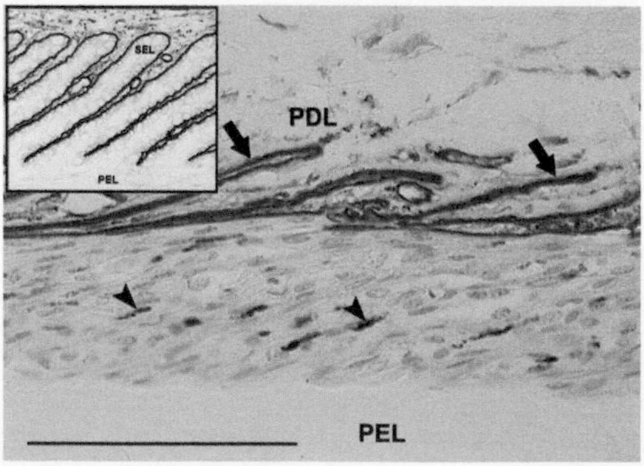

Fig. 7. Grade 3 histologic laminitis (type IV collagen immunostain). Only remnants (*arrowheads*) of the basement membrane remain between the now disorganized SELs. Most of the lamellar epidermal cells have coalesced into an amorphous mass no longer effectively attached to any connective tissue. The remainder of the lamellar BM lies free, in strands (*arrowed*), among the connective tissue of the primary epidermal lamella (PDL). Inset shows normal lamellae stained the same way. Bar = 10 μm.

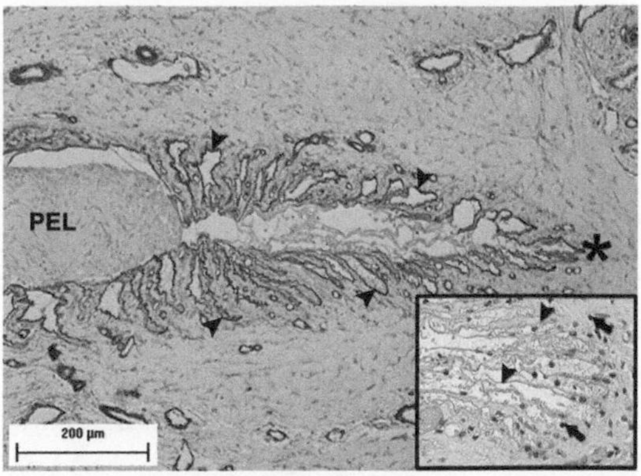

Fig. 8. Grade 3 histologic laminitis (type IV collagen immunostain). The basement membrane of the lamellar interface and blood vessels is highlighted by the type IV collagen immunostaining. The tip of the primary epidermal lamella (PEL) has completely detached from its basement membrane and is an unattached amorphous mass. Collapsed tubes of basement membrane, now empty of epidermal cells, are still attached to connective tissue (*arrowheads*). The PEL has moved 0.61 mm from its normal position in the sublamellar dermis (asterisk), a distance that may be measureable on a radiograph. The inset shows a similar lamellar tip, PAS stained. There are numerous invading leukocytes on both sides of the SEL basement membrane.

are not universally present in sections made from tissues in the early stages of laminitis. The vessels in the primary dermal lamella, even the smallest, are predominantly open, without evidence of microvascular thrombi.

Leukocytes, Inflammation and Laminitis

It is rare to detect leukocytes in the lamellar tissues of normal horses.[22] However, extravasation of leukocytes into the perivascular lamellar dermis occurs in grain starch,[2] oligofructose (see **Fig. 8**; **Fig. 9**),[15] black walnut extract,[22,23] and the hyperinsulinemic[19,24] induced forms of laminitis.

Because leukocytic infiltration of tissues is associated with inflammation, the discovery that leukocytic infiltration is common to most, if not all, forms of laminitis has reemphasized an inflammatory pathway to laminitis development. There is molecular evidence that inflammatory mediators may activate many of the processes known to damage the lamellar interface.[25,26] Polymorphonuclear leukocytes are rich in matrixmetalloproteinase-9 (MMP-9) and their presence within lamellar epidermal compartments in grade 3 histopathology[2] (see **Fig. 8**; **Fig. 10**) suggests that this BM membrane–degrading enzyme may have a pathologic role in disease development.

Neutrophils produce reactive oxygen species and proinflammatory cytokines that probably contribute to cellular damage within the lamellar milieu.[27] Lamellar damage as well as leukocyte infiltration is readily detected by calprotectin immunostaining,[15,22] and because leukocyte infiltration precedes the expression of calprotectin in the lamellar epidermis, a role for leukocytes in initiating lamellar pathology has been suggested.[23,25] The lamellar biopsy timeline of OF-induced laminitis development shows that at 12 hours after dosing, BM degradation occurs in advance of leukocyte infiltration, thus downplaying an initiating role for leukocytes in lesion development.[15] Leukocytic infiltration seems to be more of a reaction to lamellar inflammation than a cause of it. Expression of the inflammatory cytokine interleukin-6 (IL-6) precedes leukocyte

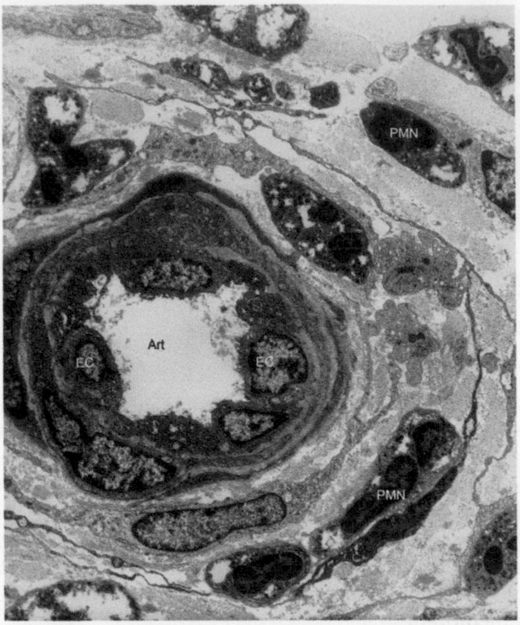

Fig. 9. Transmission electron micrograph of an arteriole (Art) in the primary dermal lamella of tissue affected by grade 3 oligofructose-induced laminitis. Numerous polymorphonuclear (PMN) leukocytes, adjacent to the arteriole, have extravasated from the vessel into the dermis.

infiltration but by itself fails to activate MMP or cause any significant weakening of the lamellar interface.[15]

The enzymatic theory of laminitis, based on the triggering of lamellar MMP activity,[28,29] challenged the alternative view that laminitis was caused by ischemia and ischemia/reperfusion injury damaging epidermal lamellae because blood flow was impeded.[30] Evidence against ischemia/reperfusion involvement in black walnut extract–induced laminitis came from studies measuring xanthine oxidase, a reactive oxygen intermediate that increases in tissues affected by ischemia and ischemia/reperfusion. Xanthine oxidase was absent in tissues with black walnut extract–induced lamellar pathology suggesting that a global lamellar hypoxic event had not

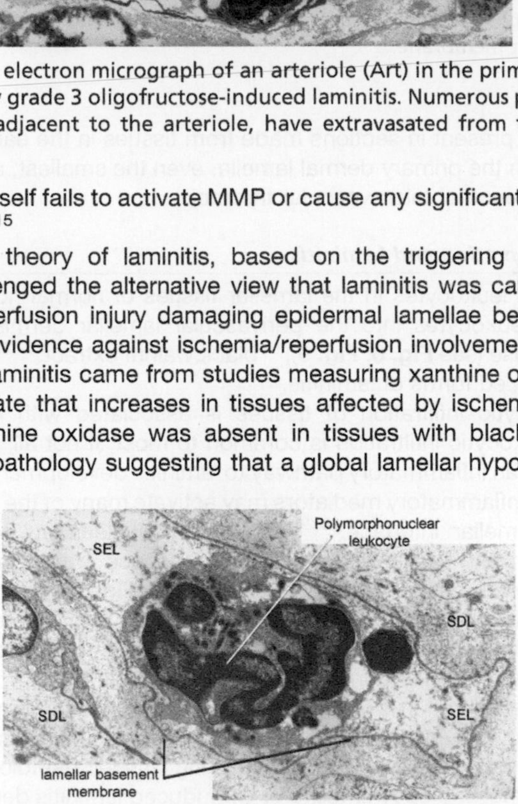

Fig. 10. Polymorphonuclear leukocytes are rich in MMP-9 and their presence within lamellar epidermal compartments in grade 3 histopathology.

occurred. Furthermore evidence from 3 independent international laboratories exists that the foot circulation during the developmental phase of carbohydrate- and now hyperinsulemia-induced laminitis is vasodilated.[31–34] Laminitis does not occur if the foot is in a state of vasoconstriction during the developmental phase, suggesting that the trigger factors only cause laminitis if they reach the lamellar tissues at a high enough concentration and for a long enough time.[31] In current laminitis therapy there is a consistent lack of efficacy of drugs addressing ischemia suggesting other pathogenic processes, such as inflammation, may be more important.

Lamellar disintegration of laminitis occurs well before clinical signs. The molecular conformation of the lamellar BM is altered 12 hours after dosing with oligofructose and a major constituent of the basement membrane, collagen IV, begins to disappear.[15] Previously, damage to the lamellar basement membrane was attributed to MMP release and activation, but new evidence places MMP activation many hours later than other molecular events.[15] An enzyme capable of modifying the proteoglycan components of lamellar basement membrane is ADAMTS-4 (a disintegrin and metalloproteinase with thrombospondin motifs). The ADAMTS-4 gene has the greatest fold increase of any gene so far discovered in laminitis development.[15,35,36] ADAMTS-4 gene expression occurs early in laminitis development and the gene product may play a central role in destabilizing proteoglycan components of the lamellar BM and thus the pathophysiology of the disease.

Equine lamellae, cultured in vitro, have tested resistant to virtually all known cytokines, tissue factors, and prostaglandins. gram-negative bacterial endotoxin, extract of black walnut (*Juglans nigra*), and even anaerobic culture conditions fail to induce lamellar separation or significant MMP activation.[37] Equine IL-6 added to cultured lamellar explants fails to activate lamellar MMPs or cause BM disruption at the lamellar interface.[15] There are some notable exceptions, however. Factors present in the supernatant of cultures of *Streptococcus bovis* (now *S lutetiensis*), isolated from the equine cecum, activate equine hoof MMP-2 and cause in vitro lamellar separation.[37] During carbohydrate overload a massive population of *S bovis* rapidly ferments carbohydrate, proliferates exponentially,[3–5] and then dies and lyses en masse. The liberated cellular components of lysed hindgut streptococci may cross the mucosal barrier of the damaged hindgut and reach the hoof lamellae hematogenously to initiate laminitis. Microbial and other factors probably associate with BMs throughout the body but only cause significant damage to lamellar basement membranes because of their uniquely equine involvement in weight bearing. On the other hand, the significant damage and leukocyte infiltration, within the mucosa of the hindgut, associated with hindgut streptococcal proliferation (see **Fig. 1**), could just as well be a source of hematogenously delivered factors that trigger lamellar BM disintegration. The actual trigger factors of oligofructose-induced laminitis remain unidentified.

The activity of tissue proteases correlates strongly with the degree of malignancy and invasiveness of lethal human tumors, such as malignant melanoma, breast, and colon cancer. Degradation of the proteoglycan present within articular cartilage caused by ADAMTS-4 is a feature of osteoarthritis. Research in these fields has generated a wide range of chemical agents capable of inhibiting enzyme activity in vitro and in vivo. One of these (Batimastat or BB-94, British Biotech, Oxford) has been shown to block the activity of lamellar MMPs in vitro and has the potential to be a useful tool in the prevention and management of acute laminitis.[38] The authors are conducting trials using the newly developed intraosseous infusion of the distal phalanx technique[39] to test whether MMP inhibitors and antiinflammatory drugs can prevent or ameliorate OF-induced laminitis.

SUMMARY

In acute laminitis, the SADP fails at the lamellar dermal/epidermal interface. A grading system for the histopathology of laminitis is based on the consistent pattern of histologic changes to the SELs, basal cells, and BM that occur as carbohydrate-induced laminitis develops. Excess carbohydrate in the equine hindgut undergoes rapid fermentation as hindgut, gram-positive bacteria *Streptococcus bovis* and *Streptococcus equinus* (now *Streptococcus lutetiensis*) rapidly proliferate. During the development of oligofructose-induced laminitis low concentrations of endotoxin are detected and may be sufficient to activate platelets, which in turn could activate leukocytes and thus contribute to lamellar inflammatory pathways. Grades 1 to 3 histologic laminitis reflect increasing separation and lysis of the lamellar BM. Because the BM is the key structure bridging the epidermis of the hoof to the connective tissue of the distal phalanx, wholesale loss and disorganization of the lamellar basement membrane leads to the pathology of hoof and bone that characterizes the acute and early chronic stages of laminitis. Leukocytic infiltration of lamellar tissues is common to most, if not all, forms of laminitis and has reemphasized an inflammatory pathway to laminitis development. During carbohydrate overload the massive population of *S bovis* suddenly dies and lyses en masse. The liberated cellular components of lysed hindgut streptocooci may cross the mucosal barrier of the damaged hindgut and reach the hoof lamellae hematogenously to initiate laminitis. Alternatively, the damage and leukocyte infiltration within the mucosa of the hindgut could just as well be a source of hematogenously delivered factors that trigger lamellar BM disintegration. The actual trigger factors of carbohydrate-induced laminitis remain unidentified.

REFERENCES

1. Obel N. Studies of the histopathology of acute laminitis: Almqvist and Wilcsells Bottrykeri Ab Uppsala [PhD thesis]. 1948.
2. Pollitt CC. Basement membrane pathology: a feature of acute equine laminitis. Equine Vet J 1996;28:38–46.
3. Milinovich GJ, Burrell PC, Pollitt CC, et al. Microbial ecology of the equine hindgut during oligofructose-induced laminitis. ISME J 2008;2:1089–100.
4. Milinovich GJ, Trott DJ, Burrell PC, et al. Fluorescence in situ hybridization analysis of hindgut bacteria associated with the development of equine laminitis. Environ Microbiol 2007;9:2090–100.
5. Milinovich GJ, Trott DJ, Burrell PC, et al. Changes in equine hindgut bacterial populations during oligofructose induced laminitis. Environ Microbiol 2006;8:885–98.
6. van Eps AW, Pollitt CC. Equine laminitis induced with oligofructose. Equine Vet J 2006;38:203–8.
7. Bailey SR, Adair HS, Reinemeyer CR, et al. Plasma concentrations of endotoxin and platelet activation in the developmental stage of oligofructose-induced laminitis. Vet Immunol Immunopathol 2009;129:167–73.
8. MacKay RJ, Clark CK, Logdberg L, et al. Effect of a conjugate of polymyxin B-dextran 70 in horses with experimentally induced endotoxemia. Am J Vet Res 1999;60:68–75.
9. Raisbeck MF, Garner HE, Osweiler GD. Effects of polymyxin B on selected features of equine carbohydrate overload. Vet Hum Toxicol 1989;31:422–6.
10. Morresey PR, MacKay RJ. Endotoxin-neutralizing activity of polymyxin B in blood after IV administration in horses. Am J Vet Res 2006;67:642–7.

11. Semrad SD, Hardee GE, Hardee MM, et al. Low-dose flunixin meglumine – effects on eicosanoid production and clinical signs induced by experimental endotoxemia in horses. Equine Vet J 1987;19:201–6.
12. Weiss D, Evanson O, MacLeay J, et al. Transient alteration in intestinal permeability to technetium Tc99m diethylenetriaminopentaacetate during the prodromal stages of alimentary laminitis in ponies. Am J Vet Res 1998;59:1431–4.
13. Sprouse RF, Garner HE, Green EM. Plasma endotoxin levels in horses subjected to carbohydrate induced laminitis. Equine Vet J 1987;19:25–8.
14. Croser EL, Pollitt CC. Acute laminitis: descriptive evaluation of serial hoof biopsies. 52nd Annual Convention of the American Association of Equine Practitioners. San Antonio (TX), December 2–6, 2006. p. 542–6.
15. Visser MB. Investigation of proteolysis of the basement membrane during the development of equine laminitis. School of Veterinary Science [PhD thesis]. Brisbane: The University of Queensland; 2009.
16. Hanly BK, Stokes AM, Bell AM, et al. Use of serial laminar tissue collection via biopsy in conscious healthy horses. Am J Vet Res 2009;70:697–702.
17. Pollitt CC, Daradka M. Equine laminitis basement membrane pathology: loss of type IV collagen, type VII collagen and laminin immunostaining. Equine Vet J Suppl 1998;26:139–44.
18. Nourian AR, Baldwin GI, van Eps AW, et al. Equine laminitis: ultrastructural lesions detected 24–30 hours after induction with oligofructose. Equine Vet J 2007;39: 360–4.
19. Nourian AR, Asplin KE, McGowan CM, et al. Equine laminitis: ultrastructural lesions detected in ponies after prolonged hyperinsulinaemia. Equine Vet J 2009;41:671–7.
20. Van Eps AW, Pollitt CC. Equine laminitis model: lamellar histopathology 7 days after induction with oligofructose. Equine Vet J 2009;41:735–40.
21. Pollitt CC, Molyneux GS. A scanning electron microscopical study of the dermal microcirculation of the equine foot. Equine Vet J 1990;22:79–87.
22. Faleiros RR, Nuovo GJ, Belknap JK. Calprotectin in myeloid and epithelial cells of laminae from horses with black walnut extract-induced laminitis. J Vet Intern Med 2009;23:174–81.
23. Black SJ, Lunn DP, Yin C, et al. Leukocyte emigration in the early stages of laminitis. Vet Immunol Immunopathol 2006;109:161–6.
24. De Laat MA, McGowan CM, Sillence MN, et al. Equine laminitis: induced by 48 h hyperinsulinaemia in Standardbred horses. Equine Vet J 2009;41. DOI: 10.2746/042516409X042475779.
25. Loftus J, Black S, Pettigrew A, et al. Early laminar events involving endothelial activation in horses with black walnut- induced laminitis. Am J Vet Res 2007; 68:1205–11.
26. Belknap JK, Giguere S, Pettigrew A, et al. Lamellar pro-inflammatory cytokine expression patterns in laminitis at the developmental stage and at the onset of lameness: innate vs. adaptive immune response. Equine Vet J 2007;39:42–7.
27. Belknap J. Pathophysiology of equine laminitis. American College of Veterinary Internal Medicine Proceedings. 2007. p. 148–50.
28. Kyaw Tanner M, Pollitt CC. Equine laminitis: increased transcription of matrix metalloproteinase-2 (MMP-2) occurs during the developmental phase. Equine Vet J 2004;36:221–5.
29. Kyaw-Tanner MT, Wattle O, van Eps AW, et al. Equine laminitis: membrane type matrix metalloproteinase-1 (MMP-14) is involved in acute phase onset. Equine Vet J 2008;40:482–7.

30. Hood DM, Grosenbaugh DA, Mostafa MB, et al. The role of vascular mechanisms in the development of acute equine laminitis. J Vet Intern Med 1993;7:228–34.
31. Pollitt CC, Davies CT. Equine laminitis: its development coincides with increased sublamellar blood flow. Equine Vet J Suppl 1998;26:125–32.
32. Robinson NE, Scott JB, Dabney JM, et al. Digital vascular responses and permeability in equine alimentary laminitis. Am J Vet Res 1976;37:1171–6.
33. Trout DR, Hornof WJ, Linford RL, et al. Scintigraphic evaluation of digital circulation during the developmental and acute phases of equine laminitis. Equine Vet J 1990;22:416–21.
34. deLaat MA, McGowan CM, Sillence MN, et al. Equine laminitis: induced by 48 hours of hyperinsulinaemia in standardbred horses. Equine Vet J 2009. DOI: 10.2746/042516409X042475779.
35. Coyne MJ, Cousin H, Loftus JP, et al. Cloning and expression of ADAM related metalloproteases in equine laminitis. J Vet Immunol 2009;129:231–41.
36. Budak MT, Orsini JA, Pollitt CC, et al. Gene expression in the lamellar dermis-epidermis during the developmental phase of carbohydrate overload-induced laminitis in the horse. Vet Immunol Immunopathol 2009;131:86–9.
37. Mungall BA, Kyaw-Tanner M, Pollitt CC. In vitro evidence for a bacterial pathogenesis of equine laminitis. Vet Microbiol 2001;79:209–23.
38. Pollitt CC, Pass MA, Pollitt S. Batimastat (BB-94) inhibits matrix metalloproteinases of equine laminitis. Equine Vet J 1998;26:119–24.
39. Nourian AR, Mills PC, Pollitt CC. Development of an intraosseous infusion method to access the lamellar circulation in the standing, conscious horse. Vet J 2009, in press. DOI: 10.1016/j.tvjl.2009.05.008.

Microbial Events in the Hindgut During Carbohydrate-induced Equine Laminitis

Gabriel J. Milinovich, BAgSc, PhD[a,b,*],
Athol V. Klieve, BAgSc, MRurSc, PhD[c,d],
Christopher C. Pollitt, BVSc, PhD[a,e],
Darren J. Trott, BVMS, PhD[a]

KEYWORDS

• Laminitis • Oligofructose • *Streptococcus* • Hindgut

The ability of equids to survive on pasture-based diets can be largely attributed to the evolutionary development of a highly adapted gastrointestinal system and the bacterial suite within. Horses derive most of their energy requirements from absorption of volatile fatty acids (VFAs), predominantly acetate, propionate, and butyrate, produced from microbial fermentation of ingesta in the hindgut.[1] These VFAs, in particular, have major roles in the health and homeostasis of the host. Acetate constitutes an energy source for many tissues, including the heart, muscle tissue, and the brain; propionate is a major precursor for gluconeogenesis, and butyrate provides an energy source for colonocytes and may play a role in the regulation and differentiation of gut epithelia.[1] In addition to provision of nutrients, maintenance of a healthy hindgut microbiota is essential to other major aspects of the host's health, including stimulation of a functional immune response, protection from pathogens, production and neutralization of toxins, and gene expression in host epithelial tissue.[2]

[a] Australian Equine Laminitis Research Unit, School of Veterinary Science, The University of Queensland, St Lucia, Queensland 4072, Australia
[b] Department of Genetics in Ecology, University of Vienna, Althanstrasse 14, Vienna 1090, Austria
[c] Schools of Animal Studies and Veterinary Science, The University of Queensland, Gatton Campus, Gatton, Queensland 4343, Australia
[d] Animal Research Institute, Agri-Science Queensland, Department of Employment, Economic Development and Innovation, Locked mail bag number 4, Moorooka, Queensland, Australia
[e] The Laminitis Institute, University of Pennsylvania School of Veterinary Medicine, New Bolton Center, Kennett Square, PA, USA
* Corresponding author. Department of Genetics in Ecology, University of Vienna, Althanstrasse 14, Vienna 1090, Austria.
E-mail address: g.milinovich@gmail.com

Vet Clin Equine 26 (2010) 79–94
doi:10.1016/j.cveq.2010.01.007 vetequine.theclinics.com

Gastrointestinal disease constitutes the single leading cause of mortality in the horse,[1] but only limited work has been conducted to determine the microbial structure and function of the normal equine hindgut. Even less work has been conducted into establishing how the alterations in these complex communities translate into pathology in an anatomically remote location, often with catastrophic consequences, as is seen in the foot during carbohydrate-induced laminitis. The distinct lack of research into the microbial basis of this disease is surprising considering the monetary value of horses, the economic contributions by the equine industries, the strong bonds formed between horses and their owners, the frequency at which laminitis occurs, and the poor prognosis for animals suffering this condition.[3] However, this lack of research is most likely attributable to the complexity of the equine hindgut and the inherent difficulties encountered in studying such a microbial system.

The development of effective treatment and prevention strategies for laminitis induced by carbohydrate overload is impeded by a lack of understanding of basic physiologic mechanisms,[4] particularly those linking changes in hindgut microbiota populations with histological and clinical evidence of laminitis development in the hoof. Laminitis is not merely a foot disease; it is a systemic syndrome, the manifestation of which is pathology in the foot,[5] and proponents of the hemodynamic and enzymatic theories of laminitis generally accept that the trigger factor for this specific type of laminitis originates in the hindgut immediately following acute carbohydrate overload.[6] Understanding the series of microbial events occurring in the equine hindgut during this developmental phase of laminitis would therefore provide foundational data to determine the downstream events that culminate in lamellar separation. This article focuses on research that has been performed to determine the changes in the microbial populations of the equine hindgut during the development of laminitis following acute alimentary carbohydrate overload.

THE DEVELOPMENT OF EXPERIMENTAL MODELS FOR INDUCING EQUINE LAMINITIS

More than half of laminitis cases are believed to result from exposure to an excessive amount of dietary carbohydrate, in the form of lush pasture or through ingestion of excess grain.[3] Lamellar separation, and the lameness that is characteristic of laminitis, is the result of a complex process initiated via the laminitis trigger factor (LTF), which derives from the hindgut.[7–10] The recognition of the gastrointestinal tract as the most likely source of the LTF necessitated the development of a reliable means for experimentally inducing laminitis, mimicking exposure to high levels of dietary carbohydrates. The studies of the histopathology of acute laminitis by Obel[11] used rye and a bolus of colibacilli culture to induce laminitis in 9 horses, an adaptation of the methodology of Åkerblom.[12] Using this protocol, Obel[11] successfully induced laminitis in 8 of the 9 horses; however, few other details of this induction method were published, except that it resulted in "violent diarrhea and a considerable rise in temperature and pulse rate." Since the study by Obel,[11] 3 further models for reliably inducing laminitis of alimentary origin have been developed and these constitute an integral step in determining the pathophysiology of this disease.

Starch-induced Laminitis

The first of these 3 models was the starch-induction model.[13] Starch constitutes the major storage carbohydrate of grains and some plants, particularly C4 plants and legumes.[14] This model achieved experimental induction of laminitis by administration of a bolus dose (17.6 g/kg body weight) of 85% starch and 15% wood cellulose flour prepared as gruel and administered directly into the stomach, via a stomach tube, and was reported to have successfully induced Obel[11] grade III laminitis in 11 of the 12 horses used within 48 hours of starch administration. However, the starch-induction model is associated with high incidences of colic and mortality.[15,16] Induction with starch remains a clinically relevant induction model, best reflecting laminitis resulting from horses consuming excess grain.

Black Walnut–induced Laminitis

Ingestion of shavings of black walnut (*Juglans nigra*), a tree species native to North America and prized for its dark-colored timber, is known to result in laminitis.[17] Bedding material containing black walnut shavings is the most common source of exposure, and an induction model using a black walnut extract (BWE) has been developed.[18] BWE inductions reportedly resulted in the development of laminitis in 12 of 12 horses within 8 to 12 hours of administration of BWE; inductions were accompanied by mild side effects and did not induce colic.[16] Studies to determine the compound within black walnut responsible for causing laminitis initially focused on juglone (5-hydroxy-1,4-naphthaquinone).[19] However, synthesized juglone was not able to consistently induce laminitis when administered orally, intravenously, or topically, and, to date, the compound within BWE that is responsible for initiating laminitis remains to be identified.[19] Exposure to BWE induces several pathologic events in the horse before lamellar separation, including vascular alterations, emigration of leukocytes to the lamellae, inflammatory mediator signaling, and matrix metalloproteinase (MMP) accumulation.[20] In addition, BWE exposure has been shown to induce eosinophilic colitis with an associated transmucosal resistance (determined in vitro),[21] a characteristic hypothesized to facilitate the passage of endotoxin or other vasoactive agents into the circulation.[22] There are few data available pertaining to the effect of BWE on the microbial community of the equine hindgut. BWE-induced laminitis does not induce metabolic acidosis or colic, as does the carbohydrate overload model,[16] suggesting a different mode of action. Furthermore, laminitis resulting from exposure to black walnut is less common than that from exposure to high levels of carbohydrates. Although the BWE-induction model constitutes an excellent model for studying the hemodynamic alterations associated with laminitis,[16] it is not ideal for studying the changes in microbial hindgut populations associated with laminitis caused by exposure to excess dietary carbohydrates.

Oligofructose-induced Laminitis

A model designed to mimic laminitis resulting from ingestion of lush pasture has been developed.[15] Fructans (β-D-fructose polymers with terminal glucose monomers) were first proposed to contribute to the onset of laminitis, in the same manner as starch.[23] Fructans are synthesized from sucrose by plants and some species of fungi and bacteria,[24] and, along with starches, constitute the predominant nonstructural plant polysaccharides. These compounds constitute the predominant storage carbohydrate of temperate plants (C3 plants), and are stored in the vegetative tissues of the plant until required.[14] In temperate grasses, starch may account for as little as 10% to 15% of the total stored carbohydrates, the remainder being sucrose and fructans. In certain climatic conditions, fructans can rapidly accumulate in grasses reaching concentrations of up to 50% of the total dry matter content.[25] The model of van Eps and Pollitt[15] used a commercial fructan extracted from the roots of chicory (*Cichorium intybus*) as short-chain, inulin-like (β2,1-linked), fructose polymers (oligofructose), rather than starch, as a means of experimentally inducing laminitis. Oligofructose was administered to horses, via a nasogastric tube, at a dose rate reflecting a theoretical maximal daily consumption from temperate grasses growing in exceptional climatic conditions for fructan production (7.5, 10 and 12.5 g/kg body weight).[14,15] The investigators reported that oligofructose reliably induced laminitis, with lameness typically observed 24 to 36 hours post oligofructose administration (POA), did not induce excessive gas production or colic, and had a reduced risk of mortality compared with the starch model.[15]

The oligofructose-induction laminitis model provides a reliable and reproducible means of experimentally inducing laminitis, mimicking that caused by exposure to lush pasture. However, it is not without criticism. Oligofructose polymers are β2,1-linked, whereas the fructans commonly found in grasses, levans, are predominantly β2,6-linked.[26] Although structurally similar, this discrepancy may or may not have an influence on hindgut microbial populations. In addition, the oligofructose manufacturing process involves a partial enzymatic hydrolyzation step in which the extracted fructans are broken down to lengths of typically 10 degrees of polymerization (DP) or fewer,[27] whereas those found in plants tend to be between 30 and 50 DP.[28] Stored fructan DP are dependent on the storage location within the plant, and ambient temperature has been shown to affect the accumulation of storage carbohydrates.[29] Analyses of timothy grass (*Phleum pratense*), a temperate grass, indicated fructans of up to 50 DP were present in the leaves[30] and 260 DP in the base of the stem.[31] These results were confirmed by Thorsteinsson and colleagues[29] who showed that fructans of timothy grass generally have DP greater than 12 and a pronounced accumulation of total carbohydrate and high DP fructans in timothy grass when grown at 10/5°C (day/night) compared with a constant temperature of 20°C. The use of a carbohydrate source with fewer DP to induce laminitis may facilitate the proliferation of organisms lacking the enzymatic pathways to break down the longer fructans found in grasses. Despite these discrepancies, the reliability of this model, combined with the reduced incidence of colic and low mortality rate compared with the starch-induction model, make the oligofructose-induction model the best available means of experimentally inducing laminitis to mimic that resulting from exposure to excess carbohydrates.

TRADITIONAL MICROBIOLOGICAL STUDIES OF THE EQUINE HINDGUT MICROBIOME DURING LAMINITIS DEVELOPMENT

Gastrointestinal microbial communities are metabolically adaptable and rapidly renewable[32]; however, any factor that significantly interferes with the microbial symbiotic relationships of the gastrointestinal tract, particularly one that has such a high metabolic input to the host as does the equine hindgut, has the potential to result in severe systemic consequences. Exposure to high levels of dietary carbohydrates initiates such an event in the horse, and the development of the first reliable model for experimentally inducing laminitis by Garner and colleagues[13] (the starch-induction model) provided a means of studying microbial changes in the hindgut preceding the onset of laminitis.

Using this model, Garner and colleagues[33] noted that laminitis resulting from experimental carbohydrate overload coincided with metabolic lactic acidosis, indicated by increased plasma L-lactate levels. Carbohydrate overload was known, at the time, to induce marked bacterial and protozoal changes in ruminants that coincided with lactic acidosis.[34,35] Furthermore, other studies indicated that dietary supplementation with oats significantly increased total and viable bacterial cell numbers in the ceca of ponies.[36] These observations led to the formulation of the theory that administration of high levels of carbohydrates to horses would alter the intestinal microbiota throughout the gastrointestinal tract, which would, in turn, affect production, uptake, and metabolism of organic acids, and that this event may be involved in the laminitis process.[33] Subsequent experimentation by Garner and colleagues[7] demonstrated such a sequence of events. Using 6 cecally fistulated horses, the investigators induced laminitis via alimentary starch overload and collected cecal fluid samples at 8 and 24 hours after administration of the carbohydrate bolus. These were analyzed for changes in bacterial populations using selective bacteriology culture media. Mean lactobacilli numbers were observed to increase significantly by 8 hours, whereas streptococci, in general, and anaerobic streptococci, in particular, reportedly decreased significantly in number by this time point. This observation correlated with a significant decrease in pH. Lactobacilli numbers remained high at the 24-hour time point, whereas streptococci were observed to return to close to the control mean value, and anaerobic streptococci remained at significantly reduced numbers. Cecal fluid pH remained at a significantly decreased value at the 24-hour time point. Populations of other bacterial species, including *Clostridium* spp, *Bacillus* spp and Enterobacteriaceae were also reported to change during the time course; however, these changes were not statistically significant. Garner and colleagues[7] identified the reduction in Enterobacteriaceae populations as being notable in the laminitis development process, in addition to several other key changes in the hindgut microbiota, which the investigators hypothesized to be involved in the development of laminitis. Carbohydrate overload was observed to induce a proliferation of hindgut lactobacilli, a concurrent increase in lactate concentration, and a significant decrease in cecal pH. The decrease in pH was hypothesized to cause the lysis of several bacterial species, most notably the Enterobacteriaceae, resulting in the subsequent release of endotoxins into the equine cecum, which, together with increased lactate concentrations, were hypothesized to cause severe mucosal damage, facilitating the passage of endotoxins into the systemic circulation. This, in turn, initiated lamellar separation.

Damage to the cecal wall has been shown by histopathological analysis to occur after carbohydrate administration in the horse.[37] Mucosal damage is associated with the bacterial fermentation end products, predominantly lactate, and exposure of colonic tissue to cecal fluid incubated with corn starch in vitro increased mucosal permeability.[38] In ruminants, the introduction of starch also induces lactic acidosis. However, this process is better characterized in ruminants than in horses. Introduction of large quantities of fermentable carbohydrates into the rumen results in increased lactate production and a concomitant decrease in rumen fluid pH.[39] The development of rumen acidosis reduces substrate conversion efficiency and microbial protein production.[40] Marked changes occur in the rumen microbial composition with the rapid proliferation of *Streptococcus bovis*, which is responsible for the production of large quantities of lactate, overwhelming the capacity of lactate-utilizing organisms, such as *Megasphera elsdenii* and *Selenomonas ruminantium*, to utilize this substrate.[40,41] Lactate continues to accumulate in the rumen to concentrations at which it is inhibitory to the organism primarily responsible for its production, *S bovis*, at which point lactobacilli become established and continue to ferment the carbohydrate source, producing lactate and further reducing the pH.[41] Researchers have largely made the assumption that lactic acidosis develops in the horse in the same manner as it does in the ruminant, despite the horse being a hindgut fermenter. Furthermore, this seems to contradict the results of Garner and colleagues[7] who reported streptococcal numbers to decrease significantly by 8 hours after starch administration, rather than increase as is reported in ruminants. However, subsequent reports indicate that streptococci do proliferate early in the laminitis process in the horse, and become established as the dominant hindgut microorganism.[10] These results have led to the development of much interest in *S bovis* as a possible source of LTFs and the subsequent speculation that this organism may be the causative agent of laminitis.

Although still limited, there is more information pertaining to the hindgut lactobacilli in the scientific domain than is available for the streptococci. These data have been produced through the identification of the association between lactic acidosis and laminitis[33] and the recognition of the need to determine the organisms responsible for the formation of lactate in the equine hindgut.[42] Subsequent to the publication of the study of Garner and colleagues,[33] increased blood D-lactate concentrations have also been associated with the development of carbohydrate-induced laminitis.[43] Al Jassim and colleagues[42] produced a collection of 72 nonstreptococcal, lactate-producing microorganisms from 2 horses with oligofructose-induced laminitis and 4 horses maintained on a roughage diet. Samples were collected at various points throughout the gastrointestinal tract post mortem, cultured on selective media, and isolates collected and analyzed for the ability to produce D- and L-lactate. Streptococci were excluded from this experiment on the grounds that, although *S bovis* and *S equinus* are predominant lactic acid bacteria of the equine hindgut, they are homofermentative, producing only L-lactate, whereas laminitis is reported to be characterized by increased blood D-lactate concentrations, which indicates a role for D-lactate–producing microorganisms in the development of laminitis. Of the 72 isolates collected, 25 produced 1 or both of the lactate isomers analyzed. Most of the isolates found to produce lactate were most closely related, by 16S rRNA gene sequence analysis, to *Lactobacillus salivarius*, *L mucosae* and *L delbrueckii*. Four isolates collected in this experiment were found to be most closely related to *Mitsuokella jalaludinii*. These isolates were the most prolific D-lactate–producing organisms of those analyzed and were collected from high dilutions (10^7–10^8), suggesting that *M jalaludinii* may be a significant contributor to D-lactate accumulation in the horse.

A number of studies have reported the equine digital vasculature to be acutely sensitive to amines, particularly the biogenic amine serotonin, which is commonly found in enterochromaffin cells and platelets.[44–46] These observations have led to the hypothesis that laminitis is caused by hemodynamic alterations initiated by the exposure of the digital circulation to amines.[46] Cecal fluid has been shown to contain a wide range of amines in high concentrations (>1 μM), and the investigators concluded that release of these into the circulation of the horse could have effects on vascular function.[47] Furthermore, cecal fluid concentrations of several identified amines were shown to be in higher concentration in horses maintained on spring/summer grass than in those maintained on winter grass. Addition of corn starch and inulin (a type of fructan) to cecal fluid, in vitro, also resulted in increased production of several of these amines, and corresponded with a decrease in pH, speculated to be caused by microbial fermentation of the added substrates. The finding of increased concentrations of vasoactive amines in cecal fluid supplemented with a readily fermentable carbohydrate source[48] and in the cecal fluid of horses maintained on spring/summer grass diets,[47] combined with the knowledge that these compounds have vasoactive properties and that increased lactate concentrations increase the permeability of the colon,[38] support the hypothesis that these compounds may be involved in the laminitis process. All of the amines identified in these studies have previously been found in foodstuffs, produced through the microbial decarboxylation of amino acids.[47,48] Despite the recognition of the apparent source of these compounds, microbiological analysis was not included in either of these publications; however, the investigators suggested that, as *S bovis* and *Lactobacillus* spp are reported to proliferate in the early stages of carbohydrate-induced laminitis, and as these organisms have the ability to produce amines from amino acids, they are the most likely source of the increased amine concentrations. In a subsequent publication, Bailey and colleagues[47] reported on changes in *Streptococci, Lactobacilli*, and gram-negative anaerobe populations corresponding to the in vitro study discussed earlier. Addition of corn starch and inulin resulted in significant increases in *Streptococci* and *Lactobacilli* populations and a concurrent significant pH decrease, but did not have a significant effect on gram-negative anaerobes. The investigators collected approximately 100 streptococci and lactobacilli isolates and screened them for the ability to decarboxylate 1 or more of the amino acids tryptophan, tyrosine, phenylalanine, isoleucine, and valine. Of the isolates analyzed, 26 had the ability to decarboxylate amino acids. Basic local alignment search tool (BLAST) analysis of partial 16S rRNA gene sequences assigned these organisms to *S bovis* (n = 4), *L mucosae* (n = 16), *L reuteri* (n = 2), *L salivarius* (n = 2), *L delbrueckii* (n = 1) and *L fermentum* (n = 1). These findings support the investigators' previous postulation that the increase in amines previously reported in these samples[48] was caused, at least in part, by streptococci and lactobacilli.[8] Dietary oligofructose supplementation has also been shown, in vivo, to significantly increase equine hindgut amine concentrations,[49] supporting the assertions of Bailey and colleagues.[48] As with the in vitro study of Bailey and colleagues,[48] the in vivo study of Crawford and colleagues[49] attributed the increase in these amines to bacterial decarboxylation of amino acids; however, the study did not attempt to correlate changes in amine concentrations with specific bacterial population shifts. The studies of Bailey and colleagues[8,47,48] and Crawford and colleagues[49] have further implicated the hindgut bacteria, particularly streptococci and lactobacilli, in the laminitis process, albeit on circumstantial evidence.

Allisonella histaminiformans, a novel organism isolated from the rumen of grain-fed cattle and the cecum of a horse, has been hypothesized to have a possible role in the development of laminitis in cattle and horses.[50] The investigators reported this organism is able to use histidine as its sole energy source, resulting in the production of histamine, and hypothesized that the histamine produced by this organism may induce laminitis in the same manner as for other amines discussed earlier. *A histaminiformans* is reported to be able to convert more than 95% of the available histidine (50 mM) to histamine in vitro,[50] and preliminary data from a subsequent publication indicated that cell numbers in cattle were dependent on diet.[51] No further information exists pertaining to *A histaminiformans* cell numbers in the horse or whether these organisms proliferate during the laminitis process.

Using the oligofructose-induction system developed by van Eps and Pollitt,[15] Milinovich and colleagues[52] induced laminitis in 5 horses, and fecal samples were collected at 8-hourly intervals from induction to 48 hours. Samples were cultured anaerobically on a nonselective medium to determine total anaerobe numbers and, by using a novel habitat-simulating medium (incubated equine cecal fluid agar; IECA), organisms with the ability to utilize oligofructose as a growth substrate (termed oligofructose-utilizing organisms; OUOs), were enumerated and identified. One hundred and fifty-six OUOs were collected and identified in this study and bacteria of the *S bovis/equinus* complex were found to be the predominant OUO present in equine feces before the onset of laminitis. Most of these isolates were most closely related to *S infantarius* subsp *coli* (previously named *S bovis*; currently *S lutetiensis*); however, other streptococci, including: *S gallolyticus* subsp *gallolyticus*, *S gallolyticus* subsp *macedonicus*, and a novel species subsequently named *S caballi*,[53] were also isolated. After the onset of laminitis, *Escherichia coli* were shown to become established as the predominant OUO cultivatable from equine feces. Furthermore, despite previous publications reporting the proliferation of lactobacilli during the onset of laminitis,[7,8] only 4 lactobacilli with the ability to utilize oligofructose as a growth substrate were isolated in this experiment.

MODERN MOLECULAR MICROBIAL ECOLOGY TOOLS AND THEIR APPLICATION TO LAMINITIS

One of the key limiting factors in previous studies on the microbial ecology of equine laminitis was that, until recently, culture was the only technique available to quantify changes in complex microbial ecosystems. Gastrointestinal microbial ecology has its foundations in traditional microbiology, with early work based on culture. However, culture has serious limitations; the human large intestine is host to more than 500 bacterial species, but only around 25% of these organisms are able to be cultured.[54] Likewise, it is estimated that as little as 30% of the equine cecal microbiota are cultivatable.[55] As a solution to this, modern microbial ecology has embraced molecular methodologies and adapted many technologies developed for other means for use in this field.[56] In doing so, microbial ecology has established itself as a progressive and innovative scientific discipline.[57] Most of the techniques developed have focused on, but not been limited to, small subunit rRNA genes, particularly the 16S rRNA gene, or rRNA itself.[58] The application of these DNA-based community analysis tools to samples of gastrointestinal contents collected serially during the course of laminitis development has provided a means of accurately and efficiently monitoring whole bacterial community profiles, enumerating organisms or groups of organisms of interest, and directly visualizing groups of cells with common phylogenetic traits, thereby furthering knowledge of this disease.

Fluorescence in situ hybridization (FISH) was among the first of these methods used to study changes in bacterial populations of the equine hindgut during laminitis development.[52,59,60] FISH allows rapid detection of organisms of interest from within complex microbial communities through the application of fluorescently labeled oligonucleotide probes targeted to signature regions of rRNA.[61,62] FISH allows microorganisms of interest to be visualized within the complex microbiome in which they reside (feces or cecal fluid in the case of laminitis) by fluorescence microscopy. Milinovich and colleagues[60] used FISH to visualize changes in bacterial populations proposed to have a role in the development of laminitis in paired cecal fluid and fecal specimens collected from 5 horses at 4-hour intervals. Changes in the abundance of targeted bacterial populations monitored in this study were correlated with the development of histologic signs of laminitis through the collection and analysis of serial hoof biopsies, harvested at 6-hour intervals.[63] This study clearly showed several key features in the microbiological alterations of the equine hindgut associated with laminitis development. First, FISH showed a rapid and early proliferation of hindgut streptococci (collectively termed the equine hindgut streptococcal species; EHSS). EHSS were observed to increase significantly ($P = .0421$) in relative frequency in the cecum by 8 hours POA and to remain at significantly increased levels until 24 hours POA. However, large increases in EHSS relative frequencies were discernable by as early as 2 hours POA (**Fig. 1**) and EHSS relative frequencies were observed in excess of 60% of the total bacterial population (preinduction relative frequencies were typically <10%) in all 5 horses before the development of histology consistent with the onset of laminitis. Of the organisms specifically targeted in this study, EHSS were the only organisms that consistently proliferated in the hindgut before the development of histologic signs of laminitis. None of the other organisms specifically targeted with FISH probes in this study (Enterobacteriaceae, *A histaminiformans*, *Enterococcus*

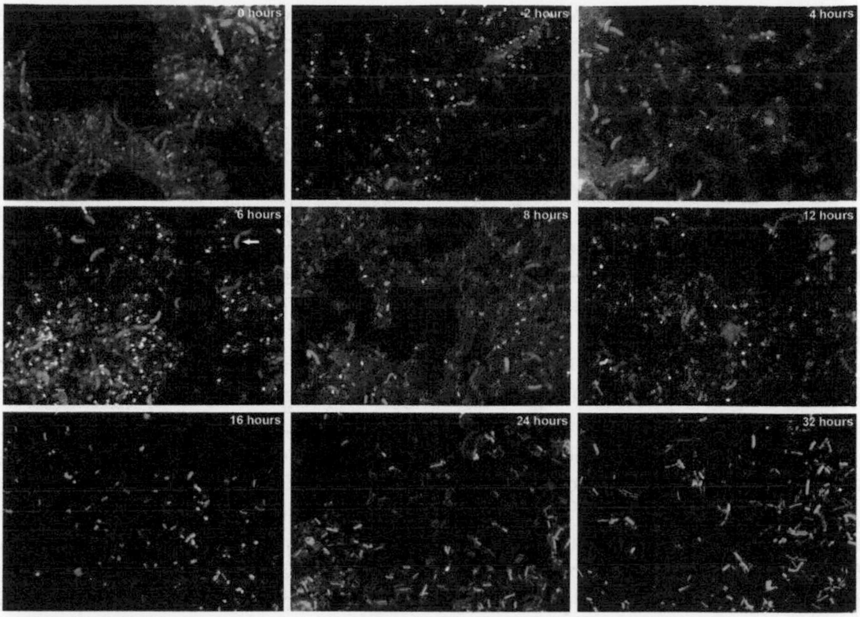

Fig. 1. FISH results for equine cecal fluid from horse 4 during the course of oligofructose-induced laminitis at 0, 2, 4, 6, 8, 12, 16, 24 and 32 hours POA. Probes: EUBMIX fluorescein isothiocyanate (FITC)–hybridized bacterial cells (*green*); dually labeled EUBMIX FITC/Sb127 CY3–hybridized bacterial cells (*yellow/orange*); and dually labeled EUBMIX FITC/Lab158 CY5–hybridized bacterial cells (*cyan*). The arrow in the 6 hours POA micrograph indicates unidentified large, curved rods. (*Reproduced from* Milinovich GJ, Trott DJ, Burrell PC, et al. Fluorescence in situ hybridization analysis of hindgut bacteria associated with the development of equine laminitis. Environ Microbiol 2007;9(8):2090–100; with permission.)

spp, *Lactobacillus* spp, *Bacteroides fragilis*, *M jalaludinii*, and *Clostridium difficile*) were shown to establish significant populations in the equine hindgut before the onset of the disease. However, lactobacilli were more discernable in feces than in cecal fluid, suggesting that lactobacilli have a proclivity for the distal regions of the hindgut, and significant increases in cecal fluid Enterobacteriaceae were observed, albeit after the establishment of EHSS as the dominant microorganism (in all 5 horses) and after the development of histologic evidence of laminitis in 2 of the 5 horses. The FISH results of this publication correlated well with the previous, culture-based, publication,[52] which reported oligofructose-utilizing *E coli* to proliferate late in the laminitis developmental process, and added further support to the previous implication of hindgut streptococci as the causative agent of equine laminitis.[10]

Denaturing gradient gel electrophoresis (DGGE) was the first DNA fingerprinting approach successfully applied in microbial ecology.[64] An adaptation of a technique developed to detect point mutations,[65] DGGE is able to produce DNA fingerprints of complex microbial populations, allowing the detection of similarities and differences between samples/communities or monitoring of changes occurring within a community over time. Polymerase chain reaction (PCR)–amplified products, typically variable regions of the 16S rRNA gene of less than 500 bp, from a community sample are passed, by electrophoresis, through a polyacrylamide gel that has been cast with an increasing denaturant gradient, typically formamide and urea. As the amplicons migrate into increasingly concentrated denaturants, they denature. Denaturation of amplicons is dependent on guanine and cytosine (GC) composition; single-stranded

DNA migrates at a slower rate than double-stranded DNA because of the increased interaction between nucleotides and the gel matrix, and, as the amplicons become increasingly denatured, migration through the gel is slowed.[56] Amplicons with higher GC content will, typically, remain double stranded for longer than those with a low GC content and migrate further through the gel. To prevent complete separation of the 2 strands a GC clamp, a 5' tail consisting of approximately 40 GC residues, is incorporated into one of the PCR primers. Once the electrophoresis is complete, bands are visualized by staining the gel, usually with ethidium bromide or by silver staining,[66] providing a fingerprint of the microbial community.

DGGE was used by Milinovich and colleagues[59] to reanalyze cecal fluid samples described in the FISH-based publication.[60] Before the publication of this study, no culture-independent studies analyzing changes in the equine hindgut microbiome during the development of laminitis had been published (the FISH study of Milinovich and colleagues[60] relied on bacterial isolate 16S rRNA gene sequence data for probe design and selection, which has the potential to introduce bias). The DGGE results of this study were used to select or design quantitative real-time PCR (qPCR) assays allowing quantification of bacterial groups of interest. This study corroborated the results of the previous FISH[60] and culture-based[52] studies but also provided further insight into the laminitis development process.

EHSS have been clearly and consistently shown by DGGE and qPCR to become established in the equine hindgut as the predominant microorganism before the onset of laminitis. However, the EHSS qPCR results[59] showed some discrepancies with the previous FISH results[60] for these organisms (**Fig. 2**). FISH and qPCR exhibited good congruence between 0 and 16 hours POA. However, after this time point, relative frequencies of EHSS by FISH declined rapidly, whereas qPCR quantifications remained at, or close to, their maximum values until the final time point at 36 hours POA. The qPCR assay targeted the 16S rRNA gene, whereas FISH targets the 16S rRNA in intact whole cells. This discrepancy suggests that the EHSS are undergoing lysis, which would allow detection by qPCR, but not by FISH. It is proposed that the en masse lysis of an organism in such high abundance before the onset of laminitis could result in the release of toxic cellular components that may constitute the elusive LTF.[59] A recent publication by Letarov and Kulikov[67] suggests that EHSS lysis may occur under the control of bacteriophages.

Temperate phages are not only capable of a vegetative life cycle, which results in intracellular proliferation of the virus, cell death, and lysis, but they can also integrate their DNA into the bacterial chromosome and can be transferred vertically.[68] In gastrointestinal environments, temperate phages are common. Klieve and colleagues[69] concluded that temperate phages were widespread among the bacteria of the rumen, and reported that 25% of culturable rumen bacterial isolates contained temperate phages. In the horse hindgut, Kulikova and colleagues[70] detected more than 60 morphologically distinct phage types. Temperate and lytic phages are well known among gastrointestinal streptococci.[69,71–74] Phage-encoded proteins can also turn benign commensal bacteria into pathogens; these phage-encoded proteins include many of the most potent bacterial toxins thus far discovered, including botulinum, cholera, diphtheria, and Shiga toxins.[75] Other virulence determinants are also found on temperate phage genomes. Although some virulence determinant genes are constitutively expressed, many are only expressed during vegetative phage multiplication, when the temperate state has been lifted by environmental, physiologic, or chemical induction.[68] Induction often affects all members of a bacterial population, resulting in widespread lysis of the population and the release of considerable toxin or other virulence factors. Such a situation could explain the sequence of events

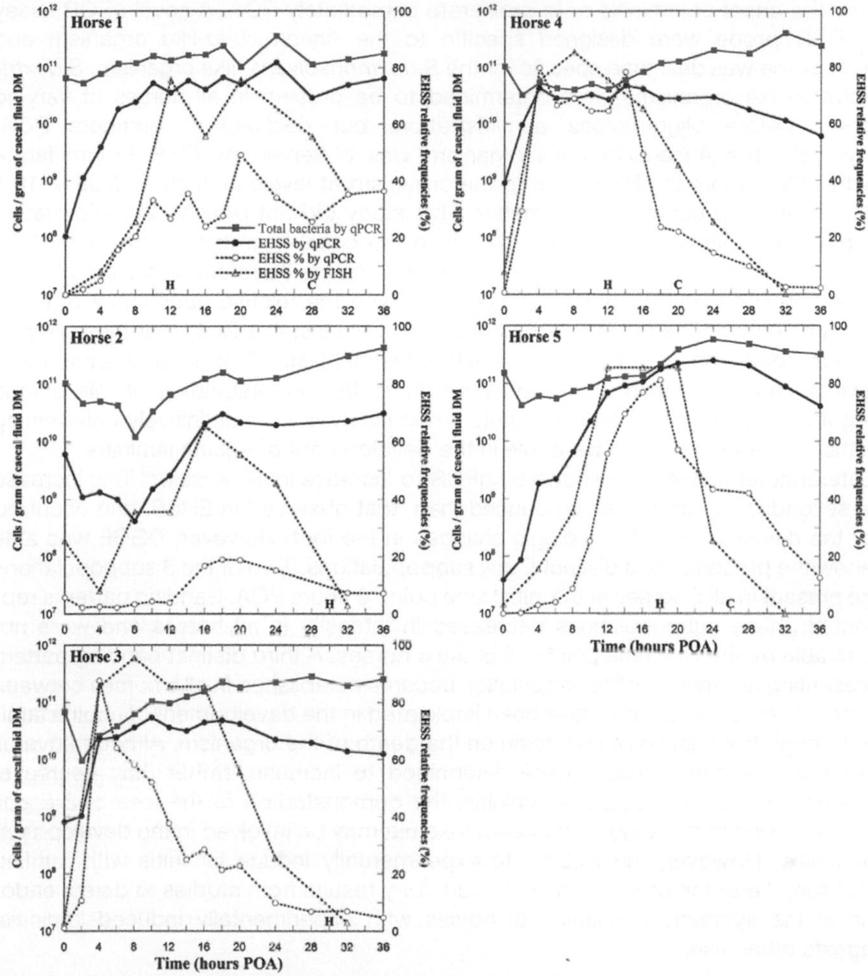

Fig. 2. Cecal fluid qPCR results for total bacteria and EHSS (*left y axis*) and relative frequencies for Sb127-hybridizing microorganisms by FISH and EHSS by qPCR (*right y axis*) for horses 1 to 5 (*top to bottom*). The time points at which histologic (H) and clinical (C) signs of laminitis were initially observed are indicated above the *x* axis. Horses 2 and 3 were initially observed to exhibit clinical signs of laminitis at 38 and 43 hours POA, respectively. (*Reproduced from* Milinovich GJ, Burrell PC, Pollitt CC, et al. Microbial ecology of the equine hindgut during oligofructose-induced laminitis. ISME J 2008;2(11):1089–100; with permission.)

observed with EHSS populations in the cecum of horses immediately before the onset of laminitis, suggesting a role for temperate phages in this syndrome. This theory is supported by previous studies that showed the ability of streptococcal culture supernatants to induce equine lamellar explant separation.[10]

As in previous studies, lactobacilli were shown by DGGE only to constitute a small proportion of the total cecal microbiome during the developmental phase of laminitis. DGGE also identified 2 previously undescribed groups of organisms in the horse hindgut: an *Anaerovibrio*-like bacterium (see **Fig. 1**: unidentified large, curved rods denoted by arrow) and an organism similar to *Succinivibrio dextrinosolvens*. These organisms were determined to constitute a high proportion of the cecal microbiome before the onset of laminitis or to proliferate immediately POA. A novel qPCR assay and FISH probe were designed specific to the *Anaerovibrio*-like organism and a FISH probe was designed specific for the *S dextrinosolvens*–like organism. *S dextrinosolvens*–like organisms were determined to be present in all horses at varying degrees before oligofructose administration, but declined in numbers POA. Conversely, the *Anaerovibrio*-like organism was observed by FISH to proliferate rapidly POA, whereas qPCR showed the organism at levels as high as 6.56×10^{10} cells per gram of cecal fluid dry matter. This study did not provide any information regarding the role of these organisms within the cecal microbiome; however, they form a large fraction of the total cecal microbiota and are therefore significant contributors to equine cecal function. Furthermore, given the relative abundance of these organisms early in the developmental phase of laminitis, it is likely that these organisms are commensals of the equine gastrointestinal tract. Proper identification and characterization of these organisms will add to the understanding of this unique hindgut microbial system and constitute a necessary step in definitively determining whether these organisms have a role in the development of equine laminitis.

Enterobacteriaceae were shown by qPCR to increase in all horses.[59] This increase was secondary to, and less pronounced than, that observed in EHSS, and occurred after the development of pathologic changes in the foot. However, DGGE was able to show the presence of 3 distinct *E coli* subpopulations. Two of the 3 subpopulations were present in all 5 horses at the initial time point, 0 hours POA. Banding patterns representing these subpopulations decreased in intensity in all horses and were not observable by the final time point in 4 of the 5 horses. A third distinct banding pattern representing another *E coli* subpopulation became established in all 5 horses between 16 and 24 hours POA. *E coli* have been implicated in the development of equine laminitis through the release of endotoxin on the death of the organism. Although overall Enterobacteriaceae numbers were determined to increase, rather than decrease, throughout the development of laminitis, the demonstration of the loss of 2 *E coli* subpopulations could suggest that endotoxemia may be involved in the development of laminitis. However, the inability to experimentally induce laminitis with purified endotoxin,[76] and the production of contradictory results from studies to detect endotoxin in the systemic circulation of horses with experimentally induced laminitis, suggests otherwise.[6]

SUMMARY

Equine laminitis constitutes the most serious foot disease of the horse, often resulting in death or necessitating euthanasia. First described in 350 BC, laminitis has long been recognised as an affliction of horses, as has the association of this condition with the ingestion of carbohydrates.[77] Despite the long held recognition of the importance of carbohydrate-induced laminitis, numerous gaps still persist in our knowledge of the pathophysiological mechanisms of this disease. Recent research, particularly that pertaining to changes in the hindgut microbiome following carbohydrate overload and its association with laminitis, has filled a number of these knowledge gaps. There is now substantial evidence implicating the rapid growth and lysis of EHSS as the precipitating event. The mechanisms by which changes in the hindgut microbiota initiate lamellar separation in the hoof, however, remain to be determined and none of the studies discussed above have been able to definitively demonstrate the exact cause. These studies do, however, provide the foundations on which to base future work to determine the source of LTF(s) and their mechanism of action; data which will definitively demonstrate both the causative organism and the pathophysiological mechanisms by which dietary exposure to high levels of carbohydrates initiates laminitis in the horse.

REFERENCES

1. Daly K, Stewart CS, Flint HJ, et al. Bacterial diversity within the equine large intestine as revealed by molecular analysis of cloned 16S rRNA genes. FEMS Microbiol Ecol 2001;38:141–51.
2. Daly K, Shirazi-Beechey SP. Design and evaluation of group-specific oligonucleotide probes for quantitative analysis of intestinal ecosystems: their application to assessment of equine colonic microflora. FEMS Microbiol Ecol 2003;44(2):243–52.
3. USDA. Lameness and laminitis in US horses. National Animal Health Monitoring System. Fort Collins (CO): USDA: APHIS:VS, CEAH; 2000. N318.0400.
4. Bailey SR. The pathogenesis of acute laminitis: fitting more pieces into the puzzle. Equine Vet J 2004;36(3):199–203.
5. Hood DM. Laminitis as a systemic disease. Vet Clin North Am Equine Pract 1999; 15(2):481–94, viii.
6. Bailey SR, Marr CM, Elliott J. Current research and theories on the pathogenesis of acute laminitis in the horse. Vet J 2004;167(2):129–42.
7. Garner HE, Moore JN, Johnson JH, et al. Changes in the caecal flora associated with the onset of laminitis. Equine Vet J 1978;10(4):249–52.
8. Bailey SR, Baillon ML, Rycroft AN, et al. Identification of equine cecal bacteria producing amines in an *in vitro* model of carbohydrate overload. Appl Environ Microbiol 2003;69(4):2087–93.
9. Elliott J, Bailey SR. Gastrointestinal derived factors are potential triggers for the development of acute equine laminitis. J Nutr 2006;136(Suppl 7):2103S–7S.
10. Mungall BA, Kyaw-Tanner M, Pollitt CC. *In vitro* evidence for a bacterial pathogenesis of equine laminitis. Vet Microbiol 2001;79(3):209–23.
11. Obel N. Studies on the histopathology of acute laminitis [PhD thesis]. Uppsala, Sweden: Almqvist and Wiksells Boktryckeri AB; 1948.
12. Åkerblom E. Über die ätiologie und pathogenese der futterrehe beim pferd. Skand Arch Physiol Suppl 1934;68:1–168.
13. Garner HE, Coffman JR, Hahn AW, et al. Equine laminitis of alimentary origin: an experimental model. Am J Vet Res 1975;36(4 Pt 1):441–4.
14. Longland AC, Byrd BM. Pasture nonstructural carbohydrates and equine laminitis. J Nutr 2006;136(Suppl 7):2099S–102S.
15. van Eps AW, Pollitt CC. Equine laminitis induced with oligofructose. Equine Vet J 2006;38(3):203–8.
16. Galey FD, Whiteley HE, Goetz TE, et al. Black walnut (*Juglans nigra*) toxicosis: a model for equine laminitis. J Comp Pathol 1991;104(3):313–26.
17. Uhlinger C. Black walnut toxicosis in ten horses. J Am Vet Med Assoc 1989; 195(3):343–4.
18. Minnick PD, Brown CM, Braselton WE, et al. The induction of equine laminitis with an aqueous extract of the heartwood of black walnut (*Juglans nigra*). Vet Hum Toxicol 1987;29(3):230–3.
19. True RG, Lowe JE. Induced juglone toxicosis in ponies and horses. Am J Vet Res 1980;41(6):944–5.
20. Loftus JP, Black SJ, Pettigrew A, et al. Early laminar events involving endothelial activation in horses with black walnut-induced laminitis. Am J Vet Res 2007; 68(11):1205–11.

21. McConnico RS, Stokes AM, Eades SC, et al. Investigation of the effect of black walnut extract on *in vitro* ion transport and structure of equine colonic mucosa. Am J Vet Res 2005;66(3):443–9.
22. Merritt A. Where does the subject of black walnut extract-induced laminitis fit into a colic symposium? Equine Vet J 2005;37(4):289–91.
23. Longland AC, Cairns AJ. Fructans and their implications in the aetiology of laminitis. Paper presented at: the 3rd International Conference on Feeding Horses. Ringstead, UK, 2007.
24. Roberfroid MB, Delzenne NM. Dietary fructans. Annu Rev Nutr 1998;18:117–43.
25. Cairns AJ, Longland AC. Sugar in grasses – an overview of sucrose and fructan accumulation in temperate grasses. Paper presented at: International Research Conference on Equine Laminitis. Stoneleigh, Warwickshire, UK, 1998.
26. Sims IM, Pollock CJ, Horgan R. Structural analysis of oligomeric fructans from excised leaves of *Lolium temulentum*. Phytochemistry 1992;31(9):2989–92.
27. Van Loo J. How chicory fructans contribute to zootechnical performance and well-being in livestock and companion animals. J Nutr 2007;137(Suppl 11):2594S–7S.
28. Vijn I, Smeekens S. Fructan: more than a reserve carbohydrate? Plant Physiol 1999;120:351–9.
29. Thorsteinsson B, Harrison PA, Chatterton NJ. Fructan and total carbohydrate accumulation in leaves of two cultivars of timothy (*Phleum pratense* Vega and Climax) as affected by temperature. J Plant Physiol 2002;159:999–1003.
30. Cairns AJ, Nash R, Carvalho MM, et al. Characterization of the enzymatic polymerization of 2,6-linked fructan by leaf extracts from timothy grass (*Phleum pratense*). New Phytol 1999;142:79–91.
31. Grotelueschen RD, Smith D. Carbohydrates in grasses. III. Estimation of the degree of polymerization of the fructosans in the stem bases of timothy and bromegrass near seed maturity. Crop Sci 1968;8:210–2.
32. Zoetendal EG, Cheng B, Koike S, et al. Molecular microbial ecology of the gastrointestinal tract: from phylogeny to function. Curr Issues Intest Microbiol 2004;5(2):31–47.
33. Garner HE, Hutcheson DP, Coffman JR, et al. Lactic acidosis: a factor associated with equine laminitis. J Anim Sci 1977;45(5):1037–41.
34. Allison MJ, Robinson IM, Dougherty RW, et al. Grain overload in cattle and sheep: changes in microbial populations in the cecum and rumen. Am J Vet Res 1975;36(2):181–5.
35. Hungate RE, Dougherty RW, Bryant MP, et al. Microbiological and physiological changes associated with acute indigestion in sheep. Cornell Vet 1952;42(4):423–49.
36. Kern DL, Slyter LL, Weaver JM, et al. Pony cecum vs. steer rumen: the effect of oats and hay on the microbial ecosystem. J Anim Sci 1973;37(2):463–9.
37. Krueger AS, Kinden DA, Garner HE, et al. Ultrastructural study of the equine cecum during onset of laminitis. Am J Vet Res 1986;47(8):1804–12.
38. Weiss DJ, Evanson OA, Green BT, et al. *In vitro* evaluation of intraluminal factors that may alter intestinal permeability in ponies with carbohydrate-induced laminitis. Am J Vet Res 2000;61(8):858–61.
39. Harmon DL, Britton RA, Prior RL, et al. Net portal absorption of lactate and volatile fatty acids in steers experiencing glucose-induced acidosis or fed a 70% concentrate diet ad libitum. J Anim Sci 1985;60(2):560–9.
40. Klieve AV, Hennessy D, Ouwerkerk D, et al. Establishing populations of *Megasphaera elsdenii* YE 34 and *Butyrivibrio fibrisolvens* YE 44 in the rumen of cattle fed high grain diets. J Appl Microbiol 2003;95(3):621–30.

41. Nocek JE. Bovine acidosis: implications on laminitis. J Dairy Sci 1997;80(5): 1005–28.
42. Al Jassim RA, Scott PT, Trebbin AL, et al. The genetic diversity of lactic acid producing bacteria in the equine gastrointestinal tract. FEMS Microbiol Lett 2005;248(1):75–81.
43. Rowe JB, Lees MJ, Pethick DW. Prevention of acidosis and laminitis associated with grain feeding in horses. J Nutr 1994;124(Suppl 12):2742S–4S.
44. Baxter GM, Laskey RE, Tackett RL, et al. *In vitro* reactivity of digital arteries and veins to vasoconstrictive mediators in healthy horses and in horses with early laminitis. Am J Vet Res 1989;50(4):508–17.
45. Bailey SR, Elliott J. Plasma 5-hydroxytryptamine constricts equine digital blood vessels *in vitro*: implications for pathogenesis of acute laminitis. Equine Vet J 1998;30(2):124–30.
46. Bailey SR, Menzies-Gow NJ, Marr CM, et al. The effects of vasoactive amines found in the equine hindgut on digital blood flow in the normal horse. Equine Vet J 2004;36(3):267–72.
47. Bailey SR, Marr CM, Elliott J. Identification and quantification of amines in the equine caecum. Res Vet Sci 2003;74(2):113–8.
48. Bailey SR, Rycroft A, Elliott J. Production of amines in equine cecal contents in an *in vitro* model of carbohydrate overload. J Anim Sci 2002;80(10): 2656–62.
49. Crawford C, Sepulveda MF, Elliott J, et al. Dietary fructan carbohydrate increases amine production in the equine large intestine: implications for pasture associated laminitis. J Anim Sci 2007;85(11):2949–58.
50. Garner MR, Flint JF, Russell JB. *Allisonella histaminiformans* gen. nov., sp. nov. A novel bacterium that produces histamine, utilizes histidine as its sole energy source, and could play a role in bovine and equine laminitis. Syst Appl Microbiol 2002;25(4):498–506.
51. Garner MR, Gronquist MR, Russell JB. Nutritional requirements of *Allisonella histaminiformans*, a ruminal bacterium that decarboxylates histidine and produces histamine. Curr Microbiol 2004;49(4):295–9.
52. Milinovich GJ, Trott DJ, Burrell PC, et al. Changes in equine hindgut bacterial populations during oligofructose-induced laminitis. Environ Microbiol 2006;8(5): 885–98.
53. Milinovich GJ, Burrell PC, Pollitt CC, et al. *Streptococcus henryi* sp. nov. and *Streptococcus caballi* sp. nov.: two novel streptococci isolated from the hindgut of horses with oligofructose-induced laminitis. Int J Syst Evol Microbiol 2008; 58(1):262–6.
54. Duncan SH, Louis P, Flint HJ. Cultivable bacterial diversity from the human colon. Lett Appl Microbiol 2007;44(4):343–50.
55. Mackie RI, Wilkins CA. Enumeration of anaerobic bacterial microflora of the equine gastrointestinal tract. Appl Environ Microbiol 1988;54(9):2155–60.
56. Felske A, Osborn AM. DNA fingerprinting of microbial communities. In: Osborn AM, Smith CJ, editors. Molecular microbial ecology. New York: Taylor & Francis; 2005. p. 65–96.
57. Lopez-Garcia P, Moreira D. Tracking microbial biodiversity through molecular and genomic ecology. Res Microbiol 2008;159(1):67–73.
58. Dahllof I. Molecular community analysis of microbial diversity. Curr Opin Biotechnol 2002;13(3):213–7.
59. Milinovich GJ, Burrell PC, Pollitt CC, et al. Microbial ecology of the equine hindgut during oligofructose-induced laminitis. ISME J 2008;2(11):1089–100.

60. Milinovich GJ, Trott DJ, Burrell PC, et al. Fluorescence *in situ* hybridization analysis of hindgut bacteria associated with the development of equine laminitis. Environ Microbiol 2007;9(8):2090–100.
61. Amann RI. Fluorescently labelled, ribosomal-RNA-targeted oligonucleotide probes in the study of microbial ecology. Mol Ecol 1995;4:543–53.
62. Daims H, Stoecker K, Wagner M. Fluorescence *in situ* hybridisation for the detection of prokaryotes. In: Osborn AM, Smith CJ, editors. Molecular microbial ecology. New York: Taylor & Francis; 2005. p. 213–39.
63. Croser EL, Pollitt CC. Acute laminitis: descriptive evaluation of serial hoof biopsies. Paper presented at: 52nd Annual Convention of the American Association of Equine Practitioners. San Antonio, TX, 2006.
64. Muyzer G, de Waal EC, Uitterlinden AG. Profiling of complex microbial populations by denaturing gradient gel electrophoresis analysis of polymerase chain reaction-amplified genes coding for 16S rRNA. Appl Environ Microbiol 1993; 59(3):695–700.
65. Fischer SG, Lerman LS. Length-independent separation of DNA restriction fragments in two-dimensional gel electrophoresis. Cell 1979;16(1):191–200.
66. Kocherginskaya SA, Cann IKO, Mackie RI. Denaturing gradient gel electrophoresis. In: Makkar HPS, McSweeney CS, editors. Methods in gut microbial ecology for ruminants. Dordrecht, Netherlands: International Atomic Energy Agency, Springer Academic Press; 2005. p. 119–28.
67. Letarov A, Kulikov E. The bacteriophages in human- and animal body-associated microbial communities. J Appl Microbiol 2009;107:1–13.
68. Ackerman HW, DuBow MS. General properties of bacteriophages. Boca Raton (FL): CRC Press; 1987.
69. Klieve AV, Hudman JF, Bauchop T. Inducible bacteriophages from ruminal bacteria. Appl Environ Microbiol 1989;55(6):1630–4.
70. Kulikova EE, Isaeva AS, Rotkina AS, et al. [Diversity and dynamics of bacteriophages in horse feces]. Mikrobiologiia 2007;76(2):271–8 [in Russian].
71. Iverson WG, Millis NF. Lysogeny in *Streptococcus bovis*. Can J Microbiol 1976; 22(6):853–7.
72. Klieve AV, Bauchop T. Phage resistance and altered growth habit in a strain of *Streptococcus bovis*. FEMS Microbiol Lett 1991;64(2–3):155–9.
73. Klieve AV, Heck GL, Prance MA, et al. Genetic homogeneity and phage susceptibility of ruminal strains of *Streptococcus bovis* isolated in Australia. Lett Appl Microbiol 1999;29(2):108–12.
74. Tarakanov BV. [Biological properties of *Streptococcus bovis* bacteriophages isolated from lysogenic cultures and sheep rumen]. Mikrobiologiia 1976;45(4): 695–700 [in Russian].
75. Skurnik M, Pajunen M, Kiljunen S. Biotechnological challenges of phage therapy. Biotechnol Lett 2007;29(7):995–1003.
76. Clark ES, Moore JN. The effects of slow infusion of a low dosage of endotoxin in healthy horses. Equine Vet J Suppl 1989;7:33–7.
77. Wagner IP, Heymering H. Historical perspectives on laminitis. Vet Clin North Am Equine Pract 1999;15(2):295–309.

Black Walnut Extract: An Inflammatory Model

James K. Belknap, DVM, PhD

KEYWORDS

- Laminitis • Treatment • Non-steroidal anti-inflammatory drugs
- Inflammation • Digital blood flow

The 2 primary experimental models to study the pathophysiology of equine laminitis have been the carbohydrate (CHO) overload models (both the traditional wood starch and the more recent oligofructose models), and the black walnut extract (BWE) model of laminitis. The BWE model was developed after the discovery that horses bedded on shavings from black walnut trees commonly developed laminitis.[1,2] The first investigators who consistently induced laminitis with black walnut shavings established that it was only the heartwood of the tree that was "laminitogenic," and that juglone, previously proposed as the compound responsible for inducing laminitis, was not the inducing substance as it is not present in the heartwood.[3] This report established the BWE model used from that point forward. The use of this model involves soaking 2 g/kg of body weight of black walnut heartwood shavings (from a tree harvested in the fall of the year) in 7 to 8 L of water for 12 hours, followed by filtering and nasogastric (NG) administration.[3] In the original study, 8 of 10 horses showed Obel Grade 3 to 4 lameness within 12 hours of administration, with 7 of 8 affected horses fully recovering over 6 days and 1 requiring euthanasia due to severity of the signs. Two horses did not develop laminitis; this lack of response in approximately 20% of the horses (usually termed "nonresponders") is fairly consistent in the author's experience. The first investigative work with the model concerned assessment of digital blood flow, in which the investigators used scintigraphic detection of technetium-labeled macroaggregated albumin to report decreased laminar blood flow 12 hours after BWE administration.[4] The same group established a developmental stage now used in many studies in which they described neutropenia occurring 4 hours following BWE administration.[5] Further studies of digital blood flow in the BWE model followed, using both an extracorporeal perfusion model[6] and a Doppler ultrasound technique[7] to report a small decrease in digital blood flow (much less than in the CHO model) at the same developmental stage, most likely because of venoconstriction in the digital

Department of Veterinary Clinical Sciences, College of Veterinary Medicine, Ohio State University, Columbus, OH 43210, USA
E-mail address: james.belknap@cvm.osu.edu

Vet Clin Equine 26 (2010) 95–101
doi:10.1016/j.cveq.2009.12.007
vetequine.theclinics.com
0749-0739/10/$ – see front matter. Published by Elsevier Inc.

microvasculature.[8] Laminar signaling events have also been studied at an earlier developmental stage in which laminae were harvested 1.5 hours post BWE administration to investigate initiating signaling events.[9] At the 1.5-hour and 4-hour (onset of leucopenia) developmental stages, the animals exhibited no signs of digital pathology (eg, no foot warmth, no increased digital pulse, and no lameness), despite numerous inflammatory events already occurring at these prodromal time points (discussed later).[9–12]

Although early reports suggested that inflammation did not play a role in laminitis because of a reported lack of laminar leukocytes upon histologic examination of the affected laminae,[13] inflammatory events were investigated in the late 1990s in the BWE model because inflammatory injury was reported to be a major component of organ failure in humans with systemic sepsis/endotoxemia and were therefore hypothesized to play a role in laminar injury and failure in the septic/endotoxemic horse.[14,15] One of the first events that occurs in distant organ injury in sepsis is a systemic inflammatory response in which products ranging from bacterial wall components to mitochondrial components of injured/dead host cells from the original infected/traumatized tissue (termed pathogen-associated molecular pattern molecules [PAMPs] and damage-associated molecular pattern molecules [DAMPs], respectively) are absorbed into the systemic circulation, resulting in inflammatory signaling both in circulating and fixed leukocytes (ie, Kupffer cells in the liver, pulmonary intravascular macrophages in the lung) exposed to circulating blood.[16,17] The fixed macrophages bind some of the circulating PAMPs and DAMPs and release cytokines into the circulation, the most common reported being tumor necrosis factor alpha (TNF-α) and interleukin-1 beta (IL-1β). The combination of circulating PAMPs, DAMPs, and cytokines leads to stimulation of the endothelium resulting in adhesion molecule and chemokine expression on the surface of the endothelial cells of the microvasculature of target organs. These endothelial events, combined with stimulation of circulating leukocytes, lead to adhesion of leukocytes (especially to the post capillary venules in tissues) and subsequent migration into the tissues where they cause tissue injury and cellular dysfunction and death due to the production of reactive oxygen and nitrogen species, proteases, and cytokines.[15,18] Investigators have hypothesized that BWE leads to absorption of lipopolysaccharide (LPS), but have been unable to detect circulating LPS in the model.[6] Because of the rapidity of the inflammatory response (many peak changes occurring within 1.5 hours of NG administration), it is more likely that there is a PAMP-like molecule in BWE that is directly absorbed through the small intestines; this theory is supported by a recent study in which LPS-like stimulation of equine monocytes by BWE was not neutralized by polymyxin B (indicating that a product that acts like LPS but is not LPS [ie, does not bind to polymyxin B] is present).[19] It is also possible that a recently reported peroxide-like effect of BWE in plasma may stimulate inflammatory signaling in the circulation (D Hurley, personal communication, 2009). Evidence of a systemic inflammatory response in the BWE model includes the reported activation of leukocytes at developmental and early lameness stages in the model,[20] and the inflammatory gene expression reported to occur in target visceral organs (lung and liver) of human sepsis in the BWE-treated horse.[21] Although the expression of most cytokines was less in the lungs and liver than in the laminae of the same horses, TNF-α, which is not increased in the laminae (discussed later), was increased in lungs and liver, most likely due to expression of the fixed macrophages in these organs.[17] Thus, the lungs and liver may contribute to the systemic inflammation and digital pathology in the BWE model (and in the clinical case) by the release of cytokines such as TNF-α into the circulation.[15]

The adhesion and migration of circulating leukocytes into target tissue/organs in sepsis relies on the activation of the endothelium resulting in expression of adhesion molecules and chemokines. Adhesion molecules, termed selectins, are important in initial association of leukocytes with the endothelial surface and rolling along the surface, whereas firm adhesion resulting in extravasation of the leukocyte into the tissue results from interactions of adhesion molecules such as ICAM-1 with integrins on the leukocyte surface. Chemokines (cytokines that bind to leukocytes, are chemoattractant for leukocytes, and activate leukocytes) are expressed onto and bind to heparin sulfate side chains on the luminal endothelial surface, where rolling leukocytes are exposed to them and become further activated. In the BWE model, there is an early and massive induction of laminar adhesion molecule and chemokine gene expression, with greater than 100-fold increases in chemokine levels such as IL-8/CXCL8 and Groα/CXCL1 by 1.5 hours post BWE administration.[9,22] Induction of E-selectin (120-fold increase) and ICAM-1 (56-fold increase) gene expression also peaks at the 1.5-hour time point, then decreases precipitously in expression by the onset of lameness.[9] Thus, the endothelium undergoes an early and marked activation in the BWE model, conducive for adhesion and extravasation of leukocytes into the laminar interstitium.

In sepsis, the neutrophil is usually discussed as the primary type of leukocyte involved in organ injury,[14] although mononuclear cells ranging from macrophages to monocytes and lymphocytes are also involved.[23,24] In the first report concentrating on laminar leukocyte emigration in laminitis, an antibody to an equine surface aminopeptidase (CD13) was used as a marker of neutrophils and monocytes.[25] In that study, no CD13-positive cells were present in the control laminae, whereas a marked influx of cells occurred at the developmental time point and at the onset of lameness in the BWE model. The majority of the cells emigrating into the laminae were neutrophils, although some monocytes/macrophages were present.[25] A later study reported a significant influx of CD13-positive cells by 1.5 hours post BWE administration.[25] These works were supported by a following study showing that laminar myeloperoxidase, a leukocyte-specific lysosomal enzyme used as a marker for neutrophils, was increased in developmental stages and at onset of lameness in the BWE model.[26] CD13 and myeloperoxidase studies also reported an increase in neutrophils in the skin,[9,26] again indicating that a systemic inflammatory response occurs in the model. A study showing a strong correlation between laminar matrix metalloprotease (MMP)-9 concentrations and CD13-positive cell counts indicates that emigrating neutrophils are the primary source of increased laminar MMP-9 concentrations in BWE-treated horses.[27] A more recent study used immunohistochemistry for calprotectin/MAC387, a marker of all neutrophils, activated monocytes, and stressed/inflamed skin to show that leukocyte infiltration in the BWE model occurs before the onset of epithelial stress, and may therefore play a role in epithelial injury and stress in this model.[28]

In both CD13 studies, the lack of CD13-positive cells in normal laminae was interpreted as evidence that there is no normal pool of leukocytes in the laminar interstitium; this was recently proved incorrect when a large pool of CD163-positive tissue macrophages and a smaller number of CD20-positive B and CD3-positive T lymphocytes were found in the laminae.[29] The CD163-positive monocyte/macrophages were normally present in the primary and secondary dermal laminae, and were also present in the deep dermis (underlying the laminae).[29] A significant increase in CD163-positive monocytes in the laminar interstitium occurred in the developmental stages of laminitis in the BWE model, but returned to normal values by the onset of lameness.[29] Thus, there is a large pool of tissue macrophages in the laminae that can be activated to play a role in inflammatory injury, and the BWE model is characterized by an activation of the endothelium and a large influx of neutrophils and monocytes in the early developmental stages of laminitis.

Three of the most common cytokines investigated in human sepsis are IL-1β, TNF-α, and interleukin-6 (IL-6).[30] Whereas IL-1β and TNF-α are usually reported to be early response genes in sepsis (commonly peaking early in the disease process),[16] IL-6 can peak early but is usually described to undergo a more sustained expression and is the cytokine most commonly correlated with increased morbidity and mortality.[31,32] Anti-inflammatory cytokines such as interleukin-10 (IL-10) are of interest because of their possible role in keeping the inflammatory response in check, and also because IL-10 has a possible role in immune suppression which can play an extremely deleterious role in severe sepsis.[33] The first work indicating inflammatory signaling in the BWE model reported the presence of perivenular cells in the primary and secondary dermal laminae undergoing marked expression of the central proinflammatory cytokine (IL-1β).[34] Comparing the location of these cells with that of emigrating leukocytes in the BWE model,[25] it is likely that the IL-1β positive cells are extravasated neutrophils. This study was followed by several reports using a real-time quantitative polymerase chain reaction to quantitate laminar cytokine mRNA concentrations in developmental stages and at the onset of lameness in the BWE model, reporting the most marked increase in laminar IL-1β occurring at the 1.5-hour developmental time point (50-fold increase vs control horses), followed by a 30-fold and 8.7-fold increase at the developmental and onset of lameness time points, respectively.[10] IL-6 exhibits a similar pattern of laminar expression in the BWE model as described in other sepsis models in that there is an early increase (550-fold at the 1.5-hour time point) with a sustained increase (>1300-fold increase) at the onset of lameness. TNF-α, a central cytokine undergoing increased expression in most target organs in human sepsis,[18,33,35] was not increased at any time point in the laminae (and has more recently been found to not increase in CHO models of sepsis also).[10] This distinct lack of TNF-α gene expression in affected laminar tissue was suggested to occur due to the following possibilities: (1) that TNF-α, characterized as an "immediate early gene," peaked earlier than the developmental time point assessed,[10] (2) that no tissue leukocytes of mononuclear origin existed in the laminae (fixed macrophages have been reported to be potent producers of TNF-α in target organs in human sepsis),[16,18] or (3) that the reported expression of the IκB protein Molecule with Ankyrin repeats Induced by Lipopolysaccharide (MAIL), now termed IκBζ, is inhibitory for TNF-α gene expression.[10] The later study, assessing laminar gene expression at a very early time point, 1.5 hours following BWE administration, negated the first theory because IL-1β was at its highest value at this time point (approx. a 50-fold increase), but there was still no increase in TNF-α expression.[9] The second theory regarding a lack of local population of monocyte lineage cells to express TNF-α is now known to be incorrect due to the recent discovery of a large pool of monocyte lineage cells throughout the laminar dermis in normal and affected horses. The third theory, revolving around the discovery of increased MAIL/IκBζ expression in an unbiased study detecting genes uniquely expressed in the laminae at the onset of lameness, takes into account the induction of IL-6 and the inhibition of TNF-α expression by MAIL/IκBζ. This is still a possible mechanism by which TNF-α is down-regulated in laminar tissue. It is still likely that the laminar cells are exposed to circulating TNF-α because of production in the liver and lungs in the BWE model.[21]

Other studies using the BWE model have supported the role of inflammation in the disease process including a recent microarray study in which a large number of genes important in different inflammatory signaling cascades, and multiple genes important in leukocyte activation and extravasation were found to be up-regulated.[36] Other studies showed increases in laminar cyclooxygenase-2 mRNA and protein concentrations in the early developmental and lameness stages of BWE-induced laminitis.[9,12,37] Two BWE studies indicated the presence of lipid peroxidation (one of the initial [and reversible] events observed in oxidant stress) in affected laminae, with increased laminar concentrations of isoprostanes and the lipid aldehyde 4-hydroxynonenal being found in the laminar tissue.[38,39] However, we have not been able to detect more severe types of oxidant stress such as protein carbonylation in the BWE model of laminitis (Belknap and colleagues, unpublished data, 2009). One of the perplexing issues in the BWE model is how the onset of such a fulminant inflammatory process in the laminae of BWE-treated horses does not usually lead to the laminar structural failure observed in clinical cases of sepsis, in the CHO models of laminitis, and even in some of the clinical black walnut toxicity cases. A likely reason is that the BWE model is similar to the endotoxin bolus model of human sepsis, where there is a transient "supraphysiologic" inflammatory response to the rapid bolus, but rarely the onset of organ failure due to a lack of sustained inflammatory injury.[40] Thus, it is likely that, similar to a short burst of endotoxin-related activity, the one-time absorption of a toxin from a single administration of BWE results in a short-lived inflammatory response that allows a rapid recovery of the cells before irreversible damage. In models such as the traditional CHO overload model, the sloughing of the lining of the cecum (and possibly the large colon) leads to a sustained absorption of toxins and likely a sustained systemic inflammatory response,[41] increasing the chance of causing irreparable injury to the laminar cells similar to the clinical sepsis case. In the clinical black walnut case, the horse usually continues to consume the shavings over several days, again most likely allowing a sustained inflammatory injury leading to more severe structural failure.

SUMMARY

Similar to the endotoxin model of human sepsis, the BWE model of laminitis has allowed investigators to determine many of the early pathologic signaling events likely to occur in the developmental and acute clinical stages of the disease process, and has brought inflammatory injury to the forefront of laminitis research. However, these events must also be assessed in the CHO overload models, the models that more closely reflect the clinical case of laminitis. Comparison between models will not only be valuable in providing documentation that some of these events occur in all models, but may also be valuable in determining events that differ in the CHO model. This may lead to the discovery of events important in the structural laminar failure occurring in the oligofructose model thus providing valuable targets for future therapy.

REFERENCES

1. True RG, Lowe JE, Heissen J, et al. Black walnut shavings as a cause of acute laminitis. Proc Am Assoc Equine Pract 1978;24:511–6.
2. Ralston SL, Rich VA. Black walnut toxicosis in horses. J Am Vet Med Assoc 1983; 183:1095.
3. Minnick PD, Brown CM, Braselton WE, et al. The induction of equine laminitis with an aqueous extract of the heartwood of black-walnut (*Juglans nigra*). Vet Hum Toxicol 1987;29:230–3.
4. Galey FD, Twardock AR, Goetz TE, et al. Gamma scintigraphic analysis of the distribution of perfusion of blood in the equine foot during black walnut (*Juglans nigra*)-induced laminitis. Am J Vet Res 1990;51:688–95.

5. Galey FD, Whiteley HE, Goetz TE, et al. Black walnut (*Juglans nigra*) toxicosis: a model for equine laminitis. J Comp Pathol 1991;104:313–26.
6. Eaton SA, Allen D, Eades SC, et al. Digital Starling forces and hemodynamics during early laminitis induced by an aqueous extract of black walnut (*Juglans nigra*) in horses. Am J Vet Res 1995;56:1338–44.
7. Adair HS 3rd, Goble DO, Schmidhammer JL, et al. Laminar microvascular flow, measured by means of laser Doppler flowmetry, during the prodromal stages of black walnut-induced laminitis in horses. Am J Vet Res 2000;61:862–8.
8. Eaton SA, Allen DA, Eades SC, et al. Digital Starling forces and hemodynamics during early laminitis induced by an aqueous extract of black walnut (*Juglans nigra*) in horses. Vet Surg 1994;23:400–1.
9. Loftus JP, Black SJ, Pettigrew A, et al. Early laminar events involving endothelial activation in horses with black walnut-induced laminitis. Am J Vet Res 2007;68:1205–11.
10. Belknap JK, Giguere S, Pettigrew A, et al. Lamellar pro-inflammatory cytokine expression patterns in laminitis at the developmental stage and at the onset of lameness: innate vs adaptive immune response. Equine Vet J 2007;39:42–7.
11. Waguespack RW, Kemppainen RJ, Cochran A, et al. Increased expression of MAIL, a cytokine-associated nuclear protein, in the prodromal stage of black walnut-induced laminitis. Equine Vet J 2004;36:285–91.
12. Waguespack RW, Cochran A, Belknap JK. Expression of the cyclooxygenase isoforms in the prodromal stage of black walnut-induced laminitis in horses. Am J Vet Res 2004;65:1724–9.
13. Hunt RJ. The pathophysiology of acute laminitis. Compend Contin Ed Pract Vet 1991;13:1003–10.
14. Strassheim D, Park JS, Abraham E. Sepsis: current concepts in intracellular signaling. Int J Biochem Cell Biol 2002;34:1527–33.
15. Belknap JK, Moore JN, Crouser EC. Sepsis - from human organ failure to laminar failure. Vet Immunol Immunopathol 2009;129:155–7.
16. Chensue SW, Terebuh PD, Remick DG, et al. In vivo biologic and immunohistochemical analysis of interleukin-1 alpha, beta and tumor necrosis factor during experimental endotoxemia. Kinetics, Kupffer cell expression, and glucocorticoid effects. Am J Pathol 1991;138:395–402.
17. Warner AE, DeCamp MM, Molina RM, et al. Pulmonary removal of circulating endotoxin results in acute lung injury in sheep. Lab Invest 1988;59:219–30.
18. Bhatia M, Moochhala S. Role of inflammatory mediators in the pathophysiology of acute respiratory distress syndrome. J Pathol 2004;202:145–56.
19. Hurley DJ, Berghaus LJ, Hurley KA, et al. The in vitro effects of aqueous black walnut extract on the function of equine mononuclear cells. Am J Vet Res, in press.
20. Hurley DJ, Parks RJ, Reber AJ, et al. Dynamic changes in circulating leukocytes during the induction of equine laminitis with black walnut extract. Vet Immunol Immunopathol 2006;110:195–206.
21. Stewart AJ, Pettigrew A, Cochran AM, et al. Indices of inflammation in the lung and liver in the early stages of the black walnut extract model of equine laminitis. Vet Immunol Immunopathol 2009;129:254–60.
22. Faleiros RR, Leise BB, Westerman T, et al. In vivo and in vitro evidence of the involvement of CXCL1, a keratinocyte-derived chemokine, in equine laminitis. J Vet Intern Med 2009;23:1086–96.
23. Tslotou AG, Sakorafas GH, Anagnostopoulos G, et al. Septic shock; current pathogenetic concepts from a clinical perspective. Med Sci Monit 2005;11:RA76–85.

24. Lunn DP, Hurley DJ. The role of leukocyte biology in laminitis. Vet Immunol Immunopathol 2009;129:158–60.
25. Black SJ, Lunn DP, Yin C, et al. Leukocyte emigration in the early stages of laminitis. Vet Immunol Immunopathol 2006;109:161–6.
26. Riggs LM, Franck T, Moore JN, et al. Neutrophil myeloperoxidase measurements in plasma, laminar tissue, and skin of horses given black walnut extract. Am J Vet Res 2007;68:81–6.
27. Loftus JP, Belknap JK, Black SJ. Matrix metalloproteinase-9 in laminae of black walnut extract treated horses correlates with neutrophil abundance. Vet Immunol Immunopathol 2006;113:267–76.
28. Faleiros RR, Nuovo GJ, Belknap JK. Immunolocalization of the DAMP protein calprotectin in myeloid and epithelial cells in laminae of horses with BWE-induced laminitis. J Vet Intern Med 2009;23:174–82.
29. Faleiros RR, Nuovo GJ, Flechtner AD, et al. Mononuclear leukocytes in the laminae of normal horses and those with black walnut extract-induced laminitis. J Vet Intern Med 2009;23:784.
30. Thijs LG, Hack CE. Time course of cytokine levels in sepsis. Intensive Care Med 1995;21(Suppl 2):S258–63.
31. Remick DG, Bolgos G, Copeland S, et al. Role of interleukin-6 in mortality from and physiologic response to sepsis. Infect Immun 2005;73:2751–7.
32. Gold JR, Perkins GA, Erb HN, et al. Cytokine profiles of peripheral blood mononuclear cells isolated from septic and healthy neonatal foals. J Vet Intern Med 2007;21:482–8.
33. Cavaillon JM, Annane D. Compartmentalization of the inflammatory response in sepsis and SIRS. J Endotoxin Res 2006;12:151–70.
34. Fontaine GL, Belknap JK, Allen D, et al. Expression of interleukin-1beta in the digital laminae of horses in the prodromal stage of experimentally induced laminitis. Am J Vet Res 2001;62:714–20.
35. Hadjiminas DJ, McMasters KM, Peyton JC, et al. Tissue tumor necrosis factor mRNA expression following cecal ligation and puncture or intraperitoneal injection of endotoxin. J Surg Res 1994;56:549–55.
36. Noschka E, Vandenplas ML, Hurley DJ, et al. Temporal aspects of laminar gene expression during the developmental stages of equine laminitis. Vet Immunol Immunopathol 2009;129:242–53.
37. Blikslager AT, Yin CL, Cochran AM, et al. Cyclooxygenase expression in the early stages of equine laminitis: a cytologic study. J Vet Intern Med 2006;20:1191–6.
38. Noschka E, Moore JN, Peroni JF, et al. Thromboxane and isoprostanes as inflammatory and vasoactive mediators in black walnut heartwood extract induced equine laminitis. Vet Immunol Immunopathol 2009;129:200–10.
39. Yin C, Pettigrew A, Loftus JP, et al. Tissue concentrations of 4-HNE in the black walnut extract model of laminitis: indication of oxidant stress in affected laminae. Vet Immunol Immunopathol 2009;129:211–5.
40. Buras JA, Holzmann B, Sitkovsky M. Animal models of sepsis: setting the stage. Nat Rev Drug Discov 2005;4:854–65.
41. Krueger AS, Kinden DA, Garner HE, et al. Ultrastructural study of the equine cecum during onset of laminitis. Am J Vet Res 1986;47:1804–12.

Acute Laminitis: Medical and Supportive Therapy

Andrew W. van Eps, BVSc, PhD

KEYWORDS

• Acute • Laminitis • Horse • Medical • Treatment

Acute laminitis has been defined as the period beginning with the onset of clinical signs (increased hoof temperature, increased digital pulse amplitude, shifting of weight, lameness) and ending with either resolution of the clinical signs or progression to chronic laminitis (displacement of the distal phalanx within the hoof capsule or after 72 hours of continuous clinical signs).[1] For the purposes of treatment, the acute phase may be more appropriately viewed as the initial clinical period of laminitis that may last for up to 7 days before any improvement or progression (clinical or radiographic) is apparent. Acute laminitis may arise as a secondary problem during treatment of a separate disease, or it may be the primary presenting complaint. Horses with clinical and subclinical chronic laminitis may also present for an acute laminitis episode.

The structural changes that occur in the lamellar tissue during acute laminitis are largely irreversible.[2] Experimental data show that histopathologic changes occur before the onset of clinical signs.[3,4] Examination of lamellar tissue from clinical cases with systemic disease (but no clinical signs of laminitis at the time of euthanasia) also suggests that damage is under way before clinical recognition of laminitis (Julie Engiles DVM, Kennett Square, PA, personal communication, November 2009). Horses with conditions associated with a high risk of laminitis development (eg, colitis, metritis, pneumonia, alimentary carbohydrate overload, severe unilateral limb lameness)[5–10] should therefore be identified and treated preemptively whenever possible.

Regardless of the primary cause, the resultant pathologic processes within the digit are similar, as is the treatment. Although the exact pathophysiology is still poorly understood, acute laminitis is characterized by pain, inflammation, enzymatic activation, vascular derangements, and lamellar destabilization.[11–15] The severity of the initial insult often determines the outcome regardless of treatment.[2] Treatment strategies should be directed at halting the progression of the disease during the developmental and acute phases. The aims of the clinician presented with a case of acute laminitis are to (1) minimize further lamellar damage, (2) provide analgesia, and (3) carefully track the progression to determine the prognosis and to make informed decisions regarding euthanasia or cessation of treatment. This article provides a summary of the recommended management for cases of acute laminitis based on currently available information.

School of Veterinary Science, The University of Queensland, Slip Road, Saint Lucia, QLD 4072, Australia
E-mail address: a.vaneps@uq.edu.au

Vet Clin Equine 26 (2010) 103–114
doi:10.1016/j.cveq.2009.12.011
0749-0739/10/$ – see front matter. Published by Elsevier Inc.

INITIAL ASSESSMENT OF THE HORSE WITH ACUTE LAMINITIS
Clinical Assessment

In some cases, a horse may present with signs of acute laminitis with no apparent predisposing cause. Therefore the initial clinical examination should include a thorough evaluation of all body systems. Horses with moderate to severe acute laminitis often have an increased resting heart rate and respiratory rate. Spontaneous sweating and a rectal temperature in the upper range of normal (or mild hyperthermia) may be apparent, although laminitis alone does not result in true pyrexia. The characteristic "saw horse" stance is common in horses in which pain is worse in the forelimbs, which is usually the case.[2] Horses with equivocal hind- and forelimb laminitis pain may have a normal stance. Differential diagnoses to consider include tetanus, rhabdomyolysis, and pleurodynia.

Careful observation at rest may reveal subtle weight shifting in the front limbs, an early clinical sign characteristic of laminitis.[2,16] Persistently increased hoof temperature is a consistent finding in horses with acute laminitis.[2] It should be noted that there is normal variation in hoof temperature throughout the day and that hoof temperature is a function of ambient temperature.[17] The coronary bands should be palpated for the presence of a depression between the proximal extent of the coronary band and the pastern (**Fig. 1**). A palpable depression at this site indicates severe downward displacement of the distal phalanx within the hoof capsule (sinking). The hooves should be examined for changes that are indicative of preexisting chronic laminitis (divergent growth rings or a dished appearance to the dorsal wall). Hoof testing may reveal a diffuse withdrawal response across the entire foot or just at the toe region, depending on the severity. In many cases there is little response to hoof testing. A withdrawal reaction to manual application of rotational force to the hoof is possibly a more reliable indicator of the presence of laminitis pain, particularly

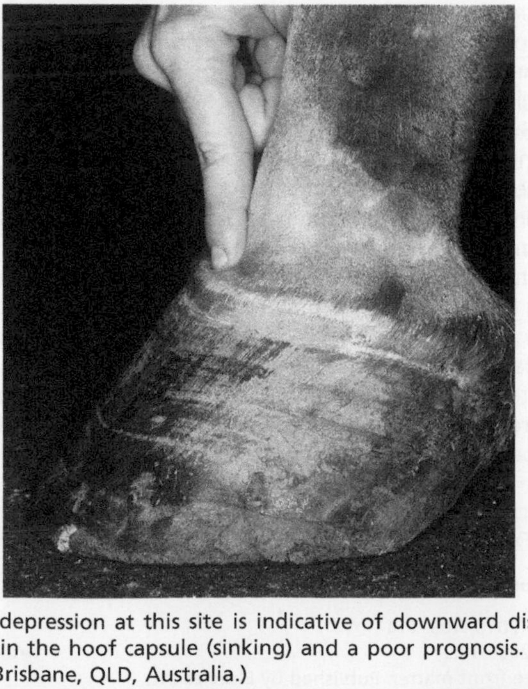

Fig. 1. A palpable depression at this site is indicative of downward displacement of the distal phalanx within the hoof capsule (sinking) and a poor prognosis. (*Courtesy of* Chris Pollitt, BVSc, PhD, Brisbane, QLD, Australia.)

in the hind limbs. The degree of lameness can be established by careful examination at the walk. Horses with mild bilateral forelimb laminitis may appear normal in the straight line, although turning on a hard surface exacerbates lameness on the inside limb in either direction. The lameness scale originally developed by Obel[16] is useful for documenting the severity of laminitis in clinical cases (**Table 1**).

Radiographic Assessment

Although there are often no detectable radiographic changes initially, it is important to obtain a baseline set of radiographs as early as possible to document progression over time. Radiographs should ideally be obtained every 3 to 4 days during the initial week after the development of clinical signs, particularly if there is no clinical improvement. Good-quality lateral-to-medial projections are usually sufficient unless there is suspicion of an additional lesion within the bone. The most important measurable parameter in acute laminitis cases is the distance between the extensor process of the third phalanx and a marker placed just below the coronary band, where the hoof wall palpably changes from hard to soft horn (**Fig. 2**).[18] This distance can vary significantly among horses (0–10 mm or more, depending on breed),[18,19] although if careful technique is used, accurate repeated measurements can be obtained, detecting even small increases in this distance (1–2 mm). Increases over 2 or more separate examinations indicate displacement of the distal phalanx within the hoof capsule. This measurement should also be consistently less in the hind feet than in the forefeet[19]; the opposite would be strong evidence for the presence of laminitis in the hind feet. The angle and distance between the outer hoof wall and distal phalanx should also be assessed.

Clinical Laboratory Tests

A complete blood count and biochemistry profile should be obtained in all cases as part of the diagnostic workup for primary disease. Acute laminitis alone does not result in any changes in routine blood parameters, apart from the presence of a stress leukogram in moderate to severe cases. Increases in levels of fibrinogen indicate inflammation associated with the primary disease or another lesion rather than the laminitis itself. Baseline values for total protein (particularly the albumin fraction) and creatinine should be obtained, as they are important parameters when monitoring for nonsteroidal antiinflammatory drug (NSAID) toxicity. Azotemia with concurrent hemoconcentration is often present because of dehydration. This condition should be corrected with fluids before commencing NSAID therapy. Azotemia that is not ameliorated with fluid resuscitation indicates preexisting renal failure, which should be taken into account when formulating the treatment plan and the prognosis.

Table 1
The lameness scale developed by Obel is useful for documenting laminitis severity

Obel Grade I	At rest the horse will alternately and incessantly lift the feet. Lameness is not evident at the walk, but a short stilted gait is noted at the trot.
Obel Grade II	The horse moves willingly at a walk, but the gait is characteristic of laminitis. A hoof can be lifted off the ground without difficulty.
Obel Grade III	The horse moves reluctantly and vigorously resists attempts to lift a forefoot.
Obel Grade IV	The horse must be forced to move and may be recumbent.

Data from Obel N. Studies of the histopathology of acute laminitis. In: Almgvist and Wilcsells Bottrykeri Ab Uppsala (thesis); 1948.

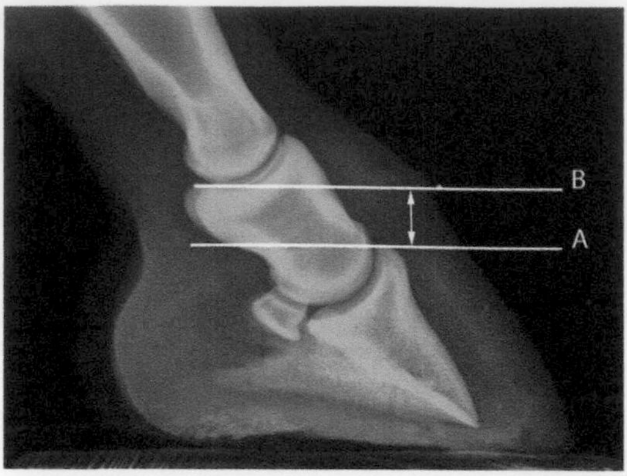

Fig. 2. There are often no radiographic changes associated with acute laminitis, although a baseline set of radiographs should be obtained as early as possible. The distance between the extensor process of the distal phalanx (A) and the coronary band (B) is the most important radiographic parameter to monitor in acute cases. Increases in this distance indicate distal displacement of the distal phalanx within the hoof capsule (sinking) and a poor prognosis. The distance and angle between the distal phalanx and outer hoof wall should also be monitored.

If there is suspicion of equine Cushing disease, the clinician should wait several days (or until the horse is stable) before determining baseline blood adrenocorticotropic hormone concentrations or performing a domperidone stimulation test,[20] as stress may interfere with the results. The low-dose dexamethasone test should be avoided during acute laminitis. Horses with acute laminitis may also have increased serum glucose and insulin concentrations (in the absence of equine metabolic syndrome).[21] If no primary cause for the laminitis is apparent, horses should also be tested for Potomac horse fever in endemic areas.

INITIAL TREATMENT OF THE HORSE WITH ACUTE LAMINITIS

A balance must be struck between minimizing mechanical trauma to the weakened lamellae, provision of adequate analgesia, aggressive treatment of the primary disease, and direct treatment of the processes causing lamellar failure.

Minimizing Mechanical Trauma

It is logical that once there is lamellar weakening, reducing the load on the suspensory apparatus between the distal phalanx and the hoof wall is a therapeutic priority. Restricting ambulation is paramount in the early stages of acute laminitis. The horse should be confined to a stall and not walked unnecessarily; diagnostic and therapeutic procedures should be performed on-site whenever possible. Extended travel for hospital referral may be detrimental during active acute laminitis. The horse should be encouraged to lie down by providing deep comfortable bedding. Tranquilizers and sedatives may encourage recumbency and reduce voluntary ambulation in horses with acute laminitis. The author commonly administers acetylpromazine (acepromazine maleate injection; 0.02–0.04 mg/kg intramuscularly or intravenously 4 times a day) for its tranquilizing effect in the first 3 to 5 days after the onset of acute laminitis.

The ideal bedding material should reduce concussion during locomotion, support the sole and frog to reduce load on the hoof wall, minimize torsion of the hoof capsule on turning, and yield under the toe to minimize breakover.[22] Sand appears to be superior to shavings or straw for this purpose. Sand conforms well to the foot and provides support to the frog and sole. Some horses seem more willing to lie down on sand if it is covered with a thin layer of straw or if a light blanket or rug is placed on the horse. Another option is bedding in deep mud or peat moss, although this is much harder to maintain. Shoes concentrate weight-bearing forces on the periphery of the foot and should be removed if present.[23] Besides weight bearing, breakover contributes to distractive forces between the distal phalanx and the hoof wall, further straining the lamellar interface. The distractive forces of breakover can be reduced by trimming the toe region and by applying various support materials to the foot itself.[22] The author prefers the application of silicone impression material (EquiFlex-Pak, Sound Horse Technologies, Inc, Unionville, PA, USA) to the sole of the foot, secured with adhesive tape. The impression material should be applied from the cranial tip of the frog caudally. The breakover point can be adjusted so that it is directly under the cranial/distal tip of the third phalanx, and the material can be molded so that the ground surface is convex, further reducing load on the hoof wall. There is a natural tendency to produce mild heel elevation with this technique, which may provide additional benefits in relieving the forces of breakover and reducing tension on the deep digital flexor tendon.[22] Any apparatus applied to the foot should be easily removable to facilitate a rapid change or to obtain radiographs. More permanent steel or aluminum shoes should be avoided during acute laminitis.

There are currently no experimental or clinical data regarding whether a total absence of weight bearing actually prevents lamellar pathology or halts the progress of pathophysiologic events in acute laminitis. Histologic analysis of lamellar tissues 7 days after experimental induction showed that there was surprisingly advanced repair of the basement membrane and little evidence of ongoing lamellar inflammation.[24] This finding suggests that if mechanical distraction and architectural derangement can be minimized during the acute insult, repair may be rapid. Absolute reduction of weight bearing on multiple limbs can be achieved only by encouraging/enforcing recumbency or providing sling support for the entire body. Forced recumbency was investigated as a potential treatment for horses with acute laminitis.[25] In this study ponies were anesthetized and allowed to recover in a stall with a lowered roof. The ponies tolerated this remarkably well and remained in sternal recumbency for up to 72 hours. Reducing weight bearing by the use of a sling is technically difficult and not well tolerated for more than short periods with existing sling technology. Horses that remain recumbent for extended periods may be supported with the use of a sling during periods when they elect to stand. Some horses readily adapt to the sling by sitting back into the device and unloading their limbs voluntarily. Many horses, however, do not use the sling in this way. In these horses, during standing periods, the sling is applied and the hoist is adjusted so that weight bearing on the front limbs is reduced while still allowing basic movement of the horse within the stall. The author has had apparent success in managing a small number of severe acute cases using this method, although it requires intensive nursing care.

Analgesia

The NSAIDs phenylbutazone (2.2 mg/kg intravenously or by mouth twice a day) or flunixin meglumine (0.5–1.0 mg/kg intravenously or by mouth twice a day) provide effective analgesia in most cases of acute laminitis. In the author's experience, the more cyclooxygenase (COX)-2-selective NSAIDs (firocoxib [Equioxx], meloxicam [Metacam]) are inferior to the non–COX-selective NSAIDs for acute laminitis pain, although they may be effective in chronic cases. In addition to analgesia, NSAIDs offer the benefit of helping to control the inflammatory processes occurring within the lamellar tissue.[12,26,27] In severe cases, where NSAIDs alone are insufficient, opioids, lidocaine, ketamine, and alpha-2 agonist drugs can be used alone or in combination to provide additional analgesia. Intravenous lidocaine infusion (1.3 mg/kg as a bolus followed by a 0.05 mg/kg/min infusion) offers excellent analgesia in many cases that are unresponsive to NSAIDs alone. In the author's experience, opioids alone do not appear particularly effective and are associated with ileus at high doses; however, the combination of lidocaine, ketamine, morphine, detomidine, and acepromazine as an intravenous infusion may be effective in severe cases.[28] Gabapentin (Neurontin) is an effective analgesic in human neuropathic and chronic pain, although more recently it has been used in acute pain to inhibit the processes of temporal summation and spinal cord "wind-up."[29,30] There are currently no data on whether gabapentin has analgesic effects in horses, although recently a neuropathic component to chronic laminitis pain has been demonstrated.[31] Gabapentin has low bioavailability in horses (16%)[32] and therefore must be used at higher doses orally (at least 5–10 mg/kg 2–3 times per day). Intravenous infusion of gabapentin may be appropriate in acute laminitis cases, although there is currently no commercially available injectable preparation. The main side effect of gabapentin administration in horses is mild sedation and tranquilization,[32] which may also be of benefit in acute laminitis cases to encourage recumbency and reduce ambulation (see article by Driessen and Bauquier elsewhere in this issue for further exploration of this topic).

Specific Pharmacologic Therapy

Evidence from experimental models and clinical cases suggests that there is a significant contribution of inflammation to the pathogenesis of developmental and acute laminitis.[12,26,27,33–38] The administration of NSAIDs is therefore indicated during acute laminitis for their antiinflammatory and analgesic properties. Pentoxifylline (Trental) exerts antiinflammatory effects via inhibition of inflammatory mediators (particularly tumor necrosis factor α) and may be useful in the treatment of acute laminitis. Corticosteroids are potent inhibitors of the COX and lipoxygenase pathways of inflammation. Their link to the development of laminitis in certain situations[39,40] has generally prohibited their use in clinical cases of acute laminitis. In horses with primary disease characterized by sepsis (colitis, pneumonia, metritis), it may be beneficial to bind circulating endotoxin through the administration of polymyxin B (3000–6000 IU/kg 3 times a day intravenously) and hyperimmune plasma (Equiplas J).[41]

Regardless of the inciting cause, enzymatic degradation of epidermal-dermal attachments by proteases (including matrix metalloproteinases [MMPs]) may contribute to ongoing lamellar failure in acute laminitis.[42–44] Traditional MMP inhibitors are prohibitively expensive for systemic use, although local delivery using the recently developed intraosseous perfusion method shows promise.[45] Recently Fugler and colleagues[46] tested a range of readily available drugs that have MMP inhibitory actions: only pentoxifylline ameliorated clinical signs in an experimental carbohydrate overload model of acute laminitis, although its antiinflammatory actions may have contributed to the favorable outcome.

It is unclear whether efforts to increase or decrease blood flow to the digit as a whole have any effect on the progression of acute laminitis, and the traditional use of vasodilatory drugs has had little or no effect. Lamellar dermal microthrombosis and increased platelet-neutrophil aggregates have been documented in the developmental and acute phases of laminitis, and microcirculatory failure may contribute to the pathogenesis of acute laminitis.[47–49] A recent report showed an apparent reduction in laminitis incidence after colic surgery in horses that were administered low-molecular-weight heparin[50]; however, the control group in this study was historical and the total incidence of laminitis low.

Horses that have developed laminitis associated with insulin resistance (equine Cushing disease or metabolic syndrome) may benefit from early intervention to increase insulin sensitivity. Exercise has been shown to prevent insulin resistance in horses[51]; however, veterinarians are often presented with cases that have already developed laminitis in which exercise is contraindicated. Initial management should include restricted access to pasture, hay, or concentrates high in nonstructural carbohydrates (NSCs). Metformin (Fortamet; Glucophage), an oral biguanide, is an insulin-sensitizing drug used in humans for several decades that may also be effective in horses. In one study, metformin administered at a dose of 15 mg/kg by mouth twice a day resulted in a subjective clinical improvement in 78% of ponies and horses affected with laminitis and insulin resistance.[52]

Cryotherapy

Continuous distal limb cryotherapy effectively ameliorates experimentally induced acute laminitis when applied continuously during the developmental phase.[53,54] There are currently no data on the efficacy of its use during acute laminitis; however, many of the same processes (inflammation and enzymatic activation) are known to continue after clinical signs have developed. Anecdotally, cooling the feet in acute cases appears to reduce the progression of laminitis and also provides some analgesia. Continuous cooling of the limbs from the metacarpus/metatarsus distally may be performed for several days after the development of clinical signs (see the article by van Eps elsewhere in this issue for further exploration of this topic).

Nutrition and Supportive Care

In horses in which the cause of the acute episode may have been consumption of pasture high in NSCs, access to such pasture should be prevented.[55] Similarly, in horses with a metabolic syndrome phenotype, access to high-NSC feeds should be prohibited.[55] It is unclear in horses that have developed laminitis secondary to other causes (weight bearing, systemic inflammatory response syndrome related) whether provision of feed high in NSC may contribute to worsening of the laminitis. In these cases, it is important to provide enough nutrition to prevent catabolism, and in some horses a capricious appetite may necessitate the provision of highly palatable feed. In any case, good-quality low-carbohydrate feed and water should be provided.

Maintaining hydration and intravascular volume is important in preventing renal tubular necrosis secondary to NSAID administration. Horses that are not drinking properly should be supplemented with water and electrolytes via nasogastric tube or intravenously. The administration of sucralfate (Carafate; 20 mg/kg by mouth 4 times a day) and/or an oral antacid (omeprazole [Gastrogard] 2.0–4.0 mg/kg once a day by mouth) may help to prevent and treat gastric ulceration that develops in conjunction with confinement and NSAID administration.[56,57] Although there is no evidence of its efficacy in horses, sucralfate may also help to prevent and treat ulceration in the right dorsal colon.

Horses that spend extended periods in recumbency are prone to decubital sores, which can be prevented by the application of a foam donut bandage to the tuber coxae. Existing sores can be treated with topical application of silver sulfadiazine or similar drugs. Recumbent horses should be monitored carefully for urine and fecal output, and the bladder and rectum evacuated if necessary.

MONITORING PROGRESSION AND FURTHER MANAGEMENT

The assessment of pain is particularly important in monitoring progression and response to treatment; so this process should be made as objective as possible.

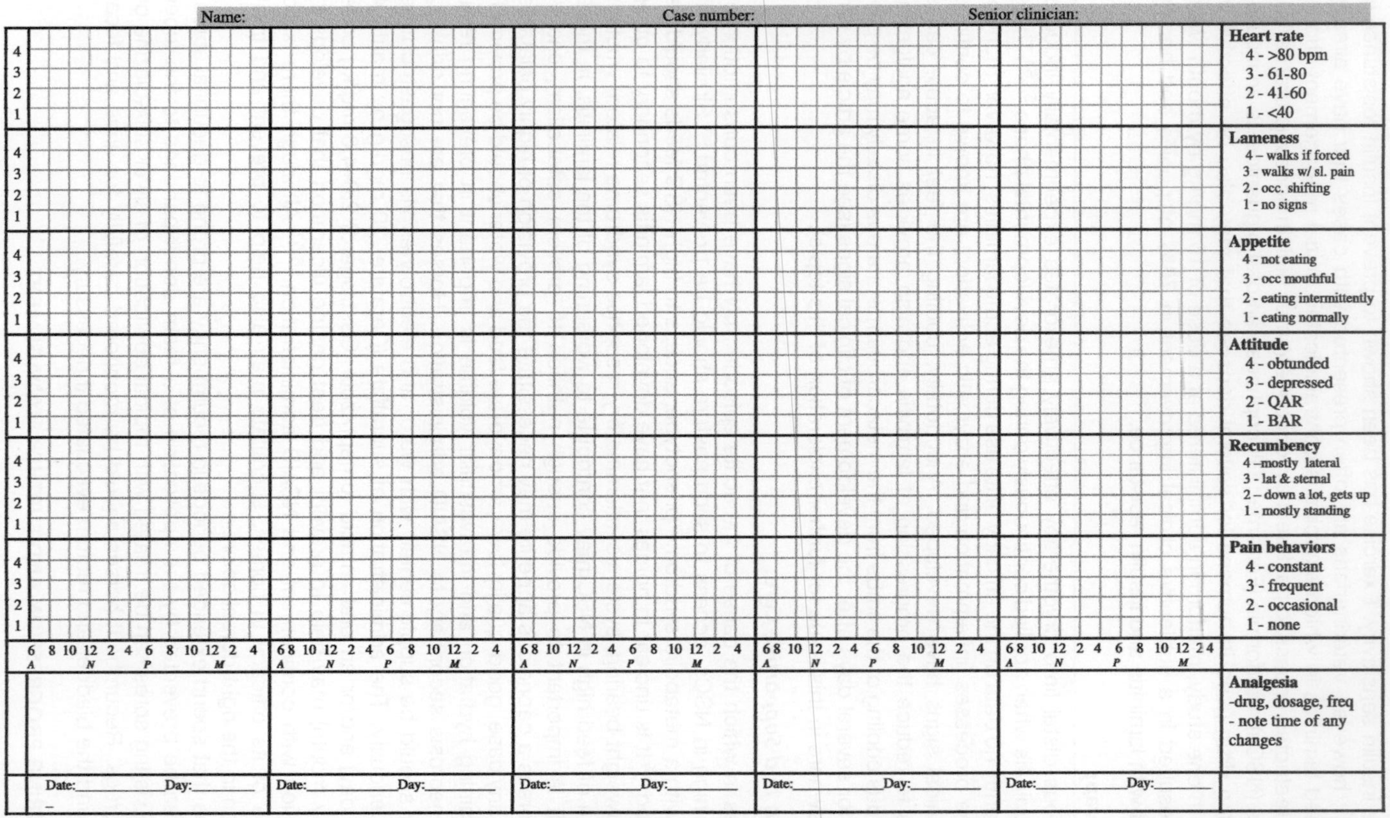

Name: Case number: Senior clinician:

	Day 1	Day 2	Day 3	Day 4	Day 5	
4 3 2 1						**Heart rate** 4 - >80 bpm 3 - 61-80 2 - 41-60 1 - <40
4 3 2 1						**Lameness** 4 – walks if forced 3 - walks w/ sl. pain 2 - occ. shifting 1 - no signs
4 3 2 1						**Appetite** 4 - not eating 3 - occ mouthful 2 - eating intermittently 1 - eating normally
4 3 2 1						**Attitude** 4 - obtunded 3 - depressed 2 - QAR 1 - BAR
4 3 2 1						**Recumbency** 4 –mostly lateral 3 - lat & sternal 2 – down a lot, gets up 1 - mostly standing
4 3 2 1						**Pain behaviors** 4 - constant 3 - frequent 2 - occasional 1 - none
	6 8 10 12 2 4 6 8 10 12 2 4 (A N P M)	6 8 10 12 2 4 6 8 10 12 2 4 (A N P M)	6 8 10 12 2 4 6 8 10 12 2 4 (A N P M)	6 8 10 12 2 4 6 8 10 12 2 4 (A N P M)	6 8 10 12 2 4 6 8 10 12 2 4 (A N P M)	
						Analgesia -drug, dosage, freq - note time of any changes
	Date:____ Day:____	Date:____ Day:____	Date:____ Day:____	Date:____ Day:____	Date:____ Day:____	

Fig. 3. An example of a pain assessment scoring sheet that incorporates clinical and behavioral parameters. The pain behaviors to be observed for frequency recording include teeth grinding, sighing, groaning, self biting, head tossing, lip quiver, yawning, tongue extrusion, licking, standing at back of stall, sour aggression, and low head carriage. (*Courtesy of* Rose Nolen-Walston, DVM, DACVIM, Kennett Square, PA.)

Lameness evaluation is the primary means of evaluating laminitis pain, although regular assessment of vital parameters, particularly heart rate, should also be performed. Behavioral assessment may provide additional evidence of the degree of pain in laminitis cases. In a recent study, certain behaviors were consistently and significantly associated with laminitis pain.[31] An example of a pain assessment scoring sheet that incorporates behavioral parameters is shown in **Fig. 3**. Although designed for a hospitalized horse, this type of system could also be adapted for use by owners caring for horses at home.

In many mild cases the clinical signs of acute laminitis resolve within 2 to 3 days. The clinician should always remember that short-term improvement in lameness that is caused by effective analgesia does not necessarily reflect any abatement of the destructive processes occurring within the lamellae or any strengthening of the lamellar interface. Analgesia should be gradually reduced in these cases in conjunction with continued treatment, confinement, and close monitoring. Horses that show no further clinical signs should still be confined and not subjected to any exercise for at least 6 weeks. Repeat radiographs should be performed 4 to 6 weeks after the initial set to document any progression and to guide the decision for resolution of athletic activity. These horses may benefit from the application of a shoe that supports the frog and heels and eases breakover (eg, a heart bar shoe or wooden clog).

In more severe cases the disease is progressive, and it becomes difficult to make a decision regarding further treatment (vs euthanasia), particularly if the horse appears to be in severe pain. In the author's experience, many moderate to severe cases of laminitis may take at least 7 days to show any improvement in clinical signs; yet these cases may still eventually have a satisfactory outcome. After more than 2 weeks of continuous clinical signs without a satisfactory response to analgesia, the likelihood of a favorable outcome is greatly reduced. Serial monitoring of radiographic parameters is vitally important in acute laminitis cases during the first week of treatment. With few exceptions, horses that have progressive distal displacement of the distal phalanx within the hoof capsule have a grave prognosis.[22,23,58] Often there may be initial evidence of mild distal displacement of the third phalanx that does not progress during subsequent examination periods. This evidence of stabilization should encourage continued treatment and close monitoring, and the prognosis in these cases is often better. Continued confinement and supportive care for several months may be necessary in more severe cases, and this care requires a significant commitment from owners and carers.

Moderate to severe cases that require ongoing treatment should have regular radiographic reassessment every 6 to 8 weeks. It is common to see progressive palmar and distal rotation of the distal phalanx within the hoof capsule from approximately 2 to 4 weeks after initial clinical signs. Trimming and therapeutic shoeing should be guided by the radiographic changes. Horses requiring continued analgesia may benefit from the reduced side effects associated with the more COX-2-selective NSAIDs (firocoxib and meloxicam). Regular monitoring of serum creatinine and albumin concentrations should be performed to check for renal and gastrointestinal side effects of prolonged NSAID use.

SUMMARY

Acute laminitis is a serious complication of many primary conditions in the horse. The progression and eventual outcome of an acute episode depends largely on the severity of the initial insult, although treatment success may be maximized by early recognition and appropriate treatment as well as preemptive management of the horse at risk. Rest, confinement, digital support, analgesia, and antiinflammatory therapy are the key aspects of treatment. Serial monitoring of pain (including response to analgesia) and radiographic parameters helps the clinician to establish the most accurate prognosis.

REFERENCES

1. Hood DM. Laminitis in the horse. Vet Clin North Am Equine Pract 1999;15:287–94.
2. Pollitt CC. Laminitis. In: Colahan PT, Merritt AM, Moore JN, et al, editors. Equine medicine and surgery. 5th edition. St Louis (MO): Mosby; 1999. p. 1521–49.
3. Nourian AR, Baldwin GI, van Eps AW, et al. Equine laminitis: ultrastructural lesions detected 24-30 hours after induction with oligofructose. Equine Vet J 2007;39:360–4.
4. Croser EL, Pollitt CC. Acute laminitis: descriptive evaluation of serial hoof biopsies. In: Proceedings of the 52nd Annual Convention of the American Association of Equine Practitioners, San Antonio (TX); 2006. p. 542–5
5. Parsons CS, Orsini JA, Krafty R, et al. Risk factors for development of acute laminitis in horses during hospitalization: 73 cases (1997–2004). J Am Vet Med Assoc 2007;230:885–9.
6. Peloso JG, Cohen ND, Walker MA, et al. Case-control study of risk factors for the development of laminitis in the contralateral limb in Equidae with unilateral lameness. J Am Vet Med Assoc 1996;209:1746–9.
7. Cohen ND, Parson EM, Seahorn TL, et al. Prevalence and factors associated with development of laminitis in horses with duodenitis/proximal jejunitis: 33 cases (1985–1991). J Am Vet Med Assoc 1994;204:250–4.
8. Cohen ND, Woods AM. Characteristics and risk factors for failure of horses with acute diarrhea to survive: 122 cases (1990-1996). J Am Vet Med Assoc 1999;214: 382–90.
9. Slater MR, Hood DM, Carter GK. Descriptive epidemiological study of equine laminitis. Equine Vet J 1995;27:364–7.
10. Alford P, Geller S, Richrdson B, et al. A multicenter, matched case-control study of risk factors for equine laminitis. Prev Vet Med 2001;49:209–22.
11. Bailey SR. The pathogenesis of acute laminitis: fitting more pieces into the puzzle. Equine Vet J 2004;36:199–203.
12. Belknap JK, Giguere S, Pettigrew A, et al. Lamellar pro-inflammatory cytokine expression patterns in laminitis at the developmental stage and at the onset of lameness: innate vs. adaptive immune response. Equine Vet J 2007;39:42–7.
13. Moore RM, Eades SC, Stokes AM. Evidence for vascular and enzymatic events in the pathophysiology of acute laminitis: which pathway is responsible for initiation of this process in horses? Equine Vet J 2004;36:204–9.
14. Pollitt CC. Equine laminitis: a revised pathophysiology. In: Proceedings of the 45th Annual Convention of the American Association of Equine Practitioners. Albuquerque, NM; 1999. p. 188–92.
15. Hood DM. The pathophysiology of developmental and acute laminitis. Vet Clin North Am Equine Pract 1999;15:321–43.
16. Obel N. Studies of the histopathology of acute laminitis. In: Almgvist and Wilcsells Bottrykeri Ab Uppsala [thesis]; 1948.
17. Mogg KC, Pollitt CC. Hoof and distal limb surface temperature in the normal pony under constant and changing ambient temperatures. Equine Vet J 1992;24:134–9.
18. Cripps PJ, Eustace RA. Radiological measurements from the feet of normal horses with relevance to laminitis. Equine Vet J 1999;31:427–32.
19. Linford RL. A radiographic, morphometric, histological and ultrastructural investigation of lamellar function, abnormality and the associated radiographic

findings for sound and foot sore thoroughbreds and horses with experimentally induced traumatic and alimentary laminitis [PhD thesis]. University of California, Davis, USA; 1987.
20. Miller MA, Pardo ID, Jackson LP, et al. Correlation of pituitary histomorphometry with adrenocorticotrophic hormone response to domperidone administration in the diagnosis of equine pituitary pars intermedia dysfunction. Vet Pathol 2008; 45:26–38.
21. van Eps AW, Pollitt CC. Equine laminitis induced with oligofructose. Equine Vet J 2006;38:203–8.
22. Parks A. Treatment of acute laminitis. Equine Vet Educ 2003;15:273–80.
23. Parks AH, Balch OK, Collier MA. Treatment of acute laminitis. Supportive therapy. Vet Clin North Am Equine Pract 1999;15:363–74.
24. Van Eps AW, Pollitt CC. Equine laminitis model: Lamellar histopathology seven days after induction with oligofructose. Equine Vet J 2009;41:735–40.
25. Wattle O, Ekfalck A, Funkquist B, et al. Behavioural studies in healthy ponies subjected to short-term forced recumbency aiming at an adjunctive treatment in an acute attack of laminitis. Zentralbl Veterinarmed A 1995;42:62–8.
26. Fontaine GL, Belknap JK, Allen D, et al. Expression of interleukin-1beta in the digital laminae of horses in the prodromal stage of experimentally induced laminitis. Am J Vet Res 2001;62:714–20.
27. Pollitt CC. Basement membrane pathology: a feature of acute equine laminitis. Equine Vet J 1996;28:38–46.
28. Abrahamsen EJ. How to manage acute pain in laminitis. In: Proceedings of the Congress of the British Equine Veterinary Association. Birmingham; 2005. p. 195–96.
29. Harding LM, Kristensen JD, Baranowski AP. Differential effects of neuropathic analgesics on wind-up-like pain and somatosensory function in healthy volunteers. Clin J Pain 2005;21:127–32.
30. Arendt-Nielsen L, Frokjaer JB, Staahl C, et al. Effects of gabapentin on experimental somatic pain and temporal summation. Reg Anesth Pain Med 2007;32:382–8.
31. Jones E, Vinuela-Fernandez I, Eager RA, et al. Neuropathic changes in equine laminitis pain. Pain 2007;132:321–31.
32. Terry RL, McDonnell SM, van Eps AW, et al. Pharmacokinetic profile and behavioral effects of gabapentin in the horse. J Vet Pharmacol Ther, in press.
33. Treiber K, Carter R, Gay L, et al. Inflammatory and redox status of ponies with a history of pasture-associated laminitis. Vet Immunol Immunopathol 2009;129: 216–20.
34. Faleiros RR, Nuovo GJ, Belknap JK. Calprotectin in myeloid and epithelial cells of laminae from horses with black walnut extract-induced laminitis. American College of Veterinary Internal Medicine. J Vet Intern Med 2009;23:174–81.
35. Faleiros RR, Leise BB, Westerman T, et al. In vivo and in vitro evidence of the involvement of CXCL1, a keratinocyte-derived chemokine, in equine laminitis. American College of Veterinary Internal Medicine. J Vet Intern Med 2009;23: 1086–96.
36. Black SJ. Extracellular matrix, leukocyte migration and laminitis. Vet Immunol Immunopathol 2009;129:161–3.
37. Blikslager AT, Yin C, Cochran AM, et al. Cyclooxygenase expression in the early stages of equine laminitis: a cytologic study. J Vet Intern Med 2006;20:1191–6.
38. Black SJ, Lunn DP, Yin C, et al. Leukocyte emigration in the early stages of laminitis. Vet Immunol Immunopathol 2006;109:161–6.
39. Harkins JD, Carney JM, Tobin T. Clinical use and characteristics of the corticosteroids. Vet Clin North Am Equine Pract 1993;9:543–62.

40. Bailey SR, Elliott J. The corticosteroid laminitis story: 2. Science of if, when and how. Equine Vet J 2007;39:7–11.
41. Sykes BW, Furr MO. Equine endotoxaemia–a state-of-the-art review of therapy. Aust Vet J 2005;83:45–50.
42. Coyne MJ, Cousin H, Loftus JP, et al. Cloning and expression of ADAM-related metalloproteases in equine laminitis. Vet Immunol Immunopathol 2009;129:231–41.
43. Kyaw-Tanner MT, Wattle O, van Eps AW, et al. Equine laminitis: membrane type matrix metalloproteinase-1 (MMP-14) is involved in acute phase onset. Equine Vet J 2008;40:482–7.
44. Kyaw-Tanner M, Pollitt CC. Equine laminitis: increased transcription of matrix metalloproteinase-2 (MMP-2) occurs during the developmental phase. Equine Vet J 2004;36:221–5.
45. Nourian AR, Mills PC, Pollitt CC. Development of intraosseous infusion of the distal phalanx to access the foot lamellar circulation in the standing, conscious horse. Vet J 2009. [Epub ahead of print].
46. Fugler LA, Eades SC, Koch CE, et al. Clinical and matrix metalloproteinase inhibitory effects of pentoxifylline on carbohydrate overload laminitis: preliminary results. In: Proceedings of the 2nd AAEP Foundation Equine Laminitis Research Workshop. West Palm Beach; 2009. p. 44.
47. Bailey SR, Adair HS, Reinemeyer CR, et al. Plasma concentrations of endotoxin and platelet activation in the developmental stage of oligofructose-induced laminitis. Vet Immunol Immunopathol 2009;129:167–73.
48. Weiss DJ, Evanson OA. Detection of activated platelets and platelet-leukocyte aggregates in horses. Am J Vet Res 1997;58:823–7.
49. Weiss DJ, Evanson OA, McClenahan D, et al. Evaluation of platelet activation and platelet-neutrophil aggregates in ponies with alimentary laminitis. Am J Vet Res 1997;58:1376–80.
50. de la Rebiere de Pouyade G, Grulke S, Detilleux J, et al. Evaluation of low-molecular-weight heparin for the prevention of equine laminitis after colic surgery. J Vet Emerg Crit Care (San Antonio) 2009;19:113–9.
51. Pratt SE, Geor RJ, McCutcheon LJ. Effects of dietary energy source and physical conditioning on insulin sensitivity and glucose tolerance in standard bred horses. Equine Vet J 2006;(Suppl):579–84.
52. Durham AE, Rendle DI, Newton JE. The effect of metformin on measurements of insulin sensitivity and beta cell response in 18 horses and ponies with insulin resistance. Equine Vet J 2008;40:493–500.
53. van Eps AW, Pollitt CC. Equine laminitis model: cryotherapy reduces the severity of lesions evaluated seven days after induction with oligofructose. Equine Vet J 2009;41:741–6.
54. van Eps AW, Pollitt CC. Equine laminitis: cryotherapy reduces the severity of the acute lesion. Equine Vet J 2004;36:255–60.
55. Geor RJ, Harris P. Dietary management of obesity and insulin resistance: countering risk for laminitis. Vet Clin North Am Equine Pract 2009;25:51–65, vi.
56. Murray MJ, Eichorn ES. Effects of intermittent feed deprivation, intermittent feed deprivation with ranitidine administration, and stall confinement with ad libitum access to hay on gastric ulceration in horses. Am J Vet Res 1996;57:1599–603.
57. Murray MJ, Haven ML, Eichorn ES, et al. Effects of omeprazole on healing of naturally-occurring gastric ulcers in thoroughbred racehorses. Equine Vet J 1997;29:425–9.
58. Hood DM. The mechanisms and consequences of structural failure of the foot. Vet Clin North Am Equine Pract 1999;15:437–61.

The Pharmacologic Basis for the Treatment of Developmental and Acute Laminitis

James K. Belknap, DVM, PhD

KEYWORDS

- Laminitis • Treatment • Nonsteroidal antiinflammatory drugs
- Inflammation • Digital blood flow

The treatment of laminitis has been fraught with confusion and controversy for several decades, mainly because of a lack of understanding of the pathophysiology of the disease process. This lack of understanding is because most earlier researchers only examined the events occurring at the onset of Obel grade 3 lameness. Study of the developmental period in different models of laminitis has shown that many events that occur in the early stages are missed if the disease is investigated only in the later stages.[1] The most common causes of laminitis in horses are (1) sepsis (ie, systemic sepsis or endotoxemia from diseases such as enterocolitis, gram-negative pleuropneumonia, acute abdomen [especially involving compromise of the large intestine]), (2) equine metabolic syndrome (ie, pasture-associated laminitis), and (3) supporting limb laminitis.[2–4] Most research has been performed using models that reflect sepsis, including the black walnut extract (BWE) model (documented to induce a systemic inflammatory response similar to sepsis)[1,5,6] and the carbohydrate overload (CHO) models (including the traditional model using wood flour/corn starch mixture[7] and the more recent model using oligofructose,[8] the primary water soluble carbohydrate in grasses). Although valuable information has been obtained from all of the different models, the scientist and clinician need to interpret the information with the knowledge of the marked differences in the models. The BWE model, described in depth by James K. Belknap elsewhere in this issue, is similar to the endotoxin bolus model used to assess organ injury in models of human sepsis. In this model, there is a rapid onset of a severe systemic inflammatory response, but the response is transient (usually a short-lived mild lameness) and rarely results in the substantial laminar injury or failure observed in clinical cases of sepsis-related laminitis. The CHO models more accurately reflect the clinical case in that (1) there is a longer developmental/prodromal stage (approximately 24 hours vs approximately

Department of Veterinary Clinical Sciences, College of Veterinary Medicine, Ohio State University, Columbus, OH 43210, USA
E-mail address: james.belknap@cvm.osu.edu

Vet Clin Equine 26 (2010) 115–124
doi:10.1016/j.cveq.2010.01.003 vetequine.theclinics.com
0749-0739/10/$ – see front matter. Published by Elsevier Inc.

12 hours in the BWE model) before the onset of lameness, and (2) the severity of laminar injury and incidence of laminar failure is similar to the clinical cases of sepsis. Importantly, the timing of events occurring in the developmental stages in the 2 models is very different, so the clinician needs to interpret the data with the differences in the models in mind.

EVENTS OCCURRING IN THE DEVELOPMENTAL AND ACUTE STAGES AT WHICH PHARMACOLOGIC THERAPY IS AIMED

The primary pathophysiologic events (many of which are still controversial) at which most therapies have been aimed include endotoxemia/systemic inflammatory response syndrome (SIRS), dysregulation of the laminar microvasculature affecting laminar blood flow, platelet adhesion/thrombosis, breakdown of the basement membrane of the laminar basal epithelial cells (LBECs, the point of failure in laminitis), and inflammatory injury to the laminae. This article discusses individually each of these events and the drugs that are used to address these events.

ENDOTOXEMIA/SIRS

The role that endotoxin plays in laminitis has remained a controversy mainly because investigators have not been able to induce laminitis with endotoxin administration, even though sepsis-related laminitis rarely occurs unless there is a gram-negative component to the disease process. Whereas it is extremely rare to have laminitis secondary to a fulminant *Streptococcus equi* infection (ie, strangles), it is a frequent occurrence in diseases of the lower respiratory tract with a gram-negative component,[9,10] in an acute metritis in which there is a polymicrobial sepsis including gram-negative organisms,[10] or in intestinal tract disease in which one or more gram-negative organisms are involved.[10] The high incidence of laminitis in diseases such as Potomac horse fever[11](caused by a rickettsial organism which does not contain endotoxin but does contain other inflammatory molecules such as lipoproteins) also suggest that endotoxin does not have to be present for laminitis to occur. Endotoxemia has been confirmed in the CHO models of laminitis.[12,13] These clinical and experimental data suggest several possibilities for why endotoxin infusions do not cause laminitis. Firstly, similar to what has been found in models of organ injury in human sepsis, endotoxin boluses and infusions do not accurately reflect the gradual ramping up of the inflammatory response that occurs in clinical cases and result in a very different inflammatory response (this fact led to the current preference of the rodent cecal ligation and puncture model over the endotoxemia model in human sepsis[14] research).[15] Secondly, there are more toxins than just endotoxin that are involved in the pathophysiologic response. In a recent study using equine epidermal epithelial cells, it was found that, in contrast to human cell studies but in congruence with the clinical picture in the horse, the equine epithelial cells responded markedly to lipopolysaccharide (LPS) but not to toxins that are more characteristic of gram-positive sepsis, including lipoteichoic acid and peptidoglycan. However, the cells underwent a response to flagellin, a molecule that is more commonly associated with gram-negative sepsis and found to be as potent at LPS in some sepsis models and that works synergistically with LPS in salmonella infections. Thirdly, similar to results reported in the human literature, injured and dying host cells release cellular proteins (especially mitochondrial proteins) that can induce a similar inflammatory response as that induced by molecules such as LPS.[2] Thus, cells injured at the source of the sepsis (ie, colon, cecum, lung) or even those injured secondarily due to the systemic inflammatory response likely release proteins that stimulate a similar inflammatory response as bacterial molecules.

POLYMYXIN B

Polymyxin B has been well established to bind endotoxin and inhibit downstream signaling in the horse and other species.[16,17] However, because of the facts discussed earlier, it is not surprising that polymyxin B, a drug that binds endotoxin and thus inhibits binding of the molecule to its receptor in host cells, failed to decrease the incidence of laminitis or signs of sepsis in the CHO model when administered alone. This study does not indicate that polymyxin B may not be helpful when used in a treatment regimen with other therapies, as endotoxin is still likely to play a role in the disease process.

HYPERIMMUNE SERUM AGAINST COMPONENTS OF ENDOTOXIN

There are conflicting reports regarding the efficacy of these products in the septic horse[17–19]; the lack of a consistent positive effect may deter the clinician from using these products.

NONSTEROIDAL ANTIINFLAMMATORY DRUGS

Although nonsteroidal antiinflammatory drugs (NSAIDs) are used as an antiendotoxic therapy, any efficacy results from the blocking of systemic and local inflammation (downstream of endotoxin); these drugs are discussed later, with other inflammatory drugs.

DYSREGULATION OF LAMINAR MICROVASCULAR BLOOD FLOW

Although there are conflicting data regarding the presence of decreased laminar blood flow in the early stages of laminitis,[20] most reports indicate that laminar blood flow is decreased in the developmental and acute clinical stages of laminitis.[21–24] Any decrease in laminar flow is likely to be a result of a postcapillary/venous constriction.[21,22] The cause of the reported venoconstriction is unknown, although laminar venules are reported to be highly sensitive (much more sensitive than laminar arteries) to vasoconstrictor substances that are likely to be present in affected laminae (including thromboxane, prostaglandin [PG] $F_2\alpha$, endothelin-1, and isoprostanes).[25,26] Although LPS administration has been reported to induce a decrease in laminar blood flow,[27] the decrease in flow is caused by an arterial constriction,[28]and, therefore, LPS is not likely the cause of any decreased digital blood flow observed in laminitis. A more likely scenario is that vasoactive substances, including PGs, thromboxane, and isoprostanes, are released by adhered platelets, the inflamed vasculature, and leukocytes adhered or extravasating into the tissues; both platelet and leukocyte adhesion occur more commonly in the venous circulation.[13,29]

Drugs for Microvascular Dysregulation

Most drugs used in the past 2 decades in attempts to increase laminar blood flow have been proved to be ineffective peripheral vasodilators in the horse[30]; acepromazine is the one vasodilator that has been demonstrated to increase flow to the entire digit.[31,32]

Nitroglycerin

Nitroglycerin applied topically to the palmarodistal limb was initially reported to be effective in ameliorating signs of lameness via increasing digital blood flow in the laminitic horse.[33] However, it was recently reported not only that nitroglycerin was ineffective in increasing digital blood flow but also that it was not even absorbed into the digital circulation (likely because it is primarily absorbed by the venous circulation draining away from the digit).[34]

Pentoxifylline

Pentoxifylline (PTX) was originally used as a hemorheologic agent to increase blood flow in compromised vasculature via increasing malleability of blood cells; the drug was found not to increase blood flow in normal horses,[30] but it has not been critically assessed in the laminitic digit. The prolonged time needed for any hemorheologic effect likely makes it an ineffective drug as a hemorheologic agent.

Isoxsuprine

Isoxsuprine has also been demonstrated to be ineffective in increasing laminar perfusion in the horse when administered orally[30]; vasodilation only occurs at doses that induce neurologic side effects.

Acepromazine

Acepromazine has been reported to effectively increase digital blood flow for a short period of time when administered intramuscularly.[32]

NSAIDs

NSAIDs may effectively block production of vasoactive prostanoids and the prostanoids with vasodilatory activities, including PGE_2 and prostacyclin; the production of both has been associated with cyclooxygenase (COX) 2 in the vascular wall.[35,36] This fact, combined with the fact that platelets are a major source of thromboxane to COX-1, indicates that a nonselective NSAID (ie, phenylbutazone or flunixin) may be a better choice (vs a COX-2 selective) in the acute stage of the disease, so as not to tilt the environment toward vasoconstriction.

PLATELET ACTIVATION/THROMBOSIS

Numerous studies have detailed platelet activation in laminitis through the demonstration of platelet-neutrophil aggregates in the bloodstream,[37,38] the demonstration of platelet adhesion in the affected laminar digit, and the activation of platelet p38 mitogen-activated protein kinase (MAPK).[13] Although large numbers of laminar microthrombi are not usually found in laminitis studies, the adhered platelets can, as described earlier, induce pathology by release of vasoactive substances.[29] The incidence of laminitis was reported to be decreased with the use of an inhibitor of platelet aggregation in one study.[38] Results from retrospective studies assessing the efficacy of unfractionated heparin in decreasing the incidence of laminitis have been conflicting.[39,40] Unfractionated heparin causes reversible agglutination of red blood cells (RBCs) in horses; these agglutinants of cells reportedly seed out in capillaries.[41] Low–molecular-weight heparin may be a better option, as it does not cause RBC agglutination and has recently been reported to result in decreased incidence of laminitis in a retrospective study of postoperative colic patients.[42]

BREAKDOWN OF THE LAMINAR BASEMENT MEMBRANE

The well-described failure of the interdigitation of the epidermal and dermal laminae at the interface of the LBECs and the basement membrane attached to the laminar dermis[43,44] has led to a great deal of interest in the involvement of matrix metalloproteases (MMPs) in the destruction of the basement membrane possibly leading to laminar failure. The in vitro inhibition of laminar separation with batimastat, an MMP inhibitor, further increased the interest in MMP inhibition as a therapy for laminitis.[45] Both MMP-2 and MMP-9 have been found in the laminae,[46,47] although whether either MMP is active in acute laminitis is not known.[48] Preliminary results of a study assessing the efficacy of tetracyclines (drugs that are clinically most used as MMP inhibitors) against equine MMPs indicate that doxycycline does not inhibit equine MMPs, and oxytetracycline, which does inhibit equine MMPs, is not effective at inhibiting laminar failure in experimentally induced laminitis (S. Eades, Louisiana State University [LSU], unpublished data, 2009). The recently reported lack of activity of laminar MMP-2 and MMP-9 in laminar tissue in the acute stage of laminitis in combination with the lack of efficacy of oxytetracycline in ameliorating the disease process questions the value of targeting MMPs in laminitis. It now seems that laminar separation, leading to laminar failure, may be more from a failure of epithelial adhesion molecules (ie, hemidesmosomes), which attach the LBECs to the BM.[49,50] Dysregulation of cell adhesion most likely follows general LBEC cytoskeletal dysfunction caused by cellular injury from events such as inflammatory and/or hypoxic injury to the LBECs.

INFLAMMATORY INJURY TO THE LAMINAE

Although for several decades the focus of antiinflammatory therapy has been the blocking of inflammatory prostanoids via the use of nonselective NSAIDs, such as flunixin meglumine and phenylbutazone, it is now known that other numerous injurious inflammatory mediators and pathways are also activated in the laminae.[2,5,51] All of the discussed inflammatory events are possible future therapeutic targets for laminitis. A similar inflammatory response occurs in the digital laminae in the early stages of laminitis as occurs in organ injury in human sepsis, including the activation of the endothelium of the laminar vasculature, leading to the expression of adhesion molecule[1,51] and chemokines,[1,5,51] both of which induce leukocytes to adhere to the endothelium and extravasate into the laminar interstitium. There is a marked laminar inflammatory mediator response including the expression of proinflammatory cytokines (ie, interleukin [IL] 1β, IL-6) and COX-2, and the likely activation of multiple inflammatory pathways, including p38 MAPK,[13,52] Jak-Stat signaling,[53] and, most likely, nuclear factor (NF) κB (indicated by downstream inflammatory molecules reported to be expressed in affected laminar tissue). In human sepsis and other inflammatory diseases, oxidative stress produced by infiltrating leukocytes and host cells with dysregulated cellular functions (due to events such as inflammatory mediator expression and hypoxia) is thought to play a major role in organ/tissue injury. Although there is evidence of initial oxidative events, including lipid peroxidation,[25,54] evidence of more severe, end-stage oxidative events, such as protein carbonylation in the BWE or CHO models of laminitis have not been found (Belknap, unpublished data, 2009). These data, combined with the fact that drugs to combat oxidative stress have not been effective in decreasing injury in human sepsis, question the role that oxidative stress plays in laminar failure. It may be more likely that other injurious mediators such as proteases and cytokines cause epithelial cell injury and dysregulation, possibly because of energy failure in the cell. This general LBEC dysfunction is likely to lead to failure of cytoskeletal and adhesion molecule dynamics discussed earlier, causing dysattachment of the LBECs from the underlying basement membrane.

NSAIDS

The most common NSAIDs used, flunixin meglumine and phenylbutazone, are effective at blocking COX production of PGH_2, the prostanoid used by the multiple PG- and thromboxane-synthase enzymes to make the different prostanoids. Both drugs can be used to address inflammatory events (such as endotoxemia) and musculoskeletal pain, although flunixin meglumine is preferred (and somewhat more effective) for treating animals still exhibiting signs of sepsis, whereas phenylbutazone is preferred (and somewhat more effective) in the animals exhibiting only musculoskeletal pain (ie, subacute or chronic case). In animals at risk of laminitis, flunixin would be the primary drug of choice. There is some evidence that, when used at high concentrations, NSAIDs can block inflammatory pathways other than the COX enzymes, thereby blocking many of the other inflammatory events discussed earlier, including proinflammatory cytokine expression.[55,56] These non-COX activities may be the reason that ponies administered low-dose flunixin (0.25 mg/kg 3 times a day) in NSAID studies appear sicker than those given the maximal dose (1.1 mg/kg 3 times a day) despite a similar degree of prostanoid blockade.[57] For this reason, the author uses flunixin meglumine at its maximal dose (1.1 mg/kg 3 times a day) for the first 2 to 3 days of therapy in animals exhibiting signs of sepsis. In animals with renal compromise, ketoprofen may be a better NSAID to use; the author uses the full dose of ketoprofen (2.2 mg/kg) 4 times a day, as it is a very safe drug[58] and does not appear to provide effective analgesia when used twice a day. In animals in the acute stage exhibiting both lameness and signs of systemic sepsis (ie, common in enterocolitis cases), some clinicians combine phenylbutazone and flunixin at lower doses. Because of toxicity concerns, animals on aggressive doses of phenylbutazone should be given a day off every 5 to7 days, with flunixin administered on that day; flunixin will not affect the clearance of phenylbutazone.

INTRAVENOUS LIDOCAINE

Because lidocaine has antiinflammatory properties, a constant rate infusion (CRI) of lidocaine is frequently used in postoperative colic cases (some antiinflammatory properties have been shown in numerous rodent models when high doses of the drug was administered as CRI). However, a recent study that used the BWE model indicated that a lidocaine CRI (at the maximal dose that can be given safely) is not antiinflammatory and appeared to cause endothelial activation.[59] Therefore, there is little reason for using this treatment modality at the moment for antiinflammatory therapy; there are likely to be analgesic effects.

DISTAL LIMB CRYOTHERAPY

Some of the efficacy of cold therapy, similar to that observed when it is used for brain trauma in humans, may be due to inhibition of inflammatory pathways including NFκB and proinflammatory cytokine signaling; this possibility is currently being investigated.

PTX

PTX has been administered for several possible effects including being a hemorheologic agent, blocking inflammatory mediator signaling (especially tumor necrosis factor α effects), and being a protease inhibitor.[60] Although the hemorheologic aspect does not appear to be true in the horse,[30] preliminary results indicate that PTX may decrease the incidence of laminar failure in an ongoing study using the CHO model of laminitis (S. Eades, LSU, unpublished data, 2009).

FUTURE THERAPIES

As more data become available regarding the importance of the different events in the ensuing laminar failure, different therapeutic targets will become available. For example, drug development to block leukocyte activation and extravasation through blockade of chemokine receptors in humans may be of value in laminitis. Many of the standard (ie, corticosteroids) and newer (ie, MAPK inhibitors) antiinflammatory drugs cause excessive immunosuppression when administered systemically and would therefore not be beneficial in animals with sepsis. However, one advantage in the horse with sepsis is that the target organ, the digit, is peripheral. Therefore, some of the more potent drugs may be administered through regional intravenous perfusion. High continuous concentrations of antibiotics may also be provided to the digit and laminae through a cannulated bone screw placed through the hoof wall into the distal phalanx.[61] If proved to be a safe method of drug administration in the laminitic digit, antiinflammatory drugs may also be administered via this technique.

REFERENCES

1. Loftus JP, Black SJ, Pettigrew A, et al. Early laminar events involving endothelial activation in horses with black walnut-induced laminitis. Am J Vet Res 2007;68:1205–11.
2. Belknap JK, Moore JN, Crouser EC. Sepsis-From human organ failure to laminar failure. Vet Immunol Immunopathol 2009;129:155–7.
3. Geor RJ, Harris P. Dietary management of obesity and insulin resistance: countering risk for laminitis. Vet Clin North Am Equine Pract 2009;25:51–65, vi.
4. Baxter GM, Morrison S. Complications of unilateral weight bearing. Vet Clin North Am Equine Pract 2008;24:621–42, ix.
5. Belknap JK, Giguere S, Pettigrew A, et al. Lamellar pro-inflammatory cytokine expression patterns in laminitis at the developmental stage and at the onset of lameness: innate vs. adaptive immune response. Equine Vet J 2007;39:42–7.
6. Hurley DJ, Parks RJ, Reber AJ, et al. Dynamic changes in circulating leukocytes during the induction of equine laminitis with black walnut extract. Vet Immunol Immunopathol 2006;110:195–206.
7. Garner HE, Coffman JR, Hahn AW, et al. Equine laminitis of alimentary origin: an experimental model. Am J Vet Res 1975;36:441–4.
8. van Eps AW, Pollitt CC. Equine laminitis induced with oligofructose. Equine Vet J 2006;38:203–8.
9. Hudson NPH, McClintock SA, Hodgson DR. Case of pleuropneumonia with complications in a Thoroughbred Stallion. Equine Vet Educ 1999;11:286–9.
10. Parsons CS, Orsini JA, Krafty R, et al. Risk factors for development of acute laminitis in horses during hospitalization: 73 cases (1997–2004). J Am Vet Med Assoc 2007;230:885–9.
11. Mulville P. Equine monocytic ehrlichiosis (Potomac horse fever): a review. Equine Vet J 1991;23:400–4.
12. Sprouse RF, Garner HE, Green EM. Plasma endotoxin levels in horses subjected to carbohydrate induced laminitis. Equine Vet J 1987;19:25–8.
13. Bailey SR, Adair HS, Reinemeyer CR, et al. Plasma concentrations of endotoxin and platelet activation in the developmental stage of oligofructose-induced laminitis. Vet Immunol Immunopathol 2009;129:167–73.
14. Liaudet L, Szabo C, Evgenov OV, et al. Flagellin from gram-negative bacteria is a potent mediator of acute pulmonary inflammation in sepsis. Shock 2003;19:131–7.

15. Buras JA, Holzmann B, Sitkovsky M. Animal models of sepsis: setting the stage. Nat Rev Drug Discov 2005;4:854–65.
16. Southwood LL. Postoperative management of the large colon volvulus patient. Vet Clin North Am Equine Pract 2004;20:167–97.
17. Durando MM, MacKay RJ, Linda S, et al. Effects of polymyxin B and *Salmonella typhimurium* antiserum on horses given endotoxin intravenously. Am J Vet Res 1994;55:921–7.
18. Garner HE, Sprouse RF, Lager K. Cross protection of ponies from sublethal *Escherichia coli* endotoxemia by Salmonella typhimurium antiserum. Equine Pract 1988;10:10–7.
19. Morris DD, Whitlock RH, Corbeil LB. Endotoxemia in horses: protection provided by antiserum to core lipopolysaccharide. Am J Vet Res 1986;47:544–50.
20. Pollitt CC, Davies CT. Equine laminitis: its development coincides with increased sublamellar blood flow. Equine Vet J Suppl 1998;26:125–32.
21. Eaton SA, Allen DA, Eades SC, et al. Digital Starling forces and hemodynamics during early laminitis induced by an aqueous extract of black walnut (Juglans nigra) in horses. Vet Surg 1994;23:400–1.
22. Allen D Jr, Clark ES, Moore JN, et al. Evaluation of equine digital Starling forces and hemodynamics during early laminitis. Am J Vet Res 1990;51:1930–4.
23. Adair HS 3rd, Goble DO, Schmidhammer JL, et al. Laminar microvascular flow, measured by means of laser Doppler flowmetry, during the prodromal stages of black walnut-induced laminitis in horses. Am J Vet Res 2000;61:862–8.
24. Hood DM, Wagner IP, Brumbaugh GW. Evaluation of hoof wall surface temperature as an index of digital vascular perfusion during the prodromal and acute phases of carbohydrate-induced laminitis in horses. Am J Vet Res 2001;62: 1167–72.
25. Noschka E, Moore JN, Peroni JF, et al. Thromboxane and isoprostanes as inflammatory and vasoactive mediators in black walnut heartwood extract induced equine laminitis. Vet Immunol Immunopathol 2009;129:200–10.
26. Peroni JF, Moore JN, Noschka E, et al. Predisposition for venoconstriction in the equine laminar dermis: implications in equine laminitis. J Appl Phys 2006;100: 759–63.
27. Ingle-Fehr JE, Baxter GM. Evaluation of digital and laminar blood flow in horses given a low dose of endotoxin. Am J Vet Res 1998;59:192–6.
28. Hunt RJ, Allen D, Moore JN. Effect of endotoxin administration on equine digital hemodynamics and starling forces. Am J Vet Res 1990;51:1703–7.
29. Robertson TP, Bailey SR, Peroni JF. Equine laminitis: a journey to the dark side of venous. Vet Immunol Immunopathol 2009;129:164–6.
30. Ingle-Fehr JE, Baxter GM. The effect of oral isoxsuprine and pentoxifylline on digital and laminar blood flow in healthy horses. Vet Surg 1999;28:154–60.
31. Hunt RJ, Brandon CI, McCann ME. Effects of acetylpromazine, xylazine, and vertical load on digital arterial blood-flow in horses. Am J Vet Res 1994;55:375–8.
32. Leise BS, Fugler LA, Stokes AM, et al. Effects of intramuscular administration of acepromazine on palmar digital blood flow, palmar digital arterial pressure, transverse facial arterial pressure, and packed cell volume in clinically healthy, conscious horses. Vet Surg 2007;36:717–23.
33. Hinckley KA, Fearn S, Howard BR, et al. Nitric oxide donors as treatment for grass induced acute laminitis in ponies. Equine Vet J 1996;28:17–28.
34. Gilhooly MH, Eades SC, Stokes AM, et al. Effects of topical nitroglycerine patches and ointment on digital venous plasma nitric oxide concentrations and digital blood flow in healthy conscious horses. Vet Surg 2005;34:604–9.

35. Krotz F, Schiele TM, Klauss V, et al. Selective COX-2 inhibitors and risk of myocardial infarction. J Vasc Res 2005;42:312–24.
36. Sanghi S, MacLaughlin EJ, Jewell CW, et al. Cyclooxygenase-2 inhibitors: a painful lesson. Cardiovasc Hematol Disord Drug Targets 2006;6:85–100.
37. Eades SC, Stokes AM, Johnson PJ, et al. Serial alterations in digital hemodynamics and endothelin-1 immunoreactivity, platelet-neutrophil aggregation, and concentrations of nitric oxide, insulin, and glucose in blood obtained from horses following carbohydrate overload. Am J Vet Res 2007;68:87–94.
38. Weiss DJ, Evanson OA, McClenahan D, et al. Evaluation of platelet activation and platelet-neutrophil aggregates in ponies with alimentary laminitis. Am J Vet Res 1997;58:1376–80.
39. Belknap JK, Moore JN. Evaluation of heparin for prophylaxis of equine laminitis: 71 cases (1980–1986). J Am Vet Med Assoc 1989;195:505–7.
40. Cohen ND, Parson EM, Seahorn TL, et al. Prevalence and factors associated with development of laminitis in horses with duodenitis/proximal jejunitis: 33 cases (1985–1991). J Am Vet Med Assoc 1994;204:250–4.
41. Mahaffey EA, Moore JN. Erythrocyte agglutination associated with heparin treatment in three horses. J Am Vet Med Assoc 1986;189:1478–80.
42. de la Rebiere de Pouyade G, Grulke S, Detilleux J, et al. Evaluation of low-molecular-weight heparin for the prevention of equine laminitis after colic surgery. J Vet Emerg Crit Care (San Antonio) 2009;19:113–9.
43. Pollitt CC. Basement membrane pathology: a feature of acute equine laminitis. Equine Vet J 1996;28:38–46.
44. Pollitt CC, Daradka M. Equine laminitis basement membrane pathology: loss of type IV collagen, type VII collagen and laminin immunostaining. Equine Vet J Suppl 1998;26:139–44.
45. Pollitt CC, Pass MA, Pollitt S. Batimastat (BB-94) inhibits matrix metalloproteinases of equine laminitis. Equine Vet J Suppl 1998;26:119–24.
46. Loftus JP, Belknap JK, Black SJ. Matrix metalloproteinase-9 in laminae of black walnut extract treated horses correlates with neutrophil abundance. Vet Immunol Immunopathol 2006;113:267–76.
47. Mungall BA, Pollitt CC. Zymographic analysis of equine laminitis. Histochem Cell Biol 1999;112:467–72.
48. Loftus JP, Johnson PJ, Belknap JK, et al. Leukocyte-derived and endogenous matrix metalloproteinases in the lamellae of horses with naturally acquired and experimentally induced laminitis. Vet Immunol Immunopathol 2009;129:221–30.
49. French KR, Pollitt CC. Equine laminitis: loss of hemidesmosomes in hoof secondary epidermal lamellae correlates to dose in an oligofructose induction model: an ultrastructural study. Equine Vet J 2004;36:230–5.
50. Nourian AR, Baldwin GI, van Eps AW, et al. Equine laminitis: ultrastructural lesions detected 24–30 hours after induction with oligofructose. Equine Vet J 2007;39: 360–4.
51. Noschka E, Vandenplas ML, Hurley DJ, et al. Temporal aspects of laminar gene expression during the developmental stages of equine laminitis. Vet Immunol Immunopathol 2009;129:242–53.
52. Eckert RE, Sharief Y, Jones SL. p38 mitogen-activated kinase (MAPK) is essential for equine neutrophil migration. Vet Immunol Immunopathol 2009;129: 181–91.
53. Tannhof E, Yin C, Pettigrew A, et al. Laminar regulation of STAT1 and STAT3 at developmental stages and at the onset of lameness in the black walnut extract model of laminitis. J Vet Intern Med 2007;21:662.

54. Yin C, Pettigrew A, Loftus JP, et al. Tissue concentrations of 4-HNE in the black walnut extract model of laminitis: indication of oxidant stress in affected laminae. Vet Immunol Immunopathol 2009;129:211–5.
55. Housby JN, Cahill CM, Chu B, et al. Non-steroidal anti-inflammatory drugs inhibit the expression of cytokines and induce HSP70 in human monocytes. Cytokines 1999;11:347–58.
56. Sagi SA, Weggen S, Eriksen J, et al. The non-cyclooxygenase targets of non-steroidal anti-inflammatory drugs, lipoxygenases, peroxisome proliferator-activated receptor, inhibitor of kappa B kinase, and NF kappa B, do not reduce amyloid beta 42 production. J Biol Chem 2003;278:31825–30.
57. Semrad SD, Hardee GE, Hardee MM, et al. Low dose flunixin meglumine: effects on eicosanoid production and clinical signs induced by experimental endotoxaemia in horses. Equine Vet J 1987;19:201–6.
58. MacAllister CG, Morgan SJ, Borne AT, et al. Comparison of adverse effects of phenylbutazone, flunixin meglumine, and ketoprofen in horses. J Am Vet Med Assoc 1993;202:71–7.
59. Williams JM, Ravis W, Loftus J, et al. Effect of intravenous lidocaine administration on leukocyte emigration in the black walnut extract model of laminitis. J Vet Intern Med 2009;23:781.
60. Dua P, Gude RP. Antiproliferative and antiproteolytic activity of pentoxifylline in cultures of B16F10 melanoma cells. Cancer Chemother Pharmacol 2006;58: 195–202.
61. Nourian AR, Mills PC, Pollitt CC. Development of intraosseous infusion of the distal phalanx to access the foot lamellar circulation in the standing, conscious horse. Vet J 2010;183(3):273–7.

Therapeutic Hypothermia (Cryotherapy) to Prevent and Treat Acute Laminitis

Andrew W. van Eps, BVSc, PhD

KEYWORDS

• Equine • Laminitis • Cryotherapy • Distal limb

Laminitis is a debilitating disease of horses that causes significant morbidity and mortality. Laminitis lesions are generally considered irreversible, and there is currently no effective treatment. Prevention of laminitis in horses considered at risk and halting the progression of acute laminitis are therefore key areas for clinicians to focus their efforts. Most laminitis cases occur as a result of metabolic disturbances in conjunction with the consumption of carbohydrate-rich pasture or hay.[1] In these cases the laminitis is often insidiously progressive and episodic, making identification of the developmental period difficult. Severe, acute laminitis is a common sequel to numerous primary diseases, including colitis, pneumonia, metritis, and rhabdomyolysis. In these cases, the developmental period is more easily predictable; therefore, prevention or early interventional treatment may be possible. Digital hypothermia during the developmental phase has been shown to ameliorate experimentally induced acute laminitis,[2,3] and has recently gained popularity in clinical cases for the prevention and treatment of acute laminitis.

Distal limb cryotherapy is commonly used in horses, particularly for the treatment of musculoskeletal injuries, although protocols are largely extrapolated from human medicine. The equine distal limb is highly resilient in the face of profound continuous hypothermia,[4] providing a unique therapeutic opportunity. The appropriate protocols aimed at preventing and treating acute laminitis differ significantly from those that are traditionally used for the treatment of athletic injury. This article reviews the effects of hypothermia on tissue, and discusses the rationale and suggested protocols for the usage of distal limb cryotherapy in the prevention and treatment of laminitis based on current information.

School of Veterinary Science, University of Queensland, Slip Road, St Lucia, QLD 4072, Australia
E-mail address: a.vaneps@uq.edu.au

Vet Clin Equine 26 (2010) 125–133
doi:10.1016/j.cveq.2010.01.002 vetequine.theclinics.com
0749-0739/10/$ – see front matter

THE EFFECTS OF HYPOTHERMIA ON TISSUE

The physiologic effects of hypothermia on tissue are complex and still poorly understood. The major effects of hypothermia on most tissues are analgesia, hypometabolism, and a vascular response.[5] Cold has a direct effect on the peripheral nerves; it reduces conduction velocity, increases the threshold for stimulation, and increases the refractory period after stimulation.[6] Hypothermia has a profound inhibitory effect on tissue metabolism: tissue metabolic rate and oxygen consumption are directly related to temperature.[7] Hypothermia has been best studied in brain tissue for its neuroprotective effects after traumatic and ischemic brain injury.[8] Cerebral metabolism decreases by 6% to 10% for each 1°C decrease in body temperature.[9–11] A reduced requirement of cooled tissue for oxygen, glucose, and other metabolites enhances the survival of cells during periods of ischemia.[12] This mechanism is believed to protect tissue on the periphery of an injury from secondary hypoxic damage,[5] and is also the basis for the use of cryotherapy in organ transplant surgery.[13] Hypothermia reduces apoptosis, mitochondrial failure, and inflammation after cerebral ischemia-reperfusion.[8] A reduction in metabolic enzymatic activity of approximately 50% has been observed with a reduction in tissue temperature of 10°C.[14] The activity of collagenases is significantly reduced at lower temperatures.[15]

Hypothermia exerts a profound anti-inflammatory effect through reduced production and activity of proinflammatory cytokines (interleukin [IL]-1β, IL-2, IL-6, and IL-8)[16–18]; increased production of anti-inflammatory cytokines (IL-10)[16,19]; reduced rolling and adhesion of leukocytes[20,21]; and reduced production of oxygen radicals by polymorphonuclear leukocytes.[22] Cryotherapy has been traditionally used to reduce inflammation in musculoskeletal injury, particularly after surgery.[5,12,23] Recently there has been interest in the profound anti-inflammatory effect of hypothermia on end-organ damage in models of sepsis and systemic inflammatory response syndrome.[16,19,24,25] Preemptive hypothermia (10°C < normal) markedly reduced the severity of acute lung injury in a rat model of sepsis by reducing neutrophil emigration, inhibiting proinflammatory cytokine activity, and increasing anti-inflammatory cytokine activity.[16] In a subsequent study, less profound hypothermia (5°C < normal), applied even after the lung was primed with neutrophilic inflammation, also decreased the severity of acute lung injury, suggesting a therapeutic role for hypothermia beyond its preventive effect.[25]

Cryotherapy causes potent local vasoconstriction.[26] This is largely mediated by sympathetic nervous control; however, a direct constrictive effect on blood vessel walls may occur, particularly at lower temperatures.[27] Periods of transient vasodilation (cold-induced vasodilation [CIVD]) may occur when temperatures are reduced to below approximately 18°C[28] A cyclic pattern of increasing and decreasing blood flow (the hunting reaction) may be noted.[29] CIVD has been studied mostly in the human hand; however, it has also been noted in the face, forearms, and feet.[30] In the human finger, CIVD seems to occur as a result of dilation of the arteriovenous anastomoses (AVAs), whereas cold-induced vasoconstriction seems to occur as a result of constriction of AVAs and the arteries supplying the finger.[31] A recent study using direct microcirculatory observation showed marked arteriolar vasoconstriction with local cooling to 8°C for 30 minutes.[32] It is generally accepted that the application of cryotherapy results in a marked net reduction in local perfusion.[8,33]

Profound whole body hypothermia (>10°C below normal) can result in severe side effects associated with cardiac, endocrine, and metabolic function.[8] Hypothermia is also associated with coagulopathy and increased risk of infection.[8] Adverse effects of locally applied cryotherapy are rare, but may include frostbite and nerve palsy.[5,34]

The temperatures and duration of exposure required to induce frostbite are unclear.[35] Nerve palsy is a rare complication of cryotherapy in human patients, and usually involves large superficial nerves.[5] Prolonged exposure to the combination of cold and moisture has been associated with the development of immersion foot and trench foot in human patients.[36] These conditions cause local swelling and pain that may progress to blistering of the skin, nerve damage, and gangrene.[37] Cryotherapy is contraindicated in humans with peripheral vascular diseases, such as Raynaud phenomenon, because of its potent vasoconstricting effect.[26]

THERAPEUTIC HYPOTHERMIA OF THE EQUINE DISTAL LIMB

Although cryotherapy is commonly used for the treatment and prophylaxis of musculoskeletal injuries in horses, there are few controlled studies evaluating the effects of cryotherapy on the equine distal limb, and treatment recommendations are largely based on extrapolation from protocols used in humans.[38–40] Distal to the carpus and tarsus, the limbs of the horse are devoid of muscle and the major blood vessels are superficial; this is seemingly ideal for inducing deep hypothermia of the foot. However, the hair coat and hoof provide a barrier to effective conduction of heat out of the limb. Also, the presence of a rich vascular network within the corium, including numerous AVAs,[37,38] means that rapid increases in net perfusion of the foot with warm blood can occur.

Numerous modalities are used for distal limb cryotherapy in horses; there are several commercially available devices for this purpose, although most are suited to short-term (30–60 minutes) applications. Published studies have used commercial cold gel wraps and cold cuffs as well as ice water immersion. A cold gel wrap (4°C) applied for 30 minutes to the metacarpal region of 10 horses resulted in a reduction in surface temperature over the dorsal metacarpal region that was sustained for 3 hours.[41] Another study compared the effects of cold water immersion and cold-pack application to the equine metacarpal region for 30 minutes.[42] This study showed a profound and sustained reduction in deep-tissue temperature during iced-water immersion (maximum reduction 16.3°C), that was far superior to cold-pack application. Continuous cryotherapy for 48 hours using iced-water immersion resulted in profound cooling of the digit (mean internal hoof temperature 5.3° $\pm$ 0.3°C) and was not associated with adverse clinical effects.[4] Further studies have since confirmed the profound cooling effects of continuous cold-water immersion for 48 hours[3] and 72 hours[2] on the digit, without apparent deleterious effects.

The application of cold to the equine distal limb generally results in profound vasoconstriction within digit. A scintigraphic study showed a significant reduction in soft-tissue perfusion when the equine digit was immersed in 4°C iced water for 30 minutes.[43] Based on hoof temperature (an indirect measure of digital perfusion),[44] digital vasoconstriction also predominates when distal limb cryotherapy is applied continuously for longer periods.[2–4] Intermittent periods of increased internal hoof temperature (up to 12°C) were noted in some horses during 72 hours of cold-water immersion.[2] These 2- to 4-hour periods of increased hoof temperature occurred 12 to 24 hours apart and often the left and right forelimbs were asynchronous. This phenomenon is similar to that noted in horses standing in natural environments that are below freezing (Chris Pollitt, BVSc, PhD, unpublished data, 2000). The increases in hoof temperature represent transient increases in perfusion, metabolism, or both,[44] and may correspond with periods of hoof growth, or clearance of metabolic waste products. The phenomenon is dissimilar to CIVD (the hunting reaction), which involves oscillations over minutes, rather than hours.[29] In the human digit it is thought to be a protective mechanism against cold-induced injury.[30] The hoof temperature fluctuations observed in the current study might be a variation of those seen in normal horses kept in climate-controlled environments.[45,46]

The equine distal limb seems to be resilient to the effects of extreme continuous hypothermia. There are no reports in the literature of complications directly related to the clinical application of distal limb cryotherapy in horses. In addition, horses show no signs of adverse effects in arctic climates where their distal limbs are continuously immersed in snow. Cold-induced pain, observed in human patients when cryotherapy is applied at 5°C or less,[23] has not been noted in horse studies. Perhaps the primary concern associated with profound digital cooling is the potential for damage to tendons and ligaments of the equine distal limb. Petrov and colleagues[47] examined the effects of hypothermia on equine superficial digital flexor tendon (SDFT) cells in vitro, and on the core tendon temperature in vivo. The mean core SDFT temperature after 60 minutes of cooling, using a commercial cooling and compression device (set at 3°C), was 10.4° ± 3.7°C, which was a mean decrease in temperature of 21.8°C over the starting point. No clinical detrimental effects were noted after the application of this protocol, and the viability of cultured tendon cells cooled to 10°C for 1 hour was not significantly different from that of cells incubated at 37°C.

USING DIGITAL HYPOTHERMIA TO HELP PREVENT LAMINITIS

Profound continuous digital hypothermia effectively ameliorates experimentally induced laminitis when applied throughout the developmental period.[2,3] Although the pathophysiology of acute laminitis remains unclear, inflammatory and enzymatic processes seem to contribute to lamellar separation.[48–56] Lamellar energy failure and ischemia-reperfusion injury are also likely to contribute to the pathogenesis of laminitis, regardless of whether they are primary or secondary events.[57–63] The profound hypometabolic and anti-inflammatory effects of hypothermia may protect lamellar tissue from these processes during the developmental phase. Cryotherapy significantly reduced the upregulation of matrix metalloproteinase-2 mRNA[3] and seems to reduce the expression of proinflammatory chemokines during the developmental phase of experimentally induced laminitis (James Belknap, DVM, PhD, unpublished data, 2009). Profound vasoconstriction may also prevent the hematogenous delivery of laminitis trigger factors.[64]

Suggested Protocol

Ideally, cryotherapy should be applied for the duration of the developmental phase. Horses with conditions associated with a high risk of laminitis development (colitis, metritis, pneumonia, alimentary carbohydrate overload)[65–69] should therefore be identified and treated preemptively whenever possible. Horses exhibiting clinical signs consistent with endotoxemia should be considered to be at a high risk of developing lamnitis.[65] Continuous application is likely to yield the best results, although the effect of intermittent cooling has not been studied. Resolution of the primary disease may be used as an indicator for timing the cessation of cryotherapy in individual cases. The author prefers to continue cryotherapy for 24 to 48 hours after the resolution of clinical and laboratory signs of systemic inflammation. Rewarming should be gradual if possible (over 12–24 hours), as rapid rewarming after therapeutic hypothermia may lead to the reinitiation of deleterious processes and loss of the protective effect.[8]

Experimental data showed a preventive effect with internal hoof temperatures around or less than 5°C, representing a decrease of 20°C or more below normal. Recent human medical-related studies suggest a superior effect when mild to moderate (10°C reduction) therapeutic hypothermia is used compared with traditional profound (>10°C reduction) hypothermia in various disease processes.[8] A critical temperature for laminitis prevention has not been established, although it is likely that even mild decreases in lamellar temperature have some beneficial effect. Accurate measurement of the actual lamellar tissue temperature is problematic. During the application of distal limb cryotherapy, hoof wall surface temperature tends to be approximately 2° to 3°C less than that measured by temperature probes buried deep within the hoof wall, adjacent to the lamellae (van Eps, unpublished data, 2008). Based on currently available data, clinical cryotherapy application should be aimed at achieving hoof wall surface temperatures that are consistently less than 10°C. This necessitates cooling the hoof directly as well as cooling the blood that enters the foot. Immersion of the limb from the upper metacarpus and metatarsus distally in an ice and water mixture effectively achieves this, although constant ice replenishment is labor intensive. Commercially available wader-style devices can be modified to include direct cooling of the hoof itself (**Fig. 1**A). Commercially available ice-pack and cold-gel applications generally do not reduce internal hoof temperature below 20°C even with regular replenishment/exchange (van Eps, unpublished data, 2008). A prototype device (see **Fig. 1**B), consisting of a membrane that recirculates refrigerated coolant, consistently reduces hoof wall surface temperature below 10°C

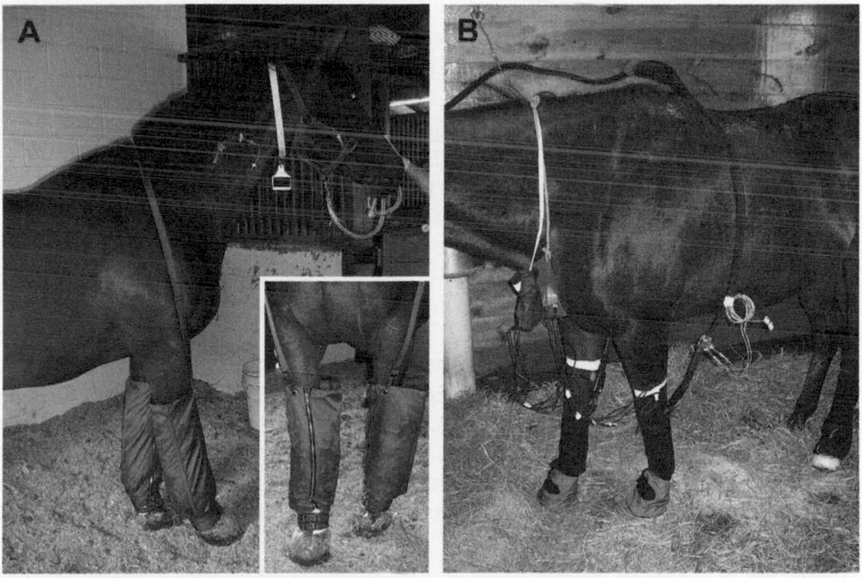

Fig. 1. Successful induction of lamellar hypothermia requires cooling of the hoof capsule as well as the limb distal to the carpus or tarsus (in order to cool blood flowing to the digit). (*A*) Modification of a commercially available wader style ice boot (Ice boot [Jack's Inc, Washington Court House, OH, USA]) to include the foot. This type of boot necessitates regular ice replenishment (every 1–2 hours, depending on ambient temperature) to achieve a consistently low temperature. (*Courtesy of* Jane Axon, BVSc, DACVIM, Scone, NSW, Australia). (*B*) A prototype membrane cooling device containing recirculating refrigerated coolant (Apex 5C [Game Ready Equine, Alameda, CA, USA]) applied to the forelimbs. This type of device may provide a convenient and controlled means of prolonged continuous cryotherapy application. (*Courtesy of* Jane Axon, BVSc, DACVIM, Scone, NSW, Australia.)

(van Eps, unpublished data, 2009). Such a device may provide a convenient and effective means of inducing effective continuous digital hypothermia in the future.

USING DIGITAL HYPOTHERMIA FOR THE TREATMENT OF ACUTE LAMINITIS

Although there are no published data regarding the efficacy of cryotherapy for the treatment of laminitis, it is rational to assume that the hypometabolic effect of hypothermia may be beneficial during the acute phase in reducing inflammation and enzymatic activity. In the author's experience cryotherapy also provides some analgesia in horses with acute laminitis. Cryotherapy should be avoided in cases where infection is suspected within the foot (subsolar abscess, septic osteitis, or seedy toe) because hypothermia reduces the natural inflammatory response to infection.[8] The author currently applies continuous distal limb cryotherapy to acute cases for up to 7 days after the first clinical signs of laminitis; however, it is unclear whether cryotherapy has any effect on the progression of laminitis, and research is required before any specific recommendations can be made.

REFERENCES

1. USDA. Lameness and laminitis in US horses. Fort Collins, Colorado, USA: USDA: APHIS:VS, CEAH, National Animal Health Monitoring System, 2000. Available at: http://www.aphis.usda.gov/vs/ceah/ncahs/nahms/equine/equine98/eq98LAME.pdf. Accessed January 5, 2010.
2. van Eps AW, Pollitt CC. Equine laminitis model: cryotherapy reduces the severity of lesions evaluated seven days after induction with oligofructose. Equine Vet J 2009;41:741–6.
3. van Eps AW, Pollitt CC. Equine laminitis: cryotherapy reduces the severity of the acute lesion. Equine Vet J 2004;36:255–60.
4. Pollitt CC, van Eps AW. Prolonged, continuous distal limb cryotherapy in the horse. Equine Vet J 2004;36:216–20.
5. Swenson C, Sward L, Karlsson J. Cryotherapy in sports medicine. Scand J Med Sci Sports 1996;6:193–200.
6. Douglas WW, Malcom JL. The effect of localized cooling on mammalian muscle spindles. J Physiol 1955;130:53–71.
7. Fuhrman GJ, Fuhrman FA. Oxygen consumption of animals and tissues as a function of temperature. J Gen Physiol 1959;42:715–22.
8. Polderman KH. Mechanisms of action, physiological effects, and complications of hypothermia. Crit Care Med 2009;37:S186–202.
9. Erecinska M, Thoresen M, Silver IA. Effects of hypothermia on energy metabolism in mammalian central nervous system. J Cereb Blood Flow Metab 2003;23:513–30.
10. Hagerdal M, Harp J, Nilsson L, et al. The effect of induced hypothermia upon oxygen consumption in the rat brain. J Neurochem 1975;24:311–6.
11. Palmer C, Vannucci RC, Christensen MA, et al. Regional cerebral blood flow and glucose utilization during hypothermia in newborn dogs. Anesthesiology 1989;71:730–7.
12. Knight KL. Metabolism and inflammation. In: Knight KL, editor. Cryotherapy in sports injury management. Champaign (IL): Human Kinetics; 1995. p. 77–84.
13. Griepp RB, Stinson EB, Shumway NE. Profound local hypothermia for myocardial protection during open-heart surgery. J Thorac Cardiovasc Surg 1973;66:731–41.

14. Zachariassen KE. Hypothermia and cellular physiology. Arctic Med Res 1991; 50(Suppl 6):13–7.
15. Harris ED Jr, McCroskery PA. The influence of temperature and fibril stability on degradation of cartilage collagen by rheumatoid synovial collagenase. N Engl J Med 1974;290:1–6.
16. Lim CM, Kim MS, Ahn JJ, et al. Hypothermia protects against endotoxin-induced acute lung injury in rats. Intensive Care Med 2003;29:453–9.
17. Westermann S, Vollmar B, Thorlacius H, et al. Surface cooling inhibits tumor necrosis factor-alpha-induced microvascular perfusion failure, leukocyte adhesion, and apoptosis in the striated muscle. Surgery 1999;126:881–9.
18. Webster CM, Kelly S, Koike MA, et al. Inflammation and NFkappaB activation is decreased by hypothermia following global cerebral ischemia. Neurobiol Dis 2009;33:301–12.
19. Scumpia PO, Sarcia PJ, Kelly KM, et al. Hypothermia induces anti-inflammatory cytokines and inhibits nitric oxide and myeloperoxidase-mediated damage in the hearts of endotoxemic rats. Chest 2004;125:1483–91.
20. Prandini MN, Neves Filho A, Lapa AJ, et al. Mild hypothermia reduces polymorphonuclear leukocytes infiltration in induced brain inflammation. Arq Neuropsiquiatr 2005;63:779–84.
21. Kamler M, Goedeke J, Pizanis N, et al. In vivo effects of hypothermia on the microcirculation during extracorporeal circulation. Eur J Cardiothorac Surg 2005;28:259–65.
22. Novack TA, Dillon MC, Jackson WT. Neurochemical mechanisms in brain injury and treatment: a review. J Clin Exp Neuropsychol 1996;18:685–706.
23. Ohkoshi Y, Ohkoshi M, Nagasaki S, et al. The effect of cryotherapy on intraarticular temperature and postoperative care after anterior cruciate ligament reconstruction. Am J Sports Med 1999;27:357–62.
24. Fujimoto K, Fujita M, Tsuruta R, et al. Early induction of moderate hypothermia suppresses systemic inflammatory cytokines and intracellular adhesion molecule-1 in rats with caerulein-induced pancreatitis and endotoxemia. Pancreas 2008;37:176–81.
25. Chin JY, Koh Y, Kim MJ, et al. The effects of hypothermia on endotoxin-primed lung. Anesth Analg 2007;104:1171–8 [tables of contents].
26. Lehmann JF, de Lateur BJ. Cryotherapy. In: Lehmann JF, editor. Therapeutic heat and cold. 4th edition. Baltimore (MD): Williams & Wilkins; 1990. p. 590–631.
27. Perkins JF, Li MC, Hoffman F, et al. Sudden vasoconstriction in denervated or sympathectomized paws exposed to cold. Am J Phys 1948;155:165–78.
28. Clarke RS, Hellon RF, Lind AR. Vascular reactions of the human forearm to cold. Clin Sci 1958;17:165–79.
29. Lewis T. Observations upon the reactions of the vessels of the human skin to cold. Heart 1930;15:177–208.
30. Daanen HA. Finger cold-induced vasodilation: a review. Eur J Appl Physiol 2003; 89:411–26.
31. Bergersen TK, Hisdal J, Walloe L. Perfusion of the human finger during cold-induced vasodilatation. Am J Phys 1999;276:R731–7.
32. Thorlacius H, Vollmar B, Westermann S, et al. Effects of local cooling on microvascular hemodynamics and leukocyte adhesion in the striated muscle of hamsters. J Trauma 1998;45:715–9.
33. Knight KL. Circulatory effects of therapeutic cold applications. In: Knight KL, editor. Cryotherapy in sport injury management. Champagne (IL): Human Kinetics; 1995. p. 107–26.

34. McGuire DA, Hendricks SD. Incidences of frostbite in arthroscopic knee surgery postoperative cryotherapy rehabilitation. Arthroscopy 2006;22:1141 e1–6.
35. Knight KL. Problems, precautions and contraindications in cold therapy. In: Knight KL, editor. Cryotherapy in sport injury management. Champagne (IL): Human Kinetics; 1995. p. 179–94.
36. DeGroot DW, Castellani JW, Williams JO, et al. Epidemiology of U.S. Army cold weather injuries, 1980–1999. Aviat Space Environ Med 2003;74:564–70.
37. Ungley CC, Channell GD, Richards RL. The immersion foot syndrome. 1946. Wilderness Environ Med 2003;14:135–41.
38. Ivers T. Cryotherapy: an in-depth study. Equine Pract 1987;9:17–9.
39. Blackwell RB. The use of cryotherapy in equine sports medicine. Equine Athlete 1991;4:1–5.
40. Ramey DW. Cold therapy in the horse. Equine Pract 1999;21:19–21.
41. Turner TA, Wolfsdorf K, Jourdenais J, et al. Effects of heat, cold, biomagnets, and ultrasound on skin circulation in the horse. In: Proceedings of the Thirty-Seventh Annual Convention of the American Association of Equine Practitioners. San Francisco (CA), 1991. p. 249–57.
42. Kaneps AJ. Tissue temperature response to hot and cold therapy in the metacarpal region of a horse. In: Proceedings of the Forty-sixth Annual Convention of the American Association of Equine Practitioners. San Antonio (TX), 2000. p. 208–13.
43. Worster AA, Gaughan EM, Hoskinson JJ, et al. Effects of external thermal manipulation on laminar temperature and perfusion scintigraphy of the equine digit. N Z Vet J 2000;48:111–6.
44. Hood DM, Wagner IP, Bru mbaugh GW. Evaluation of hoof wall surface temperature as an index of digital vascular perfusion during the prodromal and acute phases of carbohydrate-induced laminitis in horses. Am J Vet Res 2001;62: 1167–72.
45. Pollitt CC, Davies CT. Equine laminitis: its development coincides with increased sublamellar blood flow. Equine Vet J Suppl 1998;26:125–32.
46. Mogg KC, Pollitt CC. Hoof and distal limb surface temperature in the normal pony under constant and changing ambient temperatures. Equine Vet J 1992;24: 134–9.
47. Petrov R, MacDonald MH, Tesch AM, et al. Influence of topically applied cold treatment on core temperature and cell viability in equine superficial digital flexor tendons. Am J Vet Res 2003;64:835–44.
48. Belknap JK, Giguere S, Pettigrew A, et al. Lamellar pro-inflammatory cytokine expression patterns in laminitis at the developmental stage and at the onset of lameness: innate vs. adaptive immune response. Equine Vet J 2007;39:42–7.
49. Blikslager AT, Yin C, Cochran AM, et al. Cyclooxygenase expression in the early stages of equine laminitis: a cytologic study. J Vet Intern Med 2006;20:1191–6.
50. Fontaine GL, Belknap JK, Allen D, et al. Expression of interleukin-1beta in the digital laminae of horses in the prodromal stage of experimentally induced laminitis. Am J Vet Res 2001;62:714–20.
51. Johnson PJ, Tyagi SC, Katwa LC, et al. Activation of extracellular matrix metalloproteinases in equine laminitis. Vet Rec 1998;142:392–6.
52. Kyaw Tanner M, Pollitt CC. Equine laminitis: increased transcription of matrix metalloproteinase-2 (MMP-2) occurs during the developmental phase. Equine Vet J 2004;36:221–5.
53. Mungall BA, Pollitt CC. Zymographic analysis of equine laminitis. Histochemistry 1999;112:467–72.

54. Mungall BA, Pollitt CC, Collins R. Localisation of gelatinase activity in epidermal hoof lamellae by in situ zymography. Histochemistry 1998;110:535–40.
55. Waguespack RW, Cochran A, Belknap JK. Expression of the cyclooxygenase isoforms in the prodromal stage of black walnut-induced laminitis in horses. Am J Vet Res 2004;65:1724–9.
56. Waguespack RW, Kemppainen RJ, Cochran A, et al. Increased expression of MAIL, a cytokine-associated nuclear protein, in the prodromal stage of black walnut-induced laminitis. Equine Vet J 2004;36:285–91.
57. Bailey SR, Marr CM, Elliott J. Current research and theories on the pathogenesis of acute laminitis in the horse. Vet J 2004;167:129–42.
58. Hood DM, Grosenbaugh DA, Mostafa MB, et al. The role of vascular mechanisms in the development of acute equine laminitis. J Vet Intern Med 1993;7:228–34.
59. Moore RM, Eades SC, Stokes AM. Evidence for vascular and enzymatic events in the pathophysiology of acute laminitis: which pathway is responsible for initiation of this process in horses? Equine Vet J 2004;36:204–9.
60. Noschka E, Moore JN, Peroni JF, et al. Thromboxane and isoprostanes as inflammatory and vasoactive mediators in black walnut heartwood extract induced equine laminitis. Vet Immunol Immunopathol 2009;129:200–10.
61. Peroni JF, Harrison WE, Moore JN, et al. Black walnut extract-induced laminitis in horses is associated with heterogeneous dysfunction of the laminar microvasculature. Equine Vet J 2005;37:546–51.
62. Peroni JF, Moore JN, Noschka E, et al. Predisposition for venoconstriction in the equine laminar dermis: implications in equine laminitis. J Appl Phys 2006;100: 759–63.
63. Robertson TP, Moore JN, Noschka E, et al. Evaluation of activation of protein kinase C during agonist-induced constriction of veins isolated from the laminar dermis of horses. Am J Vet Res 2007;68:664–9.
64. Pollitt CC. Equine laminitis: a revised pathophysiology. In: Proceedings of the 45th Annual Convention of the American Association of Equine Practitioners. Albuquerque (NM), 1999. p. 188–92.
65. Parsons CS, Orsini JA, Krafty R, et al. Risk factors for development of acute laminitis in horses during hospitalization: 73 cases (1997–2004). J Am Vet Med Assoc 2007;230:885–9.
66. Cohen ND, Parson EM, Seahorn TL, et al. Prevalence and factors associated with development of laminitis in horses with duodenitis/proximal jejunitis: 33 cases (1985–1991). J Am Vet Med Assoc 1994;204:250–4.
67. Cohen ND, Woods AM. Characteristics and risk factors for failure of horses with acute diarrhea to survive: 122 cases (1990–1996). J Am Vet Med Assoc 1999; 214:382–90.
68. Slater MR, Hood DM, Carter GK. Descriptive epidemiological study of equine laminitis. Equine Vet J 1995;27:364–7.
69. Alford P, Geller S, Richrdson B, et al. A multicenter, matched case-control study of risk factors for equine laminitis. Prev Vet Med 2001;49:209–22.

Progression of Venographic Changes After Experimentally Induced Laminitis

Gregory I. Baldwin, BSc, BVSc[a,b,*], Christopher C. Pollitt, BVSc, PhD[c,d]

KEYWORDS

• Laminitis • Venogram • Venography • Equine • Horse

Venography (retrograde venous angiography) is a relatively simple and practical method for vascular assessment of the digits in the standing horse. The technique is a useful adjunct to routine radiography. Routine radiography allows for the quantification of distal phalanx displacement and lysis; however, on its own it provides little direct information about the digital vasculature.

In validation studies of retrograde venous therapy for the equine digit (Pollitt, personal communication, 1992), application of a tourniquet to the fetlock and infusion of a contrast medium via the lateral palmar digital vein led to the discovery of the comprehensive nature of digital venous filling. This technique was shared with Redden,[1,2] who developed the technique further and used it extensively in clinical practice. The technique has also been described by Rucker[3,4] (see the article by Amy Rucker elsewhere in this issue for further exploration of this topic).

The clinical use of the laminitis venogram has resulted in a more comprehensive understanding of the collateral pathology associated with distal phalanx displacement and abnormal hoof growth. The technique allows assessment of vascular and dermal integrity after therapeutic procedures have been used. These types of procedures vary

---

This work has been supported by grants from Rural Industries Research Development Corporation (RIRDC) and Animal Health Foundation, Missouri, USA.
[a] Australian Equine Laminitis Research Unit, School of Veterinary Science, The University of Queensland, Slip Road, St Lucia, Queensland 4217, Australia
[b] Harness Racing Queensland, Albion Park Raceway, Yulestar Street, Albion, Queensland 4010, Australia
[c] School of Veterinary Science, The University of Queensland, St Lucia, Brisbane, Queensland 4072, Australia
[d] The Laminitis Institute, University of Pennsylvania School of Veterinary Medicine, New Bolton Center, Kennett Square, PA, USA
* Corresponding author. Harness Racing Queensland, Albion Park Raceway, Yulestar Street, Albion, Queensland 4010, Australia.
E-mail address: gbaldwin@qld.harness.org.au

Vet Clin Equine 26 (2010) 135–140
doi:10.1016/j.cveq.2009.12.005 **vetequine.theclinics.com**
0749-0739/10/$ – see front matter

from remedial and weight redistribution shoeing to coronary grooving, hoof wall resections, and deep digital flexor tendon tenotomy. Performing venograms before and after these procedures not only gives an insight into the effectiveness of such procedures but also improves the clinician's and owner's understanding of the pathology affecting the case.

The use of venograms has been focused on the clinical evaluation of chronic laminitis cases. The aim of this article is to describe the venographic appearance during the transition from the clinically normal hoof to the severe chronic laminitis affected hoof in cases similar to those seen in practice.

Laminitis was induced with oligofructose (OF) as described by van Eps and Pollitt[5] and clinical trials were performed as outlined by Baldwin.[6] Only lateral to medial venograms have been considered in this article.

VENOGRAPHIC TECHNIQUE

The venographic technique was modified from that used by Redden.[2] A 23-gauge, 25-mm catheter was used in place of a butterfly needle. At least 24 hours before induction, standard-bred horses underwent venography of both the fore feet. The unshod and clinically normal horses were sedated with 40 μg/kg body weight intravenous romifidine hydrochloride (Sedivet, Boehringer Ingleheim). Permanent radio-opaque reference markers (ball bearings) were placed in the dorsal hoof wall at approximately 20 mm, 40 mm, and 60 mm distal to the coronary band with the edge of the ball bearing flush with the surface of the dorsal hoof wall. A small cylindrical opaque marker was glued to the hoof wall with its proximal end adjacent to the hairline of the coronary band. A medial and lateral abaxial sesamoid nerve block was placed using 40 mg mepivacaine hydrochloride (Mepivacaine Injection, Nature Vet). An area over the lateral digital vein on the upper pastern region was clipped and prepared for surgery. An Esmarch bandage (tourniquet) was placed around the cannon just below the knee and wrapped distally to occlude the digital artery and vein over the abaxial surface of the proximal sesamoid bones. A small incision with a number-15 scalpel blade was made in the skin over the lateral digital vein at the level of proximal pastern, ready for catheter insertion. With the limb weight bearing, the catheter was inserted in the distended vein proximal to the tortuous portion of the vein. A latex plugged extension set (15 cm) was attached once the catheter was in place. A 19-gauge hypodermic needle was inserted into the catheter plug and venous blood was allowed to flow. This evacuated air from the extension tubing. Adhesive tape was placed around the pastern to hold the catheter in place. Iodine-based contrast medium, 7500 to 9000 mg iohexol (Iopamiro 300, Schering), was infused with the limb non–weight bearing. Contrast medium was infused until either the full volume was used (30 mL) or perivenous leakage occurred due to excessive back pressure. The limb was then placed on a custom-made jig for weight bearing in lateral to medial and upright pedal views. Radiographs were acquired within 60 seconds of contrast infusion. Radiographs were obtained on mammography film using a standard 100-kV portable radiography unit. The tourniquet was removed and the catheter entry point wrapped with a sterile pressure dressing.

VENOGRAPHY OF CONTROL (NORMAL) FEET BEFORE OF DOSING

The normal vascular appearance of a lateral to medial venogram (**Fig. 1**) is the result of venous infusion of contrast medium, originating in the palmar digital vein (lateral or medial), moving retrograde through valveless veins to the capillary bed and

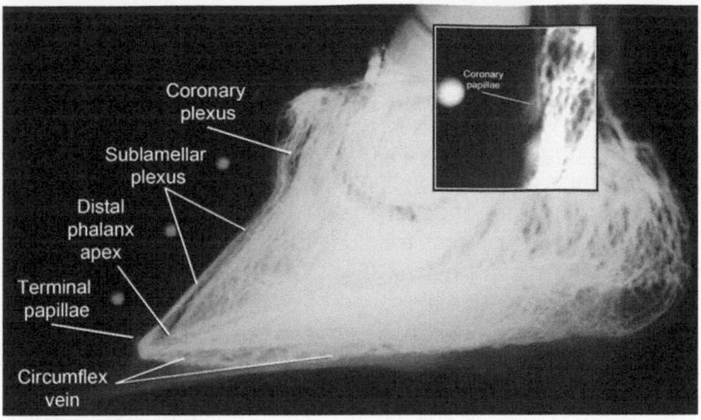

Fig. 1. Normal venogram (lateral medial projection). Radiopaque ball bearings, embedded in the midline, are flush with the surface of the dorsal hoof wall. Vessels of the coronary papillae (*inset*) are parallel to the dorsal hoof wall The distal phalanx apex is proximal to the terminal papillae and the junction of the sublamellar plexus and circumflex vein.

arteriovenous anastomoses and then into the arterial circulation. Because of the extensive number of terminal anastomoses, amongst all divisions of the circulation of the equine foot, the resultant image details the entire vascular bed distal to the area of occlusion. The foot circulation is fully vasodilated due to the nerve blocks, and the tourniquet eliminates the influence of blood pressure and cardiac output. During the procedure the foot is an independent circulatory unit. In reality the result is an angiogram rather than a venogram.

The most important areas in terms of laminitis venography are the coronary plexus, the coronary papillae, the sublamellar venous plexus, the terminal papillae, the circumflex vessels, and the soleal venous plexus (see **Fig. 1**).

The anatomic relationships of these vascular structures are altered, as laminitis drives distal phalanx displacement. The pathology associated with distal phalanx dislocation alters the pattern of the venogram.

In the normal venogram the large, dense vessels of the coronary plexus, above and below the hairline, are filled with contrast medium. The veins in the dermis of the proximal hoof wall coronary groove, adjacent to the extensor process of the distal phalanx, are similarly filled with medium and are conjoined with the sublamellar venous plexus. Arising from the coronary plexus are the vessels of the coronary papillae (inset **Fig. 1**), a row of fine vessels, tapering parallel to the dorsal hoof wall.

The sublamellar venous plexus is a column of medium thickness approximately 3 mm thick throughout its length. The distal end of the sublamellar plexus conjoins with the circumflex vessels at an angle similar to the angle formed by the dorsal and palmar cortices of the apex of the distal phalanx (approximately 50°). The circumflex vessels are distal to the apex of the distal phalanx. The vessels of the terminal papillae extend distally from the palmar surface of the circumflex vessels. The soleal venous plexus covers the palmar surface of the hoof.

VENOGRAPHY 48 HOURS AFTER OF DOSING

Horses showed clinical evidence of laminitic pain (Obel grade 2 and above) 48 hours after OF dosing and were in the acute phase of laminitis. Venograms of each horse, made before and after 48 hours of OF dosing, were compared. No venographic changes, attributable to acute laminitis, were discerned.

VENOGRAPHY 7 DAYS AFTER OF DOSING

Clear venographic changes were present when the OF-dosed horses were in the chronic phase of laminitis (ie, distal phalanx displacement had occurred). The degree of change related to the extent of distal phalanx displacement.

Of note, there was less contrast medium in the coronary plexus dorsal to the extensor process of the distal phalanx (**Fig. 2**). The sublamellar plexus was wider and had developed a blurred, dorsal margin of varying dimensions. The width of the blurred margin increased as the distance between the dorsal hoof wall and the dorsal margin of the distal phalanx increased. The sublamellar/circumflex junction was distorted and was positioned proximal to the distal phalanx apex. There was a bulge in the circumflex and soleal vessels distal to the apex of distal phalanx. The heel vasculature was relatively unchanged.

Downward displacement of the distal phalanx changes the venographic appearance of the coronary papillae. Instead of the straight, parallel arrangement seen in control horses, papillae 7 days after OF dosing were kinked (inset in **Fig. 2**).

VENOGRAPHY 6 WEEKS AFTER OF DOSING

Venograms acquired 6 weeks after OF dosing (classified as severe chronic) showed more severe contrast medium filling deficits, especially at the coronary plexus that was void of contrast (**Fig. 3**). Vessels of the sublamellar plexus were widened, distorted, and more blurred than at 7 days post dosing. The distal phalanx apex was displaced more distally and well below the distorted terminal papillae and circumflex vessels.

DISCUSSION

Chronic laminitis is associated with progressive changes to the normal anatomy of the foot, and the degree of change correlates with the severity of the disease. Greater

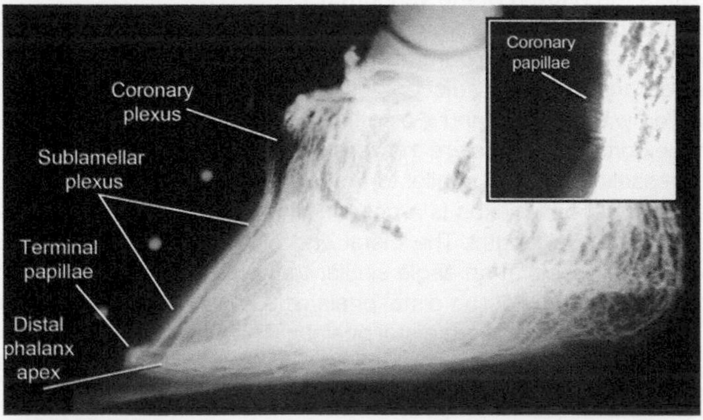

Fig. 2. Venogram taken 7 days after OF dosing to induce laminitis. There is a filling deficit in the coronary plexus, and the coronary papillae (*inset*) are kinked and no longer parallel to the dorsal hoof wall. The sublamellar plexus is wider and has a diffuse dorsal border. The margin of the distal phalanx is below the sublamellar/circumflex junction and the terminal papillae.

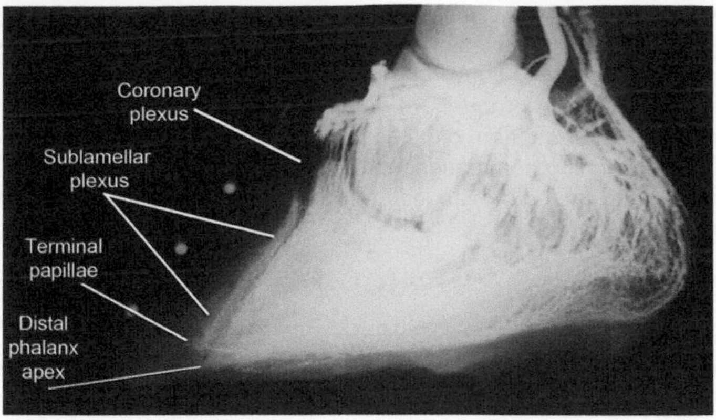

Fig. 3. Venogram taken 6 weeks after oligofructose dosing. There is no filling of the coronary plexus and the sublamellar plexus has broadened with a diffuse dorsal zone. The margin of the distal phalanx has sunk further below the sublamellar/circumflex junction and terminal papillae.

venous filling deficits and anatomic dislocation occurred in cases with the greatest downward displacement of the distal phalanx. Displacement of the distal phalanx correlated with the severity of clinical foot pain.[6]

The earliest detectable venographic changes were associated with subtle distal phalanx displacement. By definition, this occurred after the transition from the acute to the chronic phase when displacement, relative to the dorsal hoof wall, was first measurable. At the onset of the chronic phase, slight widening of the sublamellar plexus was present (7 days after OF dosing) probably resulting from distortion of the epidermal and dermal lamellar interface.

The characteristic blurred dorsal edge of the sublamellar plexus has been interpreted as contrast leakage across traumatized vessels at the time of infusion.[4] However, histopathology of chronic laminitis 7 days after OF dosing shows considerable lamellar lengthening and rearrangement of dermal anatomy, but no evidence of vascular leakage.[7] Perhaps the diffuse appearance of the contrast dorsal to the main sublamellar plexus represents contrast medium in smaller than normal, compressed vessels in a sublamellar plexus now attenuated by ongoing distal phalanx dislocation.

With greater severity of distal phalanx displacement vascular filling deficits and soft tissue distortion become more evident. A filling deficit of the coronary plexus was observed 7 days after OF dosing. The deficit enlarged with the passage of time and was virtually complete 6 weeks after dosing. Compression of the coronary dermis by deranged, inward-growing proximal hoof wall, sufficient to occlude veins, but not arteries (Pollitt, unpublished data, 2003), is the likely cause of this filling failure (see the article by Collins and colleagues elsewhere in this issue for further exploration of this topic). The progressive development of The Lamellar wedge, especially distally, seems to compress veins against the dorsal surface of the distal phalanx, resulting in reduced sublamellar plexus filling with contrast agent.

The change in orientation and kinking of the coronary papillae, associated with the downward displacement of the distal phalanx, is reflected in the abnormal dorsal, tubular hoof wall growth evident as rings in the hooves of the horses 6 weeks after OF dosing.

As displacement of the distal phalanx progressed, the apex of the bone obliterated the solar plexus, and sank below and presumably penetrated the plexus completely.

With increasing chronicity, the apex of the distal phalanx was located more distally than the junction between the sublamellar plexus and circumflex vessels (and the terminal papillae).

The results illustrate the progressive nature of severe, chronic laminitis. After the initial, single-incident induction of laminitis, the perturbations in epidermal hoof anatomy had far-reaching consequences on the adjacent dermal structures. Venography informs that pathologic changes are occurring and provides opportunities for strategic therapeutic intervention.

SUMMARY

Serial venography supplies more information about the progression of chronic laminitis than plain radiographs alone. The changes in the patterns of contrast agent filling inform on the pathologic anatomy associated with chronic laminitis development and provide valuable prognostic information. Therapeutic intervention is important if the chronic laminitic foot is to be rehabilitated. The effectiveness of therapeutic procedures such as hoof wall resection, coronary band grooving, deep digital flexor tenotomy, and therapeutic shoeing can be assessed by serial venography. If vascular filling deficits disappear then presumably the pathology associated with chronic tissue compression is also reversed. Coronary band peeling or resection restores contrast filling of the coronary plexus and encourages normal dorsal hoof wall growth (see the article by Amy Rucker elsewhere in this issue for further exploration of this topic).

Likewise, the incipient inward growth of the lamellar wedge and the resultant compression of the dermal tissues adjoining the distal phalanx, proximal to its apex, may contribute to bone lysis and pain (see the articles in this issue by Engiles and Driessen). The effectiveness of strategic hoof wall and lamellar wedge removal to prevent and treat this pathology can be monitored by venography.

ACKNOWLEDGMENTS

Thank you to Mark McGarry, Andrew Van Eps and Lester Walters for their valued contributions.

REFERENCES

1. Redden RR. The use of venograms as a diagnostic tool. Proceedings of the 7th Bluegrass Laminitis Symposium. Versailles (KY), 1993.
2. Redden RR. A technique for performing digital venography in the standing horse. Equine Vet Educ 2001;13:128–34.
3. Rucker A. The digital venogram. Equine podiatry. Philadelphia (PA): WB Saunders; 2007.
4. Rucker A. How to perform a digital venogram. 52nd Annual Convention, American Association of Equine Practitioners, 2006. p. 526–30.
5. van Eps AW, Pollitt CC. Equine laminitis induced with oligofructose. Equine Vet J 2006;38:203–8.
6. Baldwin GI. Retrograde venous angiography (venography) of the equine digit during experimentally induced acute and chronic laminitis. 47th Annual Congress, British Equine Veterinarian Association, 2008. p. 252–3.
7. Van Eps AW, Pollitt CC. Equine laminitis model: lamellar histopathology 7 days after induction with oligofructose. Equine Vet J 2009;41:735–40. DOI:10.2746/042516409X042434116.

Clinical Presentation, Diagnosis, and Prognosis of Chronic Laminitis in North America

Robert J. Hunt, DVM, MS[a,*], Robin E. Wharton, DVM[a,b]

KEYWORDS

• Chronic laminitis • EMS • Distal phalanx • Hoof wall

Chronic laminitis has long been recognized as one of the most significant clinical syndromes of horses throughout history. Thousands of horses worldwide are afflicted with the disease. In the United States, laminitis affects approximately 13% of horse operations and 2% of all horses annually.[1] The precise number of horses that progress from acute to chronic laminitis is not known, but suffice it to say that it is extremely common, and there are few equine operations and horse owners who are not eventually affected by the disease. Most horses are able to recover or compensate for the condition and remain comfortable and productive animals.

CLINICAL PRESENTATION

Laminitis has been categorized into developmental, acute, subacute, and chronic stages.[2–4] The developmental phase of laminitis is a period that follows and often overlaps a systemic or local insult. Experimental models suggest that this period is between 24 and 60 hours but in all likelihood there is a wider variation than this in the clinical setting. Acute laminitis generally lasts 24 to 72 hours before resolving or advancing. Cases that advance may become either subacute or chronic, and these 2 categories have different clinical presentations.[5,6] Subacute laminitis does not involve digital collapse. Chronic laminitis involves laminar morphologic changes resulting in digital collapse. The chronic condition can vary greatly in its clinical manifestation. Some chronic cases exhibit minimal lameness, requiring only minor routine hoof maintenance, whereas other cases exhibit unrelenting continuous pain ultimately necessitating humane destruction. This chronic categorization may be oversimplified, because there are few similarities between the horse residing at one end of the chronic spectrum, requiring only routine trimming to maintain a normal hoof capsule, and the

[a] Hagyard Equine Medical Institute, 4250 Iron Works Pike, Lexington, KY 40511-8412, USA
[b] PO Box 13304, Lexington, KY 40583-3304, USA
* Corresponding author.
E-mail address: rhunt@hagyard.com

Vet Clin Equine 26 (2010) 141–153
doi:10.1016/j.cveq.2009.12.006 vetequine.theclinics.com

horse residing at the other end of the spectrum, that is, the one that has sloughed a hoof capsule. Most chronic laminitis cases reside between these 2 extremes; with accurate recognition and implementation of an appropriate maintenance program many chronically laminitic horses may remain useful.

A thorough understanding of the clinical complex of chronic laminitis can be difficult to grasp because of the multitude of variables that affect the clinical presentation of the patient. These variables include the stage of the disease, the severity of morphologic damage of the foot, the number of feet involved, and the presence of other problems. In an attempt to address these variations, several subcategories of chronic laminitis have been described. These subcategories are defined by the relative duration of the disease, amount of laminar damage (ie, the loss of laminar integrity), the presence of sepsis, and the degree of instability of the distal phalanx/hoof wall interface, which is directly affected by the integrity of the distal phalanx, laminae, and hoof wall. Many relative descriptive terms, such as early and late, compensated and uncompensated, stable and unstable, and high, medium, and low scale, are used. The Obel[7] grading scale for the degree of lameness is also used. All these modifiers are used in an effort to describe the clinical picture of the horse according to the duration, severity of lameness, and stability of the distal phalanx/hoof wall interface.

Other classifications are based on the causes. These include road founder; grain (carbohydrate) overload; corticosteroid induction; contralateral limb laminitis; fat horse syndrome or equine metabolic syndrome (EMS); and sepsis associated with the urogenital tract (eg, retained placenta or septic metritis), respiratory system, and gastrointestinal tract (eg, proximal enteritis or colitis). It is important to ascertain the cause as there are different clinical scenarios and patterns associated with each disorder, although the end result is often a similar laminar deterioration.

A retrospective, unpublished study of laminitis cases necropsied in central Kentucky over a 10-year period yielded 8 major etiologic classifications for laminitis (University of Kentucky Livestock Disease Diagnostic Center, Wharton, Hunt, and Carter, unpublished data, 2008). This review also provided insight into the most common clinical presentations of laminitic horses. Approximately 70% of patients were female thoroughbred horses, aged 5 years or older. Most horses (87%) were euthanatized, whereas 13% died. Half of the necropsies (52%) listed laminitis as the cause of death, and 33% were due to laminitis combined with other problems (**Table 1**). Of the 585 cases reviewed (**Table 2**), the cause of laminitis was known in 332 cases or 57%. Gastrointestinal disease was most commonly associated with the development of laminitis, with only 5% of laminitis cases following colic surgeries. Musculoskeletal system problems resulted in 28% of the laminitis cases, whereas reproductive system compromise was responsible for 17%. Pituitary disease comprised 11%.

Further categorical descriptive terms are based on radiographic findings, which are enumerated and discussed in the section addressing diagnosis. These multiple categorical schemes and the complexity of the disease lead to confusion in describing a horse with chronic laminitis and understanding the pathophysiology underlying the disease process. Common salient clinical findings that should ameliorate some of this difficulty are described.

The period of initial onset of chronic laminitis is clinically important. Several dynamic changes occur during this stage, including laminar detachment and shearing, as well as displacement of the distal phalanx because of the imposed load of the horse on a compromised suspensory laminar interface.[8] Histopathologic changes within the digit during this stage are well described.[5,6] These changes result in the clinical presentation of a horse with the continuation of an acute laminitic stance of varying

Table 1
Cause of death in cases reviewed (87% euthanized)

Cause	Number	Percent (%)
Laminitis alone	304/585	52
Multiple problems with laminitis	194/585	33
Systemic problems (eg, uterine artery rupture)	28/585	5
Gastrointestinal problems	18/585	3
Musculoskeletal problems	15/585	2.5
Multiple problems without laminitis	6/585	1
Respiratory problems	4/585	1
Unknown	16/585	2.5

severity. Initially, the coronary band may be slightly thickened and edematous. Over several days to weeks, with progressive soft tissue shearing and displacement of the distal phalanx, a depression or cleft develops, which is frequently referred to as a ridge (**Fig. 1**).

During this transition from the acute to the chronic stage, pain often becomes less severe. This relative decrease in pain can be associated with loss of sensation, medication adjustments, or the horse acclimating to pain. Although it is possible that this increased comfort level is due to clinical improvement, it is a mistake to allow elevated levels of exercise or decrease supportive treatments prematurely. Another common misinterpretation made during this portion of disease progression is the failure to recognize worsening in one foot by mistaking it as an improvement in the other or to interpret a horse to have relative improvement in a primary limb lameness when it is actually developing contralateral, supporting limb laminitis. The clinician must use vigilance and thoroughness when evaluating the horse during this phase of laminitis. Attention to the precarious balance of the patient should prompt one to take extreme caution when altering medication or exercise or performing corrective procedures on the feet during this time frame.

The opposite extreme of this early chronic laminitic stage is the late- or end-stage horse, which has experienced multiple episodes of chronic pain and abscessation. There are typically periods of relative manageable comfort between a progression from digital sepsis to necrosis and deterioration of the foot. The late- or end-stage horses often prefer to lie down more frequently than the acute and early chronically

Table 2
Cause of laminitis, known in 332 of 585 cases (57%)

Cause	Number	Percent (%)
Gastrointestinal system	110/332	33
- Postcolic signs	16/332	5
Musculoskeletal system	94/332	28
Reproductive system	58/332	17
Pituitary disease	37/332	11
Respiratory system	12/332	4
Endotoxemia	12/332	4
Multiple systems	4/332	1
Drug or toxin induced	4/332	1

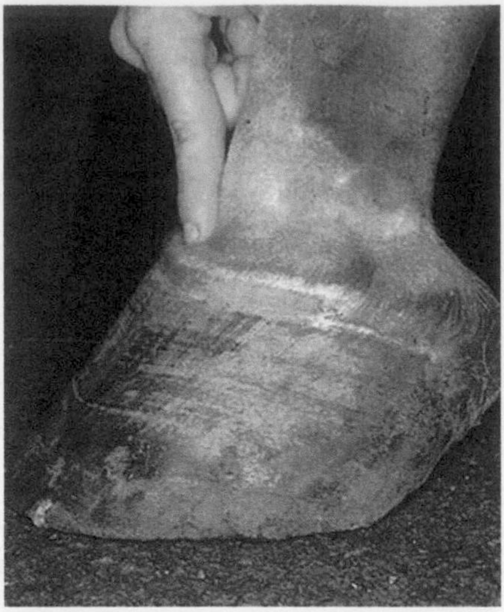

Fig. 1. Horse's foot with sinker syndrome. There is a palpable coronary band depression.

laminitic horses. Eventually minimal functional hoof remains, and sequelae develop, including limb contraction, decubital sores, and loss of body condition. These secondary problems exacerbate the difficulty of patient management and may exponentially expand the clinical manifestations of the primary disease process.

Most horses with chronic laminitis clinically lie between these early and late extremes and are typically in a compensated state regarding their overall clinical status. There may be marked gross and histologic changes as well as dramatic radiographic changes within the foot, but there is relatively little physical discomfort depending on the intended use of the horse. The horse may exist with little to no apparent lameness and only appear foot sore, especially on firm surfaces. These symptoms are generally more evident if the horse is unshod. These horses may characteristically respond to hoof tester compression over the solar region of the dorsal portion of the foot, or of the entire foot, although many horses do not display a response to hoof testers. The foot may range from normal in appearance to having a dropped, flat sole with wall separation and diverging concentric rings or having an excessively overgrown foot with a grossly thickened sole (**Fig. 2**).

The dorsal wall is frequently dished if not trimmed appropriately and the foot develops a wide and often irregular white line (**Fig. 3**).

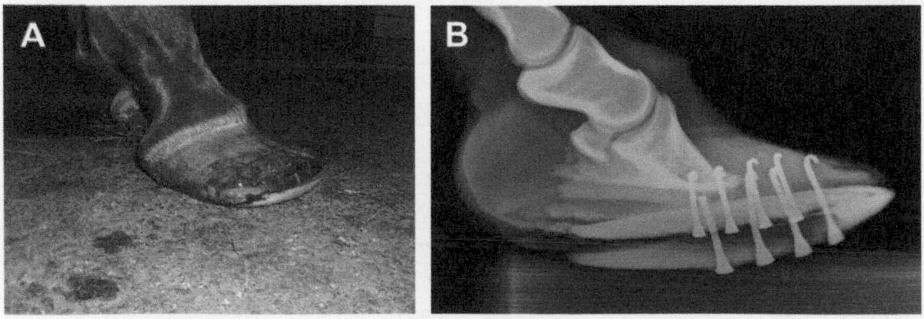

Fig. 2. (*A*) Foot with chronic laminitis demonstrating diverging concentric rings and an overgrown toe. (*B*) Radiograph of the same foot in **Fig. 2**A.

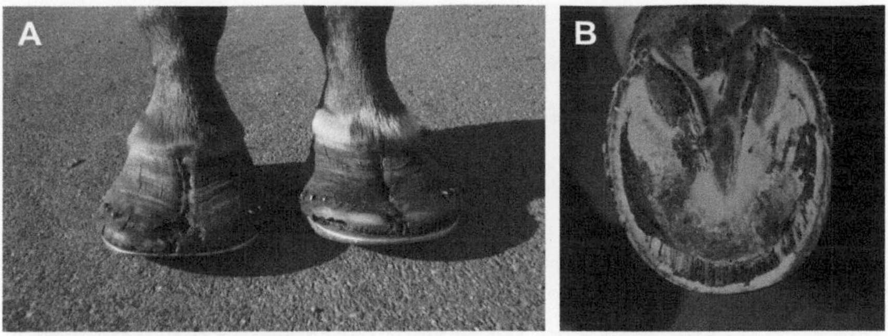

Fig. 3. (*A*) Front feet with dished dorsal walls and dorsal vertical hoof cracks associated with chronic laminitis. (*B*) Sole of a chronic laminitic foot with an irregular, thickened white line.

There may also be variations of ridging and depression at the coronary band. Eventual gross thickening of the coronary band may occur once an advanced chronic state is reached. Some gross morphologic changes observed with chronic laminitis are also observed in normal horses as they age. These changes include dropping of the sole, dorsal wall separation, and depression of the coronary band.

Horses with chronic laminitis may be more prone to recurrent episodes of laminitis resulting in progressive deterioration of the foot. They are also prone to future episodes of lameness associated with foot soreness because of abnormal laminar architecture and inferior integrity. These horses are at risk of bruising, caused by dropped soles. Digital sepsis and/or abscessation is a common sequela to foot bruising or internal injury of soft tissue and is often mistaken for recurrence of laminitis. This sequence is, in many cases, the ultimate progression of the disease and results in destruction of the chronically laminitic horse.

Differentiation of the cause of laminitis is important because different forms of laminitis appear to manifest themselves in a unique and often predictable clinical scenario. For example, laminitis as a result of retained placenta or septic metritis typically follows a course of extreme pain (Obel grade 3 or 4) for 3 to 5 days, followed by a moderate improvement. The horse then appears clinically stable (Obel grade 2) for the following 4 to 8 weeks. After this period there is commonly a recrudescence of pain accompanied by further displacement of the distal phalanx.

A horse with laminitis associated with administration of corticosteroids usually presents with a different clinical picture. These horses often undergo no displacement of the distal phalanx; however, they may remain persistently foot sore and athletically unsound. When steroid induced laminitis does result in displacement of the distal phalanx, it is generally severe and may result in sloughing of the hoof capsule in a matter of days to weeks (**Fig. 4**).

A similar clinical presentation is often associated with horses suffering from severe diarrhea or proximal enteritis, in which the severity of clinical laminitis and displacement of the distal phalanx appear to have a direct correlation. Severely toxic horses may undergo displacement of the distal phalanx to the point of detachment of the hoof capsule very rapidly. In contrast, horses with unilateral laminitis as a result of physical overload generally progress very slowly up to a certain point, with extreme displacement and instability then occurring over a relatively short period of days. Horses afflicted with metabolic syndrome may display moderate to severe pain and generally undergo displacement of the distal phalanx in a slow and insidious manner, sometimes taking months to show displacement and deterioration of the distal

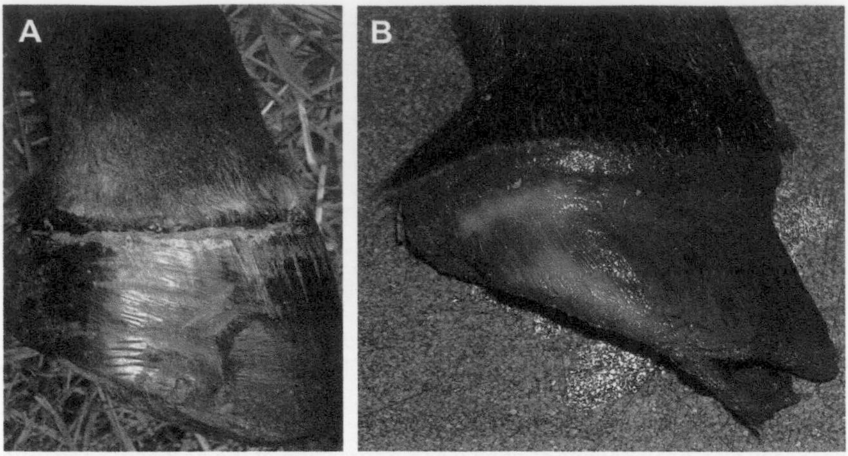

Fig. 4. Laminitic foot undergoing digital separation at the coronary band (*A*). Later the hoof capsule sloughed off exposing the entire corium of the foot (*B*).

phalanx. It is unknown if these differing clinical manifestations have dissimilar pathophysiologic events involved in the developmental stages preceding clinical laminitis. In general, the more rapidly progressive the disease, the poorer the prognosis.

EMS, also referred to as fat horse syndrome, is the result of a metabolic disturbance characterized by hyperinsulinemia and insulin resistance but is distinguishable from hypothyroidism and pars intermedia pituitary dysfunction. This syndrome is recognized in mature horses and all breeds but there seems to be an increase in incidence in Morgan, Paso Fino, Arabians, and pony breeds.[9,10] Most horses with EMS are recognized as "easy keepers" and tend to flourish on minimal rations. These horses may be generally obese or they may display localized adiposity with excessive fat deposition in the crest of the neck, in the abdomen, and around the tailhead, giving a squared appearance to the rump (**Fig. 5**). Other salient clinical features include

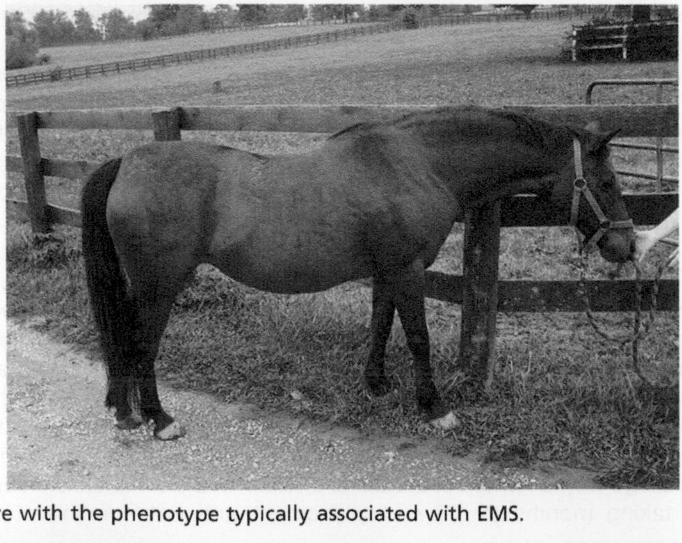

Fig. 5. Mare with the phenotype typically associated with EMS.

hyperinsulinemia and insulin resistance, as previously mentioned, as well as hypertriglyceridemia, hyperleptinemia, and hypertension.[9–13]

Horses with EMS have an affinity for the development of laminitis. This predisposition is believed to be associated with insulin resistance, which might contribute to laminitis development in 2 ways. First, the resultant elevated blood glucose levels adversely affect endothelial cells and lead to disturbances in microvascular circulation due to vasospasticity and dysregulated vascular perfusion.[10] Second, insulin resistance may impair glucose delivery to hoof keratinocytes,[14,15] therefore functionally affecting the formation of the hoof capsule.

Horses with EMS laminitis display a range of laminitic severity; however, most cases are chronic in nature. Radiographic findings are variable and do not necessarily correlate with the severity of the lameness. Severely lame horses may have minimal abnormalities assessed radiographically, whereas horses that have significant deviations from normal on radiographs may be relatively sound.

DIAGNOSIS

Accurate assessment of the whole patient is mandatory, and consideration must be given to signalment, occupation, and owner expectations. One must not only ascertain if the horse truly has laminitis but also attempt to determine the underlying cause. After such determination, there are 3 vital pieces of information to be obtained when evaluating a horse and formulating a diagnostic, therapeutic, and prognostic plan: the reason for and source of pain, the location of pain, and the degree of instability within the foot. It may take several visits and serial evaluations spread over days or weeks to accurately make this assessment.

The diagnostic evaluation to determine if chronic laminitis is present in the horse is basic and straightforward, but thoroughness cannot be overemphasized. Physical examination of the horse as a whole is mandatory and should be undertaken first. In most instances, observation of the stance and gait are strong indicators of the presence of laminitis. The characteristic, stilted, camped out front legs are believed to redistribute load to the hindquarters. Variations on this stance are likely to occur because of the presence of pain in the rear feet or variations in the location of pain in the front feet. Gait is usually easily evaluated from the walk and aids in identifying the affected feet. The patient should be observed moving in a straight line and turning in both directions. Observation of the trot may be necessary if the lameness is mild. It is not often necessary to perform nerve blocks to diagnose laminitis; however, instances of low-grade bilateral pain associated with chronic laminitis can be an exception.

After assessment of the horse's stance and ambulation, a detailed evaluation of the feet must be made. Assessment of the quality and integrity of the feet, intensity of digital pulse, and hoof capsule temperature should be made. The coronary band should be assessed for the presence of edema (swelling), depressed areas (sinking), or palpably tender areas, which may indicate abscess or separation of hoof wall. The shape and position of the sole is observed for the degree of concavity or protrusion, soft spots, or excessive thinning (**Fig. 6**). The size, shape, and integrity of the feet are especially important for monitoring change associated with progression of laminitis, once a diagnosis has been achieved.

A detailed history is imperative to address the cause of laminitis. Patient history alone frequently elucidates the underlying cause, but ancillary diagnostics can sometimes be required (eg, in metabolic syndrome laminitis). Determination of the inciting event is important for 2 reasons. First, many causes have a moderately predictable

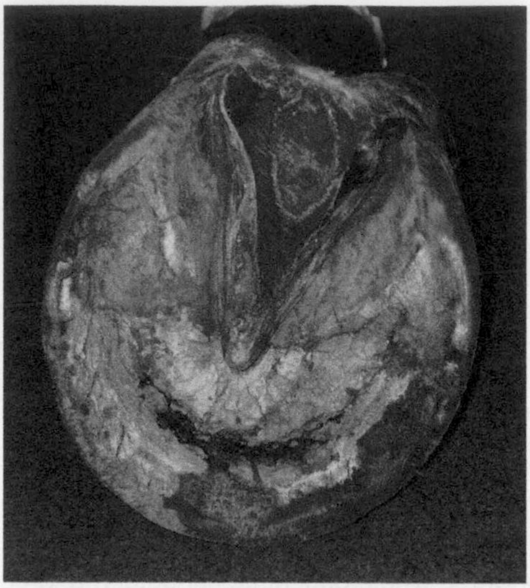

Fig. 6. Foot undergoing solar prolapse with protrusion of the distal phalanx.

course of laminitis, as discussed earlier, which can help the practitioner anticipate clinical problems that are likely to arise. Second, although some causes are finite in time, others require continued monitoring and periodic therapeutic adjustments or reveal secondary medical issues, which require attention to achieve the best possible outcome for the patient.

Once physical evaluation and the underlying cause have been addressed, the source or cause of pain within the foot should be determined. Differentiation should be made between septic and nonseptic processes, bruising, laminar shearing, ischemia, and/or bone pathology. Digital sepsis or abscessation may occur without loss of structural integrity to the laminae. The cause and stage of laminitis should be considered when assessing the source of pain, because accurate diagnosis of the source of pain is important to achieve correct therapeutic intervention. For example, a chronically laminitic horse with keratin hyperplasia resulting in an overgrown foot with seedy toe and prolapsed sole is more likely to have a subsolar abscess contributing to lameness than a horse with laminitis with radiographic evidence of sinking. Recent distal displacement pain is probably associated with laminar shearing, digital collapse, and pressure on inflamed sensitive tissue. Although both the conditions may present with significant clinical pain, treatment plans are different.

The location of pain is likewise important to determine. Hoof tester evaluation is useful when positive but a negative response does not rule out foot pain or laminitis. It is common to have a negative hoof test response in a horse with thick soles and hoof capsule. Horses with EMS also often have a negative response. Bilateral diffuse solar pain across the toe and dorsal wall is considered characteristic for laminitis; however, bilateral foot bruising may yield similar findings on a single evaluation. Focal pain anywhere in the foot is generally associated with abscess but the horse may display a laminitic gait to relieve load on the foot. Pain predominantly located in the toe, dorsal wall, and sole is managed differently than pain in the heel region or along the medial wall quarter. Variations in stance and gait are recognized when pain originates in areas other than the toe and dorsal wall. Laminitis involving the heels presents with a toe first gait or land flat footed or may have the feet camped under the body; the heels may collapse or detach at the coronary band. Collapse of the medial hoof wall is another recognized entity associated with distal displacement of the distal phalanx (**Fig. 7**). It is not fully understood at this time if this is attributable to a greater degree of lamellar damage in this region or simply regional mechanical overload along the medial wall. This is seen in some nonlaminitic horses as they age and become more pigeon toed in conformation.

The most important determinant of long-term outcome in the laminitic horse, and one of the most difficult to accurately evaluate, is the degree of instability between the distal phalanx and hoof wall. Differences in distal phalanx position between loading and non–weight bearing may provide some indication of degree of stability, but at present this is theoretical. Impending instability is difficult to determine with the current evaluation techniques, and therefore by the time active displacement is recognized instability is present. At present there are limited means by which this assessment can be made. Currently, serial radiographic evaluation is the only imaging modality with as much value as physical evaluation. In some situations, the venographic study can be useful; however, venograms are indicated for prognostic and diagnostic purposes.

Whether using conventional or digital radiography, techniques and views are well standardized.[16] Standard views, including the lateral to medial, dorsal palmar, and 45° dorsal palmar projections, should be performed routinely. Findings should be assessed with respect to the entire clinical picture. It is important to consider the stage of the disease and particularly the rate of change of the position of the distal phalanx within the hoof capsule. The radiographic study represents a static image of a dynamic model and disease and is most useful when combined with the clinical evaluation during serial sessions.

Radiographic findings include measurement of the degrees of rotational displacement of the distal phalanx away from the hoof capsule (**Fig. 8**). Measurement technique and the relative standardization allow for communication with others about a patient. Currently, other objective parameters are also assessed. These include the palmar angle of the distal phalanx, the proximal and distal horn-lamellar zone width, the extensor process-coronary band distance, and the sole depth at the tip

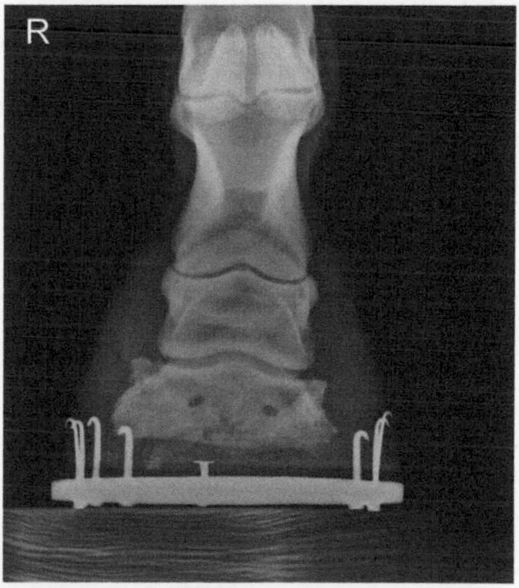

Fig. 7. Radiograph of a foot that has undergone medial sinking.

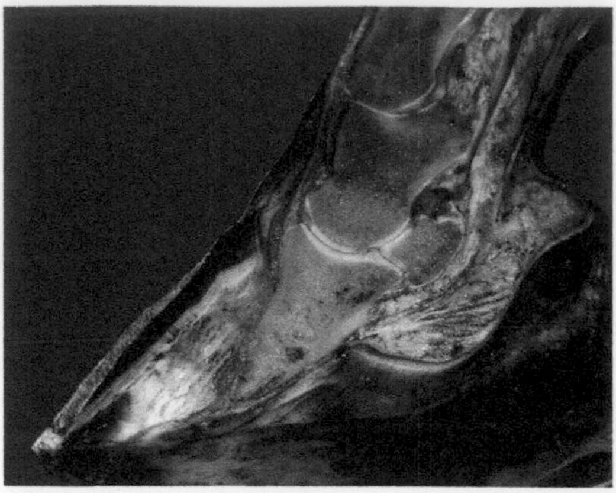

Fig. 8. Necropsied foot with rotational displacement of the distal phalanx away from the hoof wall.

and wing of the distal phalanx. Integrity of the distal phalanx should also be evaluated for proliferative or erosive changes, relative density, and porosity or pathologic fracture. Distal displacement (sinker) or medial distal displacement (medial sinker) as well as arthritis of the metacarpophalangeal joint may be evaluated via radiography. These findings all aid the diagnostic evaluation of the laminitic horse. Of the horses euthanized due to laminitis, which were included in the central Kentucky retrospective study, rotation of the distal phalanx from the hoof wall was observed in 80% of cases, distal displacement was seen in 26%, and only 1% underwent sloughing of the hoof capsule (**Table 3**) (University of Kentucky Livestock Disease Diagnostic Center, Wharton, Hunt, and Carter, unpublished data, 2008). While a single evaluation provides limited information relative to the long-term management of the patient, many of these findings and trends in their progression over time have significant prognostic value (**Fig. 9**A, B).

Digital venography has considerable usefulness at assessing the viability of the vascular supply and soft tissue structures of the foot.[17–19] A venogram that shows normal filling of the vascular space generally carries a much better prognosis than a horse with no perfusion (**Fig. 10**A, B).

Relative poor perfusion is accounted for by vascular compression, vascular damage from soft tissue disruption, possible influence of arterio-venous shunts, or technical errors associated with the procedure. Venography allows evaluation of the digital vasculature for deficits in the coronary circulation, terminal arch, dorsal papillae,

Table 3
Clinical parameters of laminitis in cases reviewed

Clinical Parameter	Number	Percent (%)
Rotation of PIII	414/516	80
Sinkers	150/585	26
Sloughed foot or feet	6/585	1
All 4 limbs affected	154/568	27
Front feet only affected	304/568	53.5
Single foot only affected	88/568	15.5

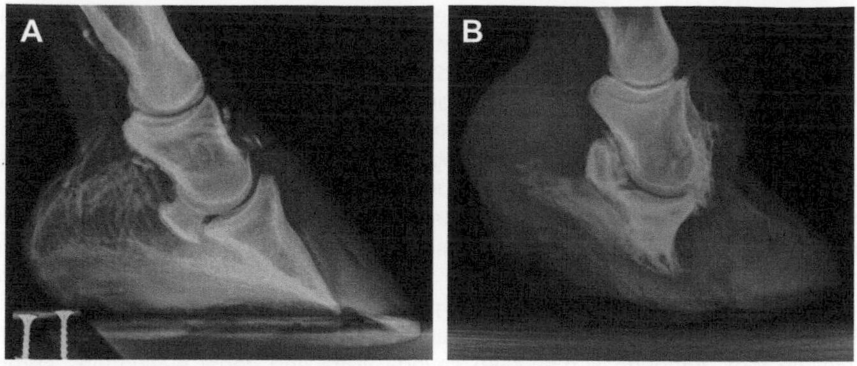

Fig. 9. Radiograph of a horse (*A*) with early severe, chronic laminitis and distal displacement of the distal phalanx (sinker). Two years later (*B*) there is severe deterioration of the distal phalanx and ankylosis of the distal interphalangeal joint associated with advanced arthritis. Note the redundant overgrown dorsal hoof wall.

bulbar circulation, and circumflex vessels. Loss of perfusion is a definite prognostic indicator when the clinical picture is somewhat ambiguous.

PROGNOSIS

Eventual functionality of the foot is determined by its structural integrity and is related to vasculature compromise, bone pathology, and the quality of the laminar/hoof wall interface; however, prognosis is also influenced by owner expectation, and few horses actually die from laminitis. Very little evidence-based research exists on prognosticating laminitic horses. Determining the long-term prognosis for a horse with chronic laminitis is in large part based on the information accumulated from the diagnostic evaluation and is somewhat controversial. This is understandable given the number of variables associated with management of the clinical patient including not only the feet but also the rest of the body with client variables superimposed. Some studies have attempted to provide clinical parameters that are useful in prognosis. One study

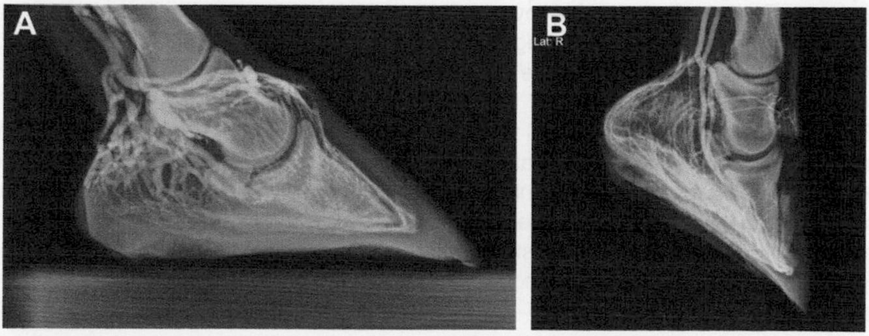

Fig. 10. (*A*) Venogram of a horse with chronic laminitis with sufficient digital vascularization. Note the extravasation of contrast medium at the distal dorsal laminar region. (*B*) Venogram of the horse in Fig. 9A. Abnormal venographic changes consist of a void in the proximal portion of the dorsal coronary and laminar vessels and leakage of the contrast medium into the distal dorsal laminar region.

used radiographic findings to correlate the degree of distal phalanx rotation to eventual soundness.[20] Baxter[21] described distal displacement of the distal phalanx and reported a poor prognosis. In another study, severity and duration of pain was shown to have a correlation with the clinical outcome and future survival.[22] As with most clinical entities, there are exceptions to every rule. The authors largely rely on clinical experience and temper this with their recognized guidelines. These general guidelines are influenced by other clinical findings such as the accompanying disease, stage of laminitis, or degree of instability within the hoof capsule. For example, a horse with chronic laminitis that has 10° to 12° of capsular rotation but is stable has a much better prognosis than a laminitic horse with 3° to 4° rotation, which has occurred over a 1-week period accompanied by severe pain.

Perhaps the most important determinant of outcome is the degree of instability within the foot. Although it may take several visits and serial evaluations spread over days or weeks to accurately assess this parameter, ultimately, one hopes to determine if the horse can continue to generate a viable and functional hoof capsule. Ability, or lack thereof, to maintain a functional, viable hoof capsule is directly correlated to the ultimate prognosis of the patient. Vascular integrity is an essential component of hoof regeneration, which may be assessed with digital venography in addition to conventional serial radiographs and clinical evaluation (see **Fig. 10**).

Client expectations and long-term intended occupation of the laminitic horse influence prognosis and vary greatly. Degree of soundness acceptable for each horse is affected by the owner's ultimate goal for the horse. An acceptable comfort level in a broodmare, and thus a good prognosis, may not meet owner expectations for a horse used in athletic endeavors. In addition, the level of care, time commitments, and financial and emotional burdens assumed by the owner affect prognosis. One level of maintenance care may be justifiable in a broodmare producing sales yearlings, whereas it is not acceptable in a retired horse. A final consideration is the level of suffering, which the horse is subjected to, with little hope of recovery to a good quality of life.

SUMMARY

Chronic laminitis is very common and affects a large number of horses in North America. The clinical presentation can vary broadly, depending on the underlying cause, the course of disease, the instability of the laminar interface, and concomitant degree of lameness. Disease progression over time may be of prognostic importance with regard to the development of degenerative morphologic changes within the foot. Etiology can often help predict the course of the disease and is therefore important to discern.

Evaluation of the horse is critical to diagnosis and consists of serial physical examinations with special attention to all structures in the foot. In addition, repeat radiographs are a valuable tool in chronicling the progress of vertical and rotational distal displacement. Venography may be beneficial by determining the vascular supply to the foot and may be of prognostic and diagnostic value. The ultimate outcome depends on the viability of the individual structures in the foot and the degree of compromise to function.

REFERENCES

1. Kane AJ, Traub-Dargatz J, Losinger WC, et al. The occurrence and causes of lameness and laminitis in the U.S. horse population. In: Proceedings of the

46th Annual American Association of Equine Pracitioners Convention. San Antonio (TX), November 26–29, 2000. p. 277–80.
2. Hood DM. Laminitis in the horse. Vet Clin North Am Equine Pract 1999;15(2): 287–94.
3. Baxter GM. Laminitis. In: Robinson NE, editor. Current therapy in equine medicine. 4th edition. Philadelphia: WB Saunders; 1997. p. 737–43.
4. Colles DM, Jeffcott LB. Laminitis in the horse. Vet Rec 1977;100:262–4.
5. Pollitt CC. Equine laminitis: a revised pathophysiology. In: Proceedings of the 45th Annual American Association of Equine Practitioners Convention. Albuquerque (NM), December 5–8, 1999. p. 188–92.
6. Hood DM. The pahtophysiology of developmental and acute laminitis. Vet Clin North Am Equine Pract 1999;15(2):321–44.
7. Obel N. Studies on the histopathology of acute laminitis [dissertation]. Uppsala (Sweden), Almqvist & Wiksells Boltryckeri AB, 1948.
8. Hood DM. The mechanisms and consequences of structural failure of the foot. Vet Clin North Am Equine Pract 1999;15(2):437–62.
9. Frank N. Insulin resistance in horses. In: 52nd Annual Convention of the American Association of Equine Practitioners. San Antonio (TX), December 2–6, 2006. p. 51–4.
10. Davis EG. Equine metabolic syndrome. In: Proceedings of the North American Veterinary Conference. Orlando (FL), January 8–12, 2005. p. 140–2.
11. Johnson PJ. The equine metabolic syndrome peripheral Cushing's syndrome. Vet Clin North Am Equine Pract 2002;18(2):271–93.
12. Bailey SR, Habershon-Butcher JL, Ransom KJ, et al. Hypertension and insulin resistance in a mixed-breed population of ponies predisposed to laminitis. Am J Vet Res 2008;69(1):122–9.
13. Treiber KH, Kronfeld DS, Hess TM, et al. Evaluation of genetic and metabolic predispositions and nutritional risk factors for pasture-associated laminitis in ponies. J Am Vet Med Assoc 2006;228(10):1538–45.
14. Pass MA, Pollitt S, Pollitt CC. Decreased glucose metabolism causes separation of hoof lamellae in vitro: a trigger for laminitis? Equine Vet J Suppl 1998; 26:133–8.
15. Mobasheri A, Critchlow K, Clegg PD, et al. Chronic equine laminitis is characterized by loss of GLUT1, GLUT4 and ENaC positive laminar keratinocytes. Equine Vet J 2004;35:248–54.
16. Park RD. Radiographic examination of the equine foot. Vet Clin North Am Equine Pract 1989;5(1):47–66.
17. D'Arpe, Bernardini D. Interpreting contrast venography in horses with controlateral laminitis. In: Proceedings of the European Society of Veterinary Orthopaedics and Traumatology. Munich (Germany), September 10–14, 2008. p. 226–33.
18. Rucker A, Redden RF, Arthur EG, et al. How to perform the digital venogram. In: 52nd Annual Convention of the American Association of Equine Practitioners. San Antonio (TX), December 2–6, 2006. p. 526–30.
19. Rucker A. The digital venogram. In: Floyd AE, Mansmann RA, editors. Equine podiatry. St. Louis (MO): Saunders Elsevier; 2007. p. 328–46.
20. Stick JA, Jann HW, Scott EA, et al. Pedal bone rotation as a prognostic sign in laminitis of horses. J Am Vet Med Assoc 1982;180(3):251–3.
21. Baxter GM. Equine laminitis caused by distal displacement of the distal phalanx: 12 cases (1976–1985). J Am Vet Med Assoc 1986;189(3):326–9.
22. Hunt RJ. A retrospective evaluation of laminitis in horses. Equine Vet J 1993; 25(1):61–4.

Pathology of the Distal Phalanx in Equine Laminitis: More Than Just Skin Deep

Julie B. Engiles, VMD[a,b,*]

KEYWORDS

- Bone modeling • Distal phalanx • Laminitis
- Osteoclasis • Osteoproliferation

Laminitis is a devastating disease of the equine foot with a varied and complicated etiopathogenesis. The equine foot, complex in both anatomy and physiology, integrates multiple organ systems, including the musculoskeletal, integumentary, nervous, immune, and cardiovascular systems. Thus, as a correlate, initiating causes of laminitis in naturally occurring disease are often multifactorial, and can be influenced by different body systems, including the gastrointestinal (eg, colitis, carbohydrate overload/enteric dysbiosis), respiratory (eg, pleuropneumonia), reproductive (eg, metritis), cardiovascular (eg, hypovolemia, vasculitis/vasculopathies, local ischemia), endocrine (eg, equine Cushing/pituitary pars intermedia dysfunction, hyperinsulinemia, "metabolic syndrome"), and musculoskeletal (eg, contralateral limb overload) systems. In addition, exposure to exogenous toxins, specifically the extract of black walnut (*Juglans nigra*), or iatrogenic administration of corticosteroids can also induce laminitis. Depending on the case, the pathogenesis of equine laminitis most likely involves an inflammatory, a toxic/enzymatic, or a metabolic process or a combination of these processes. Laminitis results in progressive pathoanatomic alterations, which disrupt the intimate connections between the distal phalanx and the cutaneous elements of the hoof wall lamellae. Often this results in the painful structural collapse of the foot and the eventual demise of the animal.

[a] Department of Pathobiology, School of Veterinary Medicine, New Bolton Center-Murphy Laboratory, University of Pennsylvania, 382 West Street Road, Kennett Square, PA 19348, USA
[b] Department of Clinical Studies, New Bolton Center, School of Veterinary Medicine, University of Pennsylvania, Kennett Square, PA, USA
* Department of Pathobiology, School of Veterinary Medicine, University of Pennsylvania, New Bolton Center-Murphy Laboratory, 382 West Street Road, Kennett Square, PA 19348.
E-mail address: engiles@vet.upenn.edu

Vet Clin Equine 26 (2010) 155–165
doi:10.1016/j.cveq.2009.12.001
vetequine.theclinics.com
0749-0739/10/$ – see front matter

Much has been done in recent years to better characterize the structural and molecular changes that occur during laminitic episodes, especially regarding black walnut extract and oligofructose induction models.[1–6] However, in naturally occurring disease, neither the origins or mechanisms that relate laminitic pain to biomechanical instability, nor the gross/radiographic pathology, nor the cellular and molecular components of inflammation are completely characterized. In addition, although systematic histopathological examination of the hoof wall lamellae has been undertaken in some forms of laminitis (mainly black walnut extract and oligofructose models), concurrent examination of the pedal bone is often neglected. In his 1987 PhD thesis dissertation, Robert Linford[7] described radiographic and some histologic bone changes associated with subclinical lamellar pathology in Thoroughbred racehorse, trauma-induced laminitis, and carbohydrate-induced laminitis models. He proposed that lamellar integrity was critical to soundness and that lamellar alterations were likely to cause bony changes in the distal phalanx. However, since then, to the author's knowledge, no further characterization of the distal phalanx has been published. Recent experimental evidence in both human and animal scientific literature indicates that subtle changes in bone occurring at the microscopic level result in profound local immunologic changes, which may not only affect and influence bone quality and fragility, but also elements of the integument (epidermis and dermis).[8,9] It should also be considered that some painful but subtle, and often radiographically occult, human syndromes involving bone (eg, bone marrow edema syndrome, regional migratory osteoporosis, occult avascular osteonecrosis) have been associated with certain inflammatory conditions or alterations in biomechanical forces.[10–12] Interestingly, histologic changes described for some of these conditions, such as pathologically active bone modeling, medullary edema, and fibromyxoid change, are similar to what is seen in the distal phalanx of laminitis horses. Given the close anatomical and physiological associations between the distal phalanx and the lamellae, and recent discoveries in the field of osteoimmunology, the equine distal phalanx should be considered, perhaps in addition to the soft tissues, both as a potential source of clinically significant pain and as a site of ongoing, "self-perpetuating" inflammation that can affect, or be affected by, the overlying epidermal and dermal soft tissues. This article describes histopathologic changes that occur within the distal phalanx in various clinical cases of laminitis. The potential mechanisms behind these changes and their implications for disease progression and therapeutic intervention are discussed.

ARCHITECTURE OF THE DISTAL PHALANX

The structural integrity of the equine digit depends on maintenance of the proper pathoanatomical relationships among the epidermal elements of the hoof wall and sole, the underlying dermis (corium), the specialized connective tissues of the digital cushion, the tendons, the ligaments, and the distal phalanx. This article focuses on the interface between the hoof wall lamellae, corium, and distal phalanx. The hoof wall lamellae are composed of rectangular plates of keratinized primary epidermal lamellae and subsets of secondary epidermal lamellae. Primary and secondary dermal lamellae, which are extensions of the specialized lamellar dermis, interdigitate with the respective epidermal lamellae (**Fig. 1**). The lamellar dermis is a highly specialized connective tissue that contains blood vessels (arterioles, venules, arteriovenous anastomoses, and capillaries) and nerves that nurture the epidermal lamellae. In addition, dense type I collagen fibers from the inner corium directly insert onto the outer cortex of the distal phalanx, which is devoid of a "true" periosteum. The collagen fibers literally

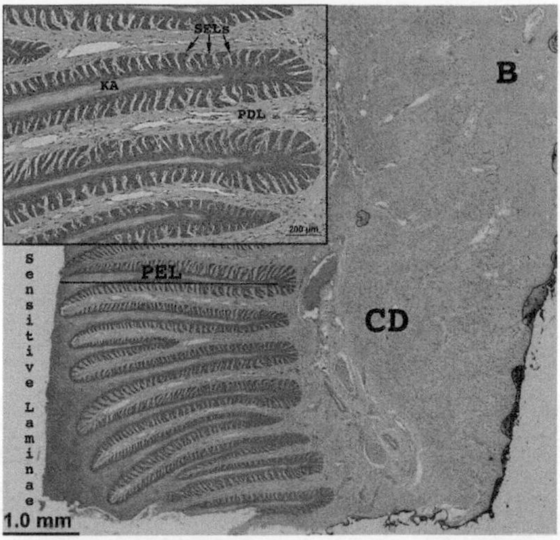

Fig. 1. Hematoxylin and eosin–stained section of the dorsal hoof wall comprising hoof wall lamellae, coronary dermis (CD), and bone of the distal phalanx (B). Higher magnification photomicrograph (*inset*) demonstrates the relationship among primary epidermal lamellae (PEL) and secondary epidermal lamellae (SELs), which interdigitate primary dermal lamellae (PDL) and secondary dermal lamellae, respectively. Primary epidermal lamellae contain a central keratinized axis (KA).

suspend the distal phalanx within the hoof capsule. This deeper connective tissue of the corium also contains mesenchymal stem cells. These cells are capable of differentiating into osteoprogenitor cells, which produce woven and lamellar compact (osteonal) bone (**Fig. 2**). Although the overall shape of the distal phalanges does not resemble that of a typical "long bone," embryonic development does involve, in addition to intramembranous bone formation, endochondral ossification with proximal growth plates. The outer cortices of the pedal bone are thin and composed of

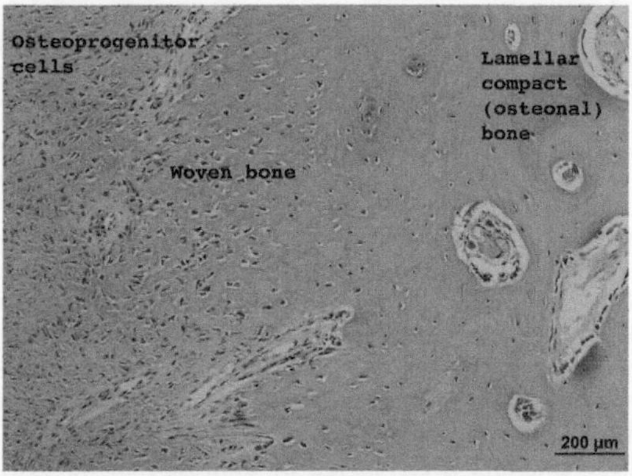

Fig. 2. Hematoxylin and eosin–stained section of dorsal cortical bone from the distal phalanx of a juvenile animal. Image shows the intramembranous ossification of the dorsal cortex of the distal phalanx. Osteoprogenitor cells of the periosteal cambium-like tissue differentiate into osteoblasts, which produce both woven and lamellar compact (osteonal) bone.

compact (osteonal) bone with vascular (osteonal) canals interspersed by concentric lamellae of bone matrix. The dorsal cortex is relatively porous, containing numerous vascular canals, which accommodate the transit of digital blood vessels that supply the hoof wall lamellae.[13] In contrast, the dorsal, solar cortex is a dense plate of bone that contains few (if any) perforating vascular channels. The distal phalanx has an inner composition of cancellous or "spongy" bone comprising interconnected plates and struts of bone trabeculae interposed by medullary spaces containing well-vascularized adipose tissue, bone marrow stromal cells, osteoblasts, and osteoclasts (**Fig. 3**).

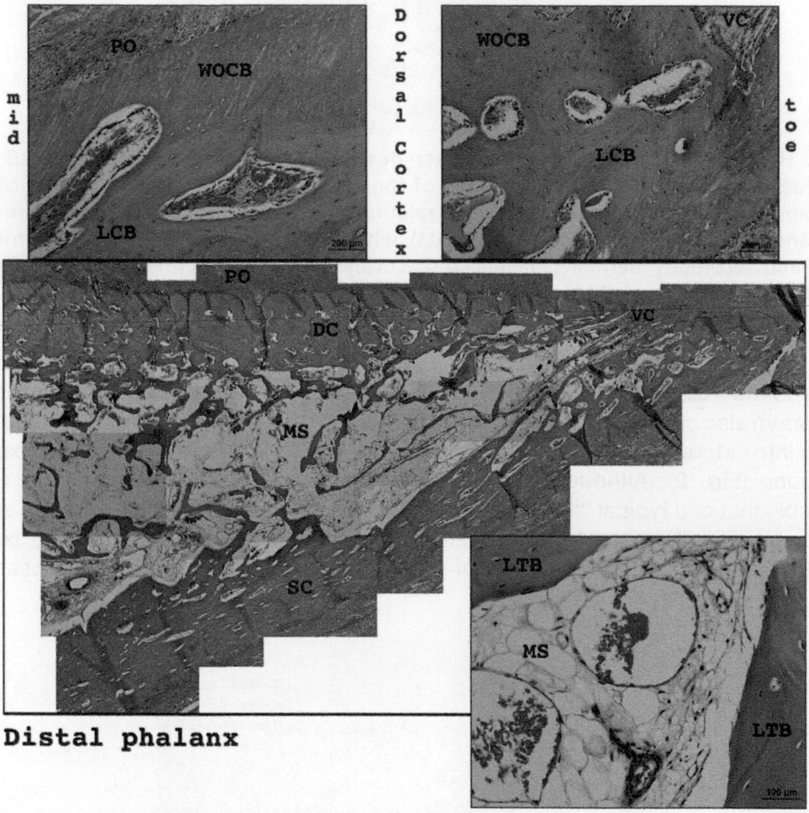

Fig. 3. Hematoxylin and eosin–stained section of decalcified bone from the distal phalanx of an adult horse with no clinical or histopathological evidence of laminitis. The distal solar margin (tip of the distal phalanx) is oriented to the right. The dorsal cortex (DC) comprises compact (osteonal) bone through which penetrate small and large vascular channels (VC) that radiate outward to supply the lamellar dermis. In contrast, the solar cortex (SC) is a dense plate of compact bone without penetrating vascular canals. Bone remodeling units are lined by polygonal osteoblasts with rare multinucleate osteoclasts. The inner medullary space (MS) of the distal phalanx is composed of adipose-rich fibrovascular stroma interspersed with anastomizing lamellar bone trabeculae. Higher magnification photomicrographs illustrate the distal region (*upper right panel*) and midregion (*upper left panel*) of the distal phalanx, as well as the medulla (*lower right panel*). LCB, lamellar compact bone; LTB, lamellar trabecular bone; PO, periosteum; WOCB, woven outer cortical bone.

BONE MICROENVIRONMENT

The microenvironment of bone is dynamic. In spite of its physical rigidity, bone is a plastic organ that not only is in a constant state of turnover ("remodeling"), but also retains the ability to transform its configuration, shape, or density in response to external stimuli ("modeling"). The terms *remodeling* and *modeling* are often interchanged. However, remodeling is typically considered a physiologic process (eg, calcium homeostasis and general bone matrix maintenance), whereas modeling occurs either during growth of the skeletal system or in response to a pathologic process (fracture, inflammation, neoplasia, metabolic conditions). Of course, the two processes overlap somewhat. As mentioned above, the skeletal system has been linked to not only the immune system, but to the integumentary, gastrointestinal, and nervous systems, through both local and systemic means. During embryologic development, Wnts, a group of secreted signaling proteins, not only regulate diverse developmental processes in embryogenesis, but also play an important role in regeneration of adult tissues, including lymphoid, colonic, integumentary/adnexal, and bone tissues.[14,15] Wnt-mediated osteoblastogenesis is mediated through its coreceptor LPR5, which in turn is regulated by vasoactive amines, mainly serotonin (5HT).[16] Neuroendocrine (enterochromaffin) cells, which are considered the main source of serotonin, can be stimulated by various mechanical or chemical stimuli (eg, bile salts, nutrients, acid, or bacterial toxins). However, serotonin and other monoamines are also produced by carbohydrate fermentation by bacteria extracted from the equine cecum.[17,18] Serotonin can be stored within platelets and thus circulated to distant sites. In addition to their potential roles as inhibitors of Wnt-mediated osteoblastogenesis, serotonin and other monoamines released from circulating equine platelets have potent vasoactive effects, especially on equine digital vessels.[19,20] Because blood supply to the dorsal hoof wall lamellae must first transit through the vascular canals of the distal phalanx, these serotonin/monoamine-mediated pathways would seem to have implications for not only the soft tissue lamellae, but also the pedal bone.[21] Considering that alterations in bone matricellular proteins in the murine microenvironment (osteopontin, SPARC [cystein-rich acidic secreted protein], tenacin C, thrombospondins) affect not only rates of bone turnover and bone modeling in fracture healing, but also neovascularization, it seems logical to consider a similar process could occur during laminitis.[22] Examinations comparing the distal phalanx in normal control specimens with the distal phalanx in various cases of laminitis, including inflammatory disease–associated and contralateral limb overload–associated laminitis, often reveals widening of the vascular canals through osteoclastic resorption and increased number and tortuosity of vascular profiles within these vascular canals. Changes to the compact and trabecular bone, as well as intermedullary spaces, are also observed. These changes suggest alterations in vascular dynamics or vascular modeling, as well as pathological bone modeling (**Fig. 4**). Linford[7] described similar changes and found a clinically significant increase in the number of radiographically apparent vascular channels ("end-on" vessels) in the center of the distal phalanx (dorsoproximal-palmarodistal projection), as well as lucency of the palmar cortex and asymmetric modeling of the solar margins of P3. When comparing the onset of clinical signs and the severity of the histologic changes at the lamellar tissues, it appears these changes can occur very quickly (within days to weeks). To prove whether these changes occur secondary to prior thrombosis, change in flow dynamics, direct molecular stimulation, or by some other mechanism requires systematic characterization of various stages and types of laminitis, both experimentally induced and naturally occurring. Already there is great promise in using relatively noninvasive techniques, such as intraosseous catheterization of the lamellar circulation, and intralamellar microdialysis to analyze the equine digital microenvironment.[21,23]

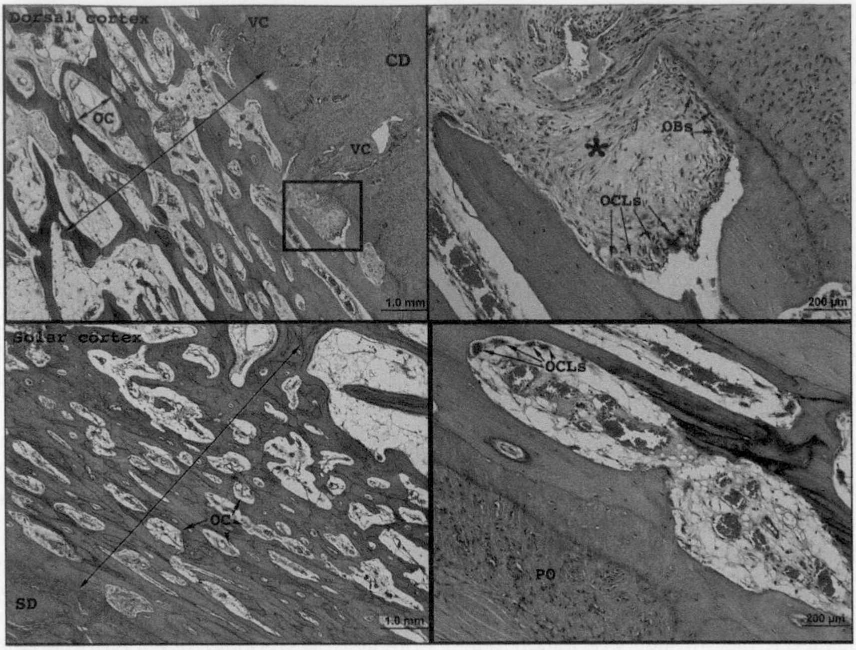

Fig. 4. Photomicrographs of hematoxylin and eosin–stained sections of decalcified bone from the dorsal cortex (*upper panels*) and solar cortex (*lower panels*) of a horse with chronic-active laminitis. There is marked increased porosity of both cortices because of osteoclastic resorption and modeling of both osteonal canals (OC) and vascular channels (VC) of the dorsal cortex. Long arrows denote cortical width. The upper right panel, a higher magnification image of the outlined box in upper left panel, shows active modeling by osteoclasts (OCLs) and osteoblasts (OBs), as well as medullary fibromyxoid proliferation (*asterisk*). The lower right panel, a higher magnification image of the outer solar cortex, depicts edema with increased numbers of small-caliber congested blood vessels and active osteoclast resorption. CD, dorsal corium; PO, periosteum; SD, solar dermis.

OSTEOIMMUNOLOGY AND INFLAMMATION-INDUCED BONE MODELING

Since the direct link between bone and the immune system was made, there has been a dramatic expansion in the field of "osteoimmunology."[24–26] Scientists recently found that RANKL (the receptor activator of nuclear factor kappa B ligand) is not only expressed on osteoblasts, but is also expressed by activated T-lymphocytes and by mammary and thymic epithelium, as well as by normal and inflamed epidermal cells.[27–32] Soluble RANKL, though not as potent an inducer of osteoclasis as RANKL bound to membranes (eg, on osteoblasts), is an effective mediator of osteoclast differentiation and activation.[26] Epidermal cells have the ability to secrete, in addition to RANKL, many other proinflammatory signaling molecules, including cytokines interleukin (IL) 1 (IL-1) alpha and beta; chemokines IL-8, CCL4 (macrophage inflammatory protein-1), and CCL20; and growth factors epidermal growth factor, granulocyte-monocyte colony stimulating factor, and nerve growth factor.[33] Not only do these factors serve as paracrine signals to activate fibroblasts, endothelial cells, T cells, and dendritic cells, resulting in prostaglandin and collagenase production, but the factors also serve as autocrine stimulators of keratinocyte proliferation and activation, resulting in release and activation of matrix metalloproteinases. Aberrant expression of nerve growth factor has been associated with alterations in sensory nerve fiber sprouting, neuropeptide production, and neuopathic pain, especially in proliferative inflammatory dermatoses, such as psoriasis, where inflammation (neurogenic or inflammatory cell–mediated) is associated with dysregulated and dysplastic proliferation of epidermal keratinocytes.[34] Laminitic horses have been observed to have, in addition to lamellar keratinocyte hyperplasia and dysplasia, alterations in type and distribution of sensory nerve fibers, neuropeptide Y, the neural injury marker activating transcription factor-3 in afferent neurons, and specific dorsal root ganglia.[35] Although the intermedullary spaces of bone are typically rich in sensory nerve fibers and could significantly contribute to laminitic pain, this has yet to be evaluated.

Inflammatory-mediated bone loss is a well-recognized clinical syndrome in both human and veterinary medicine. It is associated with common clinical entities, such as osteoarthritis, periodontitis, and osteomyelitis, but is also associated with prosthetic devices involving a combination of biomechanical, bacterial, or autoimmune disease (rheumatoid arthritis) and even endocrine disorders (type I diabetes).[36,37] Bone loss results from a shift away from osteoblastic bone formation to osteoclastic bone resorption mediated through RANKL expression by osteoblasts, osteal macrophages, bone marrow stromal cells, and activated lymphocytes.[38,39] Proinflammatory molecules, including cytokines (tumor necrosis factor–alpha, IL-1, IL-6, IL-8, IL-17, IL-23), growth factors (macrophage-specific colony-stimulating factor, vascular endothelial growth factor), reactive oxygen intermediates, and prostaglandins (PGE2), are either expressed locally or circulate regionally/systemically.[33,38–40] Endotoxin (lipopolysaccharide [LPS]) can also stimulate RANKL expression directly by osteoblasts, or indirectly through inflammatory leukocytes via toll-like receptors (TLR4), nuclear factor kappa B (NF-κB), and mitogen-activated protein kinase (MAPK) pathways.[37] In turn, RANKL, which is a potent promoter of differentiation and activator of multinucleate osteoclasts, as well as an inducer of NF-κB activation, generates a vicious "self-perpetuating" cycle of bone loss via positive feedback production of additional proinflammatory cytokines.[41] Recent scientific evidence shows that p38MAPK

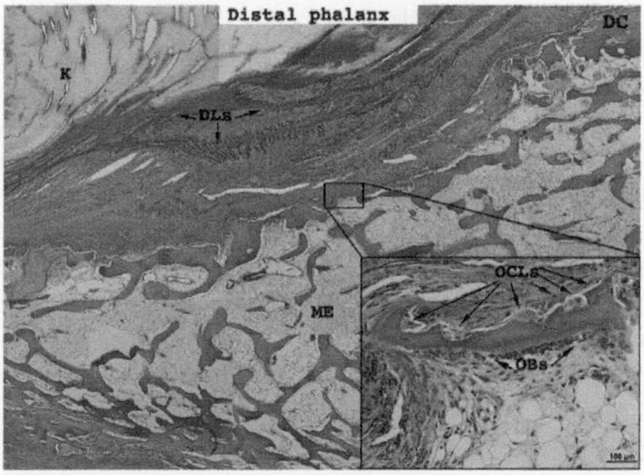

Fig. 5. Low-magnification photomicrograph of the mid- to distal portion of the distal phalanx. There is a large accumulation of orthokeratotic keratin (K), which is associated with dysplastic hoof wall lamellae (DLs). Medullary edema (ME) and fibromyxoid change is observed within the medullary spaces of the bone. There is marked modeling and loss of the compact bone of the dorsal cortex (DC), with active osteoclastic osteolysis (osteoclasts [OCLs] in *inset*) and osteoproliferation (osteoblasts [OBs] in *inset*). Since the rate/amount of bone resorption has outweighed the rate/amount of bone formation, net bone loss has occurred.

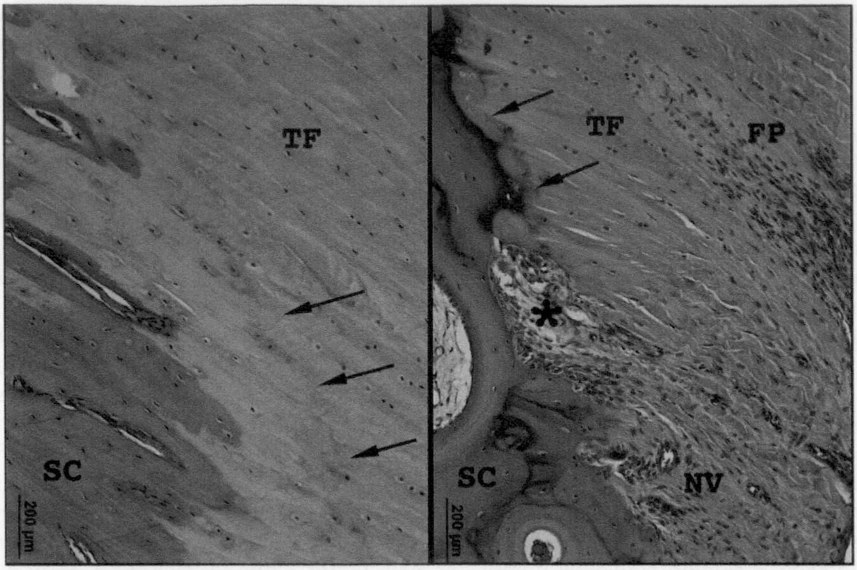

Fig. 6. Photomicrographs of the insertion of the deep digital flexor tendon in a normal horse (*left panel*) and in a horse with chronic laminitis (*right panel*). In the normal animal, regular, linear arrays of tendon fibers (TF) and their nuclei insert onto the solar cortex (SC) of the distal phalanx. Note the well-defined mineralized "tide line" of Sharpey fibers at the tendon-bone insertion interface (*arrows in left panel*). Compare these features to the laminitic horse, which demonstrates neovascularization (NV) and fibroplasia (FP) of the tendon, as well as active osteoclasis and bone modeling (asterisk) at the insertion interface with loss of the well-defined mineralized "tide line" (*arrows in right panel*).

pathways are induced in equine leukocytes when stimulated with LPS.[42] Given the specialized anatomical and physiological interactions of the epidermal, dermal, and osseous structures of the equine digit, it would seem logical that laminitic epidermal and dermal pathology could influence pedal bone pathology, and vice versa.

BIOMECHANICALLY INDUCED BONE MODELING

In addition to the above-described inflammatory mediated pathways, direct alterations in biomechanical forces contribute to bone modeling. Progressive loss of the connections between the hoof-bone interface changes tension and compressive forces, which directly influence bone modeling. Also, aberrant proliferation of dysplastic, regenerating epidermal lamellae are observed in some cases of laminitis. These form keratoma-like structures, which become a component of the chronic lamellar wedge in chronic laminitis and inevitably compress and cause distortions of the overlying bone (**Fig. 5**). This particular form of lamellar dysplasia may also serve as a significant source of pain and progressive pathology. Modeling at the insertion of the deep digital flexor tendon is also present in some cases (**Fig. 6**).

SUMMARY

In conclusion, aside from Linford's 1987 PhD thesis, descriptions of osteoporotic and osteoproliferative bone modeling in cases of laminitis are limited to radiographic and gross morphologic analyses even though such modeling is often noted.[43] At our institution, preliminary studies of laminitic digits of horses with naturally occurring disease show dramatic and active histopathologic alterations in the bone microenvironment. The author feels these findings have important implications for clinical pain, disease progression, and therapeutic intervention. Given the intimate functional anatomic associations among the epidermal lamellae, the lamellar and sublamellar dermis, and the distal phalanx, and considering recent scientific evidence pertaining to the field of osteoimmunology, evaluation of epidermal, dermal, and bony structures must be performed concurrently to fully understand the complex pathological dynamics of equine laminitis.

REFERENCES

1. Galey FD, Whiteley HE, Goetz TE, et al. Black walnut (Juglans nigra) toxicosis: a model for equine laminitis. J Comp Pathol 1991;104(3):313–26.
2. van Eps AW, Pollitt CC. Equine laminitis induced with oligofructose. Equine Vet J 2006;38(3):203–8.
3. Pollitt CC. Basement membrane pathology: a feature of acute equine laminitis. Equine Vet J 1996;28(1):38–46.
4. Black SJ, Lunn DP, Yin C, et al. Leukocyte emigration in the early stages of laminitis. Vet Immunol Immunopathol 2006;109(1–2):161–6.
5. Faleiros RR, Stokes AM, Eades SC, et al. Assessment of apoptosis in epidermal lamellar cells in clinically normal horses and those with laminitis. Am J Vet Res 2004;65(5):578–85.
6. van Eps AW, Pollitt CC. Equine laminitis model: lamellar histopathology seven days after induction with oligofructose. Equine Vet J 2009;41(8):735–40.
7. Linford RI. In: A radiographic, morphometric, histological and ultrastructural investigation of lamellar function, abnormality and the associated radiographic findings for sound and footsore Thoroughbreds and horses with experimentally induced, traumatic, and alimentary laminitis [dissertations]. CA: University of California, Davis; 1987. p. 101–18.
8. Ruppel ME, Miller LM, Burr DB. The effect of the microscopic and nanoscale structure on bone fragility. Osteoporos Int 2008;19(9):1251–65.
9. Ross FP, Christiano AM. Nothing but skin and bone. J Clin Invest 2006;116(5):1140–9.
10. Starr AM, Wessely MA, Albastaki U, et al. Bone marrow edema: pathophysiology, differential diagnosis, and imaging. Acta Radiol 2008;49(7):771–86.
11. Toms AP, Marshall TJ, Becker E, et al. Regional migratory osteoporosis: a review illustrated by five cases. Clin Radiol 2005;60(4):425–38.
12. Schweitzer ME, White LM. Does altered biomechanics cause marrow edema? Radiology 1996;198(3):851–3.
13. Nourian AR. In: Equine laminitis: ultrastructural changes, lamellar microcirculation and drug delivery [dissertations]. Queensland (Australia): University of Queensland; 2009. p. 57–74.
14. Westendorf JJ, Kahler RA, Schroeder TM. Wnt signaling in osteoblasts and bone diseases. Gene 2004;341:19–39.
15. Bennett CN, Longo KA, Wright WS, et al. Regulation of osteoblastogenesis and bone mass by Wnt10b. Proc Natl Acad Sci U S A 2005;102(9):3324–9.
16. Yadav VK, Ryu JH, Suda N, et al. Lrp5 controls bone formation by inhibiting serotonin synthesis in the duodenum. Cell 2008;135(5):825–37.
17. Sharkey KA, Mawe GM. Neuroimmune and epithelial interactions in intestinal inflammation. Curr Opin Pharmacol 2002;2(6):669–77.

18. Bailey SR, Rycroft A, Elliott J. Production of amines in equine cecal contents in an in vitro model of carbohydrate overload. J Anim Sci 2002;80(10):2656–62.
19. Elliott J, Berhane Y, Bailey SR. Effects of monoamines formed in the cecum of horses on equine digital blood vessels and platelets. Am J Vet Res 2003;64(9): 1124–31.
20. Bailey SR, Elliott J. Plasma 5-hydroxytryptamine constricts equine digital blood vessels in vitro: implications for pathogenesis of acute laminitis. Equine Vet J 1998;30(2):124–30.
21. Nourian AR, Mills PC, Pollitt CC. Development of intraosseous infusion of the distal phalanx to access the foot lamellar circulation in the standing, conscious horse. Vet J 2009. [Epub ahead of print].
22. Alford AI, Hankenson KD. Matricellular proteins: extracellular modulators of bone development, remodeling, and regeneration. Bone 2006;38(6):749–57.
23. Nourian AR, Mills PC, Pollitt CC. Development of an intra-lamellar microdialysis method for laminitis investigations in horses. Vet J 2010;183(1):22–6.
24. Arron JR, Choi Y. Bone versus immune system. Nature 2000;408(6812):535–6.
25. Lorenzo J, Horowitz M, Choi Y. Osteoimmunology: interactions of the bone and immune system. Endocr Rev 2008;29(4):403–40.
26. Nakashima T, Takayanagi H. The dynamic interplay between osteoclasts and the immune system. Arch Biochem Biophys 2008;473(2):166–71.
27. Kim NS, Kim HJ, Koo BK, et al. Receptor activator of NF-kappaB ligand regulates the proliferation of mammary epithelial cells via Id2. Mol Cell Biol 2006;26(3): 1002–13.
28. Lee HW, Park HK, Na YJ, et al. RANKL stimulates proliferation, adhesion and IL-7 expression of thymic epithelial cells. Exp Mol Med 2008;40(1):59–70.
29. Lee HW, Kim BS, Kim HJ, et al. Upregulation of receptor activator of nuclear factor-kappaB ligand expression in the thymic subcapsular, paraseptal, perivascular, and medullary epithelial cells during thymus regeneration. Histochem Cell Biol 2005;123(4–5):491–500.
30. Barbaroux JB, Beleut M, Brisken C, et al. Epidermal receptor activator of NF-kappaB ligand controls Langerhans cells numbers and proliferation. J Immunol 2008; 181(2):1103–8.
31. Loser K, Mehling A, Loeser S, et al. Epidermal RANKL controls regulatory T-cell numbers via activation of dendritic cells. Nat Med 2006;12(12):1372–9.
32. Kim N, Odgren PR, Kim DK, et al. Diverse roles of the tumor necrosis factor family member TRANCE in skeletal physiology revealed by TRANCE deficiency and partial rescue by a lymphocyte-expressed TRANCE transgene. Proc Natl Acad Sci U S A 2000;97(20):10905–10.
33. Kitaura H, Zhou P, Kim HJ, et al. M-CSF mediates TNF-induced inflammatory osteolysis. J Clin Invest 2005;115(12):3418–27.
34. Pincelli C. Nerve growth factor and keratinocytes: a role in psoriasis. Eur J Dermatol 2000;10(2):85–90.
35. Jones E, Vinuela-Fernandez I, Eager RA, et al. Neuropathic changes in equine laminitis pain. Pain 2007;132(3):321–31.
36. Motyl KJ, Botolin S, Irwin R, et al. Bone inflammation and altered gene expression with type I diabetes early onset. J Cell Physiol 2009;218(3):575–83.
37. Xu J, Wu HF, Ang ES, et al. NF-kappaB modulators in osteolytic bone diseases. Cytokine Growth Factor Rev 2009;20(1):7–17.
38. Pettit AR, Chang MK, Hume DA, et al. Osteal macrophages: a new twist on coupling during bone dynamics. Bone 2008;43(6):976–82.

39. Quinn JM, Saleh H. Modulation of osteoclast function in bone by the immune system. Mol Cell Endocrinol 2009;310(1–2):40–51.
40. Chen L, Wei XQ, Evans B, et al. IL-23 promotes osteoclast formation by up-regulation of receptor activator of NF-kappaB (RANK) expression in myeloid precursor cells. Eur J Immunol 2008;38(10):2845–54.
41. Yano S, Mentaverri R, Kanuparthi D, et al. Functional expression of beta-chemokine receptors in osteoblasts: role of regulated upon activation, normal T cell expressed and secreted (RANTES) in osteoblasts and regulation of its secretion by osteoblasts and osteoclasts. Endocrinology 2005;146(5):2324–35.
42. Neuder LE, Keener JM, Eckert RE, et al. Role of p38 MAPK in LPS induced pro-inflammatory cytokine and chemokine gene expression in equine leukocytes. Vet Immunol Immunopathol 2009;129(3–4):192–9.
43. Morgan SJ, Grosenbaugh DA, Hood DM. The pathophysiology of chronic laminitis. Pain and anatomic pathology. Vet Clin North Am Equine Pract 1999;15(2):395–417.

Equine Venography and Its Clinical Application in North America

Amy Rucker, DVM

KEYWORDS

• Laminitis • Venography • Foot • Distal phalanx

The digital venogram uses contrast radiography to assess the vascular status of the foot (**Fig. 1**). In 1992, Redden and Pollitt developed the initial technique on a standing, conscious horse.[1–3] In the nonpathologic normal foot, the venographic appearance is consistent over time.[4] As compromised tissue loses integrity, contrast pattern alterations demonstrate soft tissue pathology that cannot be assessed by traditional radiography.[5,6] The venogram is used to assess shoeing techniques, delineate margins of a keratoma, and direct surgeries of the foot. Venography is also used to determine a diagnosis in an acutely lame horse when differentials include excessive trimming with sole bruising, pedal osteitis, foot abscessation, and laminitis.[7–11] In the laminitic horse, correlation of clinical and radiographic findings with information obtained from the venogram directs treatment.[12–14] Serial venograms assess response to treatment and may stimulate tissue growth.[15]

PERFORMING THE VENOGRAM

Preparation

Clean the foot, remove shoes when appropriate, sedate the horse (Dormosedan, Pfizer Animal Health, New York, NY, USA), and perform an abaxial sesamoid nerve block (Carbocaine, Pfizer Animal Health, New York, NY, USA). Gather all radiographic equipment including 2-foot blocks of such a height that the x-ray beam is focused at the distal margin of the distal phalanx (DP). Medical supplies include a tourniquet (2.5 cm wide, 50 cm long, made from a car inner tube), tape (Elastikon, Johnson & Johnson, New Brunswick, NJ, USA), 21-gauge × 1.9-cm butterfly catheter with 30.5-cm tubing (Winged Infusion Set, Abbott Laboratories, Abbott Park, IL, USA), luer-lock injection cap, and 2 12-mL luer-lock syringes with 20-gauge × 2.5-cm needles. Each syringe is filled with diatrizoate meglumine contrast (Reno-60, Bracco Diagnostics, Princeton,

MidWest Equine, PO Box 30520, Columbia, MO 65205, USA
E-mail address: ruckeramy@hotmail.com

Vet Clin Equine 26 (2010) 167–177
doi:10.1016/j.cveq.2009.12.008

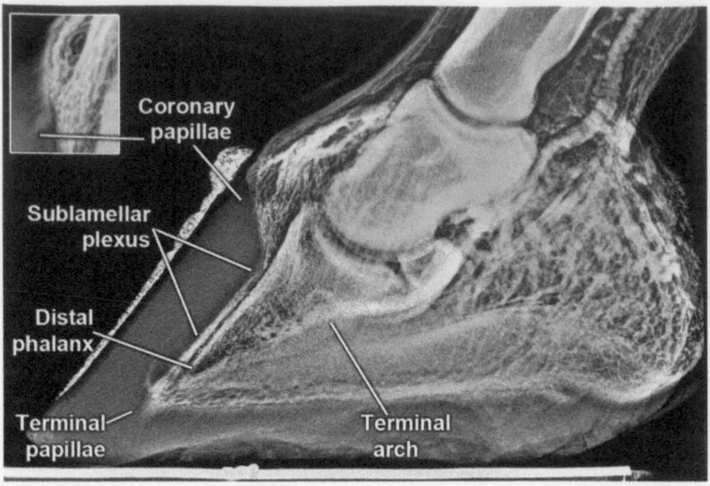

Fig. 1. Venogram of the normal, sound foot of a 400-kg American quarter horse. The coronary (*inset*), terminal, and solar papillae are oriented in the same plane as the dorsal face of the distal phalanx (DP). The sublamellar-circumflex junction is at a sharp 50° angle, similar to that of the DP's apex.

NJ, USA). Contrast volume varies; a typical 12-cm wide foot requires 20 mL contrast. If you suspect sepsis, 250 mg of amikacin may be added to each syringe.

Positioning

Stand the horse squarely on the blocks, which are oriented according to conformation. The metacarpi are vertical to the ground. The radiograph cassettes should touch the foot to avoid image magnification. Tape is placed around the fetlock at the base of the sesamoid bones, and the free end is used to anchor the tourniquet. Taking care not to distort the skin, the tourniquet is tightly applied around the sesamoid bones. The tourniquet is taped in place, with the free end of tape to be used to secure the catheter tubing post injection.

The veterinarian kneels dorsolateral to the leg with a shoulder touching the carpus. The medial arm of the veterinarian wraps around the limb in a medial-to-palmar direction and injects the contrast. The lateral hand applies light digital pressure to the catheter and vein during injection. The radiograph machine is placed lateral to the foot. The assistant is placed palmolateral.

Injection

The needle is gently threaded into the lateral vein but not advanced; blood drips freely from the tubing. The assistant attaches the injection cap and inserts the needle of the first syringe of contrast medium. The veterinarian injects the first syringe and the assistant replaces it. As the second syringe is injected, the veterinarian's medial arm partially flexes the carpus, unloading the foot, and the veterinarian then uses a shoulder to push the limb back into extension and return the foot to full weight-bearing.

Radiographs

The injection tubing is taped proximally, and a medial-lateral radiograph, followed by a dorsopalmar radiograph, is obtained. Additional informative views may follow, including an elevated heel, nonweight-bearing, grid, or oblique view. All radiographs must be taken within 45 seconds of contrast injection. A final "late" lateral is taken to examine how the contrast diffuses into nonvascular tissue. The tourniquet is loosened, the palmar digital vessels are lightly padded and taped, and the catheter is removed. The bandage remains in place for 20 to 30 minutes.

Technique Error

The most common error is inadequate volume of contrast (**Fig. 2**A). Usually this is secondary to tourniquet failure (resulting from being placed above the fetlock, or from excessive edema, hair, or tape, the first wrap of tourniquet being loose, or using a material other than an inner-tube strip). Calculate the volume of contrast needed. A warmblood breed may require 36 mL contrast, whereas a pony may require 12 mL. If the DP has penetrated the sole, contrast may run out of the foot. Inadequate volume also results from multiple venipunctures with a resultant perivascular loss of contrast. If the lateral vein cannot be identified, consider using the medial vein because it is less tortuous. However, the veterinarian must kneel directly in front of the horse, and the assistant cannot see the procedure.

If blood does not flow freely while placing the needle, back the needle out by 1 to 2 mm (the bevel may be against the wall of the vein). Do not try to advance it if the vein is tortuous. If contrast injection becomes perivascular during injection, the lateral hand feels a cool sensation, and the medial hand encounters resistance to injection. If needle position is questionable, gently aspirate and check if blood returns to the tubing. If the vein is damaged during the injection of the initial 1 or 2 mL of contrast, remove the tourniquet, place digital pressure on the vein for 10 minutes and then catheterize the medial vein. If the vein is blown after a larger volume of contrast is injected, immediately stop injecting and take radiographs to obtain as much information as possible. Wait 3 days before repeating the venogram.

Inexperienced venographers should practice on normal horses until the procedure becomes routine. All diagnostics and treatments of a laminitic horse need to be done quickly. The sedated and locally anesthetized horse should not be kept standing still on a hard surface for more than an hour.

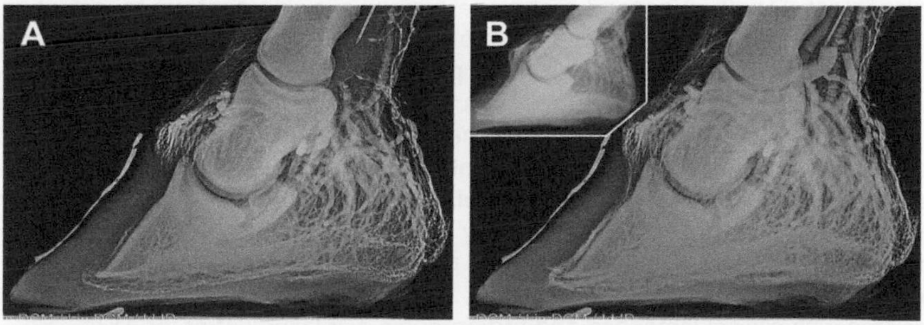

Fig. 2. (*A*) Inadequate contrast volume. Contrast has been injected into the palmar digital vein of this 550-kg thoroughbred with a 14-cm wide foot. Vessels are narrow with reduced contrast filling especially in areas of load. (*B*) Normal variation. When an adequate volume of contrast is injected (26 mL total), vessels are filled with contrast except for a mild reduction distal to the DP palmar processes. Terminal papillae are evident at the lamellar-circumflex junction, which is mildly distorted at the apex of the DP. If the tourniquet is left in place for an additional 45 seconds, contrast diffuses into the tissue (*inset*).

Rupturing a vein and causing a hematoma on a laminitis horse having compromised vasculature is not desirable. Do not remove the catheter from the vein until the tourniquet is loosened.

THE 6 AREAS OF INTEREST OF THE NORMAL VENOGRAM

Contrast is injected into the palmar digital vein, resulting in retrograde filling of the veins and arteries. The palmar digital arteries and veins enter the palmar cortex of the DP and course through the solar canal in a terminal arch. Smaller arteries and veins leave this terminal arch and pass through foraminae in the parietal surface of the DP to the sublamellar plexus and lamellar corium. The sublamellar vascular bed is evident as a distinct line within 4 mm of the DP on the dorsal, medial, and lateral aspects. The circumflex vessels are distal and peripheral to the distal margin of the DP. Terminal and sole papillae are evident within 10 mm of the DP on a foot with a heavy sole (15–20 mm depth). The lamellar-circumflex junction is distinctly shaped at a 50° angle on the lateral view (approximating the angle formed by the dorsal and palmar surfaces of the DP). Terminal papillae and sole papillae are in the same plane as the dorsal face of the DP. The coronary plexus is proximodorsal to the DP extensor process, with coronary papillae evident on the lateral view. On the dorsopalmar view, the coronary pattern is not symmetric because of differences in load and foot conformation. The heel is almost always full of vascular contrast, and is reduced only in severe cases of DP displacement.[16]

INTERPRETATION

There are variations of normal that develop from chronic foot conditions (**Fig. 2**B). Contrast is reduced in an area that is under load, for example, in the circumflex vasculature distal to the palmar processes of the DP when a horse has a negative DP palmar angle. Sole papillae are absent if the sole depth is less than 10 mm. The chronic club foot has reduced contrast distal to the DP apex, and the lamellar-circumflex junction is altered to accommodate the remodeled apex.

The most common technique-induced artifact is inadequate contrast volume (see **Fig. 2**A). Vessels are tapered and narrow in diameter. The amount of contrast seen in the image is generally reduced. This appearance is vastly different from the bluntly truncated vessels and contrast voids seen with laminitis-induced distal phalangeal displacement (**Fig. 3**). A second technique error is allowing contrast to diffuse into tissue before taking the radiograph. This error results in generalized opacity, unlike the distinct vascular alterations caused by pathology (see **Fig. 2**A, inset).

Laminitic pathology alters the appearance of the venogram even before changes are evident on plain-film radiographs.[4] As the DP dislocates, the coronary plexus, sublamellar vascular bed, and circumflex vessels distort, and may develop a reduction or absence of contrast. These findings correlate with angiographic studies in chronic laminitic horses with solar compression by the apex of the DP and coronary corium compression between the DP extensor process and coronary plexus.[16] In the research setting with induction of laminitis, the severity of changes on the venogram correlates with clinical lameness and radiographic displacement of the DP.[4]

Venous compression, and thus the contrast image beneath the hoof capsule, is affected by weight-bearing. Mechanical compression due to load is relieved when the foot is not weight-bearing. When performing the venogram, full weight-bearing images are followed by heel elevation or nonweighted images, which may contain information important for treatment and prognosis. If a normal horse is placed on a 20° heel wedge, the heel contrast is reduced, but the image of the dorsal portion

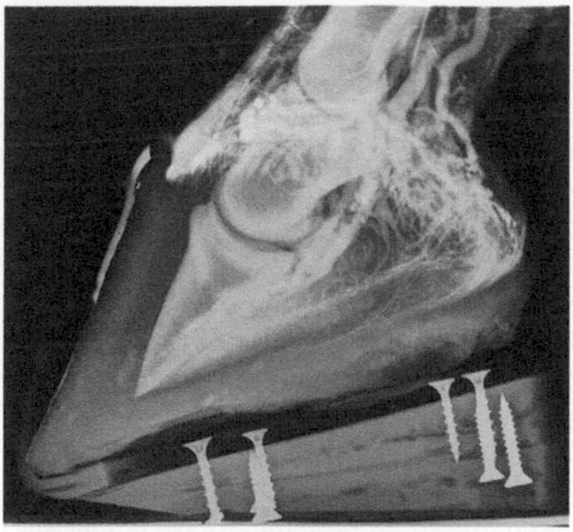

Fig. 3. The venogram of the foot of a horse with peracute, severe distal displacement (sinker) of the DP, 2 weeks after contralateral limb injury. The pathology is extensive, and the entire dorsal foot is void of contrast. Vessels are truncated at the coronary band with minimal contrast in the terminal arch and heel. This horse was euthanized.

of the foot is unchanged. However, this is not always true for a laminitic foot; elevating the heel frequently increases the amount of contrast in the dorsal foot (**Fig. 4**). Changes in the palmar angle induce changes in the contrast pattern of the venogram.[17] Often, nonweight-bearing views have areas filled with contrast that were not evident previously. With more severe pathology, even the nonweight-bearing images have contrast voids.

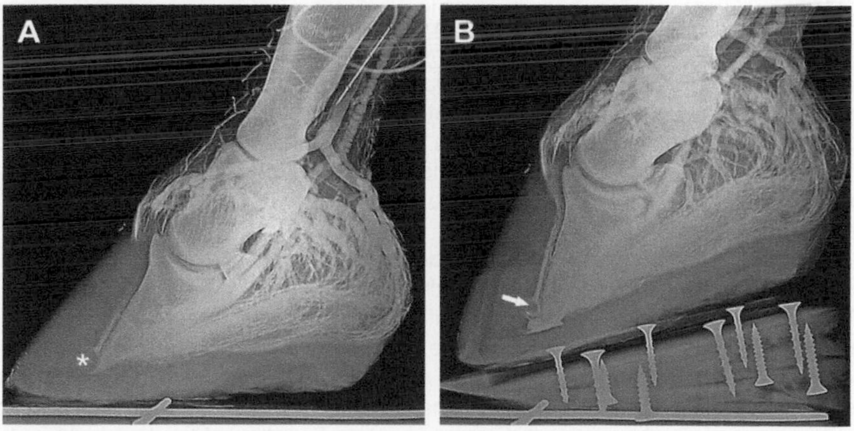

Fig. 4. Heel elevation in the laminitic foot. Laminitis of 11 weeks' duration (*A*) with remodeling of the dorsal and palmar surface of the DP apex. Contrast is absent at the coronary plexus at the level of the extensor process, proximal dorsal lamellae, lamellar-circumflex junction, and the circumflex vessels distal to the dorsal third of the DP. The supply of contrast to the dorsal sublamellar vascular bed is presumably via the DP terminal arch. When the foot is placed in a 20° elevated shoe (Ultimate, Nanric, Versailles, KY, USA), contrast returns to the coronary and dorsal sublamellar vascular bed (*B*). The distal sublamellar plexus is deformed (*arrow*), and corresponds to a zone of compression associated with bone lysis on the distal dorsal cortex of the DP (*asterisk* in *A*). A homogenous area of contrast is evident distal to the DP apex.

CLINICAL APPLICATION

Veterinarians often disagree over treatment of the laminitic horse because in such cases, progress cannot be measured by patient comfort. Using plain-film radiographs, success is indicated by increases in sole depth and continued integrity of the apex of the DP; but these can only be assessed over long periods of time. The venogram can guide treatment and ascertain progress every 3 to 7 days. If the contrast pattern does not improve, either the treatment is not working or pathology has overwhelmed any chance for tissue repair.

In clinical practice, the laminitic patient deteriorates in either of 2 ways. There could be a slow, downward spiral as small amounts of damage accumulate, creating a disaster 4 to 6 weeks after its onset. Alternatively, there could be extensive damage in the first 48 hours in the severe DP-displacement horse. Each has its distinct venogram pattern.

At the onset of cumulative damage laminitis, there is a slight widening of the sublamellar vascular bed. The sole papillae become disoriented and disappear, and the lamellar-circumflex junction is mildly distorted (**Fig. 5**A).

The author's treatment includes therapeutic shoeing, restricted exercise, nonsteroidal antiinflammatory drugs (NSAIDs), and removing the inciting cause of laminitis. The mechanical goals of the shoes are to enhance digital breakover (to relieve strain on the laminae) and increase the palmar angle to 20 degrees (to decrease strain between the DP and the deep flexor tendon).[18] The palmar rim of the DP is parallel to the top of the shoe, therefore load is transferred to the relatively unaffected heel. The venograms are repeated in 3 to 14 days. At that time, the sole papillae should be apparent and the lamellar-circumflex junction should not be distorted. In 10 days, the sole depth should have increased by 2 to 3 mm. If the foot is found as expected, eliminate the NSAIDs, continue exercise restriction and do not alter the shoeing protocol.

If the case has deteriorated, the second venogram has alterations in the appearance of the coronary plexus. As the DP descends into the capsule, the coronary papillae become oriented in a kinked, horizontal direction as they are "pulled" from the proximal hoof wall. The coronary plexus elongates and distorts and gradually decreases in width. Other changes include reduction in proximal dorsal sublamellar contrast, and absence of contrast distal to the dorsal region of the DP (**Fig. 5**B). The lamellar-circumflex junction appears bent or angulated, no longer aligned with the sharp 50° angle of the DP apex (**Fig. 5**C–F).

With further displacement of the apex distal to the circumflex vessels, contrast is absent in the circumflex vasculature and the sole corium (**Fig. 6**A).

Terminal papillae at the lamellar-circumflex junction become horizontal in orientation, and then point slightly dorsal as the junction is further distorted. If treatment does not decompress the sole corium and restore the apex proximal to the circumflex vessels, remodeling of the dorsal and palmar aspects of the DP apex occurs, and sole growth ceases. In some cases, the inappropriate orientation of the terminal papillae results in a horn growth that compresses the dorsal distal aspect of the DP (see **Fig. 4**B).[19]

Displacement of the DP apex distal to the circumflex vessels is an indication to shoe the horse at a 5° palmar angle and perform a deep flexor tenotomy. The venogram is repeated in 14 days, and improvement is expected in the appearance of the lamellar-circumflex junction (**Fig. 6**B).

The cut tendon and restored digital alignment contribute to loading of the palmar processes, lifting the apex from the sole corium. Medial listing of the DP commonly

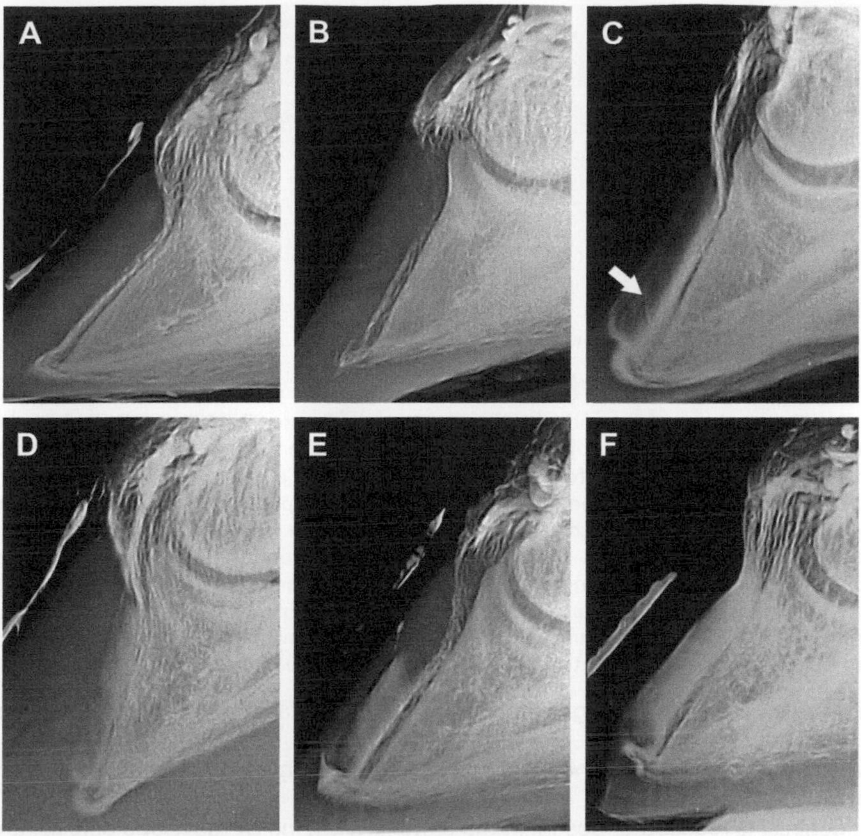

Fig. 5. In acute laminitis (*A*), sole papillae, normally outlined by contrast, are compressed, and the lamellar-circumflex junction is mildly distorted. With further pathology (*B*), the DP apex has descended to the level of the circumflex vessels, the lamellar-circumflex junction is folded, and there is no contrast distal to the DP apex. The coronary plexus is distorted and empty of contrast. The sublamellar vascular bed is widened, and contrast is absent in its proximal third. In more severe chronic laminitis with mild lameness (*C*), the coronary plexus is compressed. A feathering pattern of contrast (*arrow*) between distorted, stretched laminae and dorsal to the sublamellar plexus, denotes laminar instability. The circumflex vessels distal to the DP are compressed, there are no sole papillae, and the foot has poor sole depth. In painful, recrudescent chronic laminitis (*D*), secondary to uncontrolled hyperinsulinemia, the homogeneous appearance of contrast in the dorsal sublamellar vascular bed indicates instability. Coronary papillae are oriented in the plane of the dorsal hoof wall. In severe acute laminitis with distal displacement of the DP (*E*), the coronary plexus is distorted. The distal two-thirds of the sublamellar vascular bed has widened because the dermal and epidermal laminae have separated. The lamellar-circumflex junction has folded and the terminal papillae are at right angles to the dorsal face of P3. The DP apex has descended distal to the circumflex vessels, and contrast is void in the sole corium. Five weeks after initial presentation (*E*) and treatment with shoeing, DDF tenotomy and coronary resection, complete separation of dermal and epidermal laminae is evidenced by the homogeneous contrast in the dorsal sublamellar vascular bed (*F*). The lamellar-circumflex junction has almost returned to its normal location, and some contrast is evident distal to the DP apex. This horse returned to compete as an American saddlebred western pleasure horse. The other forefoot is shown in **Fig. 6**.

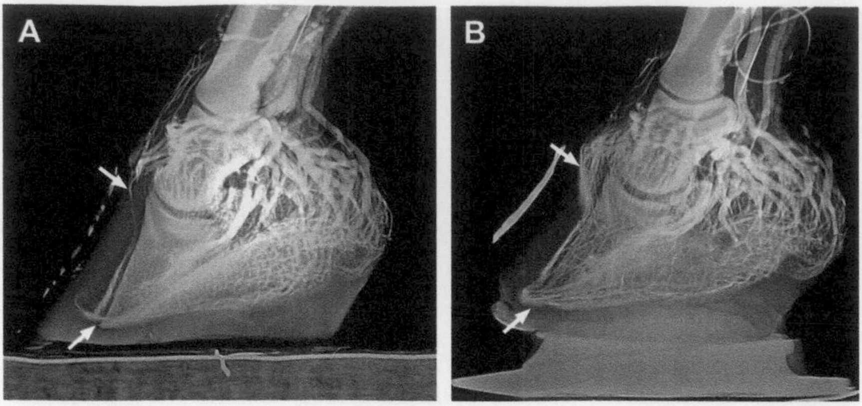

Fig. 6. (*A*) Acute laminitis secondary to equine Cushing disease. The DP apex has descended distal to the circumflex vessels (*arrow*) and contrast is absent distal to the apex (*A*). The lamellar-circumflex junction is folded, the terminal papillae are oriented in a dorsal (horizontal) direction, and a fine line of contrast extends to the periphery of the border where the dermal lamellae joined the epidermal lamellae. The sublamellar vascular bed is widened. The coronary plexus is distorted with reduced contrast (*arrow*), and coronary papillae are absent. A venogram (*B*), 6 weeks post shoeing and deep-digital-flexor tenotomy, shows that contrast has returned to the coronary plexus, and papillae are evident (*arrow*). The DP apex and the lamellar-circumflex junction have returned to a normal orientation (*arrow*). Contrast is slightly reduced distal to the DP palmar processes.

occurs. Lack of contrast filling in the coronary and lamellar corium indicates the need for hoof wall resection.

With severe pathology, contrast is absent in most of the dorsal portion of the hoof capsule (**Fig. 7**).

If contrast is reduced or absent in the terminal arch, the DP develops osteitis, and the long-term prognosis is grave. Even if treatment restores contrast filling of the corium and hoof capsule, the horse cannot survive without a functional terminal

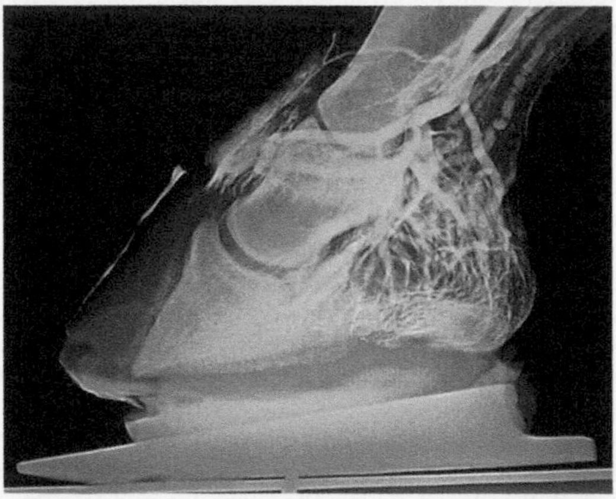

Fig. 7. Severe chronic laminitis. This patient was presented with laminitis of 2 months' duration. Shoeing and a deep-flexor tenotomy had been performed 2 weeks earlier, but there has been no improvement in the venogram and no sole growth. Contrast remains absent at the coronary plexus and distal to the DP. The dorsal sublamellar plexus and terminal arch contain little or no contrast. This venogram indicates a poor prognosis.

arch. In chronic cases of laminitis in which the DP has lysed/remodeled to the terminal arch, the horse is lame, frequently has superficial and deep digital flexor contracture, and suffers chronic draining tracts because of osteitis and soft tissue necrosis (**Fig. 8**).

Chronic hoof-capsule distortion makes it clinically difficult to identify the sources of pain on plain-film radiographs. The various reasons for pain are mechanical strain of digital breakover (especially if the toe is long), loading of the DP apex, sole necrosis, and reduced sole depth due to corium compression, osteitis, and instability of the lamellar tissue. Chronic laminitic cases that are sound have a venographic appearance similar to that of a normal horse, except that there is remodeling of the laminar-circumflex junction around the apex of the DP and some diffusion of contrast into areas of laminar disarray. The coronary papillae are oriented in the plane of the distorted dorsal-hoof wall and are no longer parallel to the dorsal face of the DP.[20] If chronic laminitic hooves do not have strong laminar attachments, the horse is usually mild to moderately lame. Contrast diffuses throughout the sublamellar corium, and the contrast in the circumflex and sole corium is reduced (see **Fig. 5**C). If a chronic laminitic horse has an acute episode of laminitis, the contrast pattern may appear similar to that of an acute case, even though the wall is greatly distorted by the lamellar wedge (see **Fig. 5**D).

When distal displacement of the DP occurs rapidly, a rectangular widening of the sublamellar vascular bed is apparent on the venogram (see **Fig. 5**E) before initial plain-film evidence of laminitis. A line of contrast delineates the original location of the peripheral margins of the dermal lamellae. An increase in dorsal wall thickness develops over several days (a 5-year-old light-breed horse's normal horn-lamellar zone of 15 mm increases to a thickness of more than 18 mm). If the dermal and epidermal laminae are completely separated, the sublamellar vascular bed appears as a homogeneous zone of contrast (see **Fig. 5**F). With further pathology, the entire foot is void of contrast (see **Fig. 3**). Vessels are truncated at the coronary band, with minimal contrast in the terminal arch and heel. This contrast pattern can occur within 24 hours of laminitis that develops secondary to metritis and within 7 days of contralateral limb load induced laminitis. Survival is enhanced if distal displacement

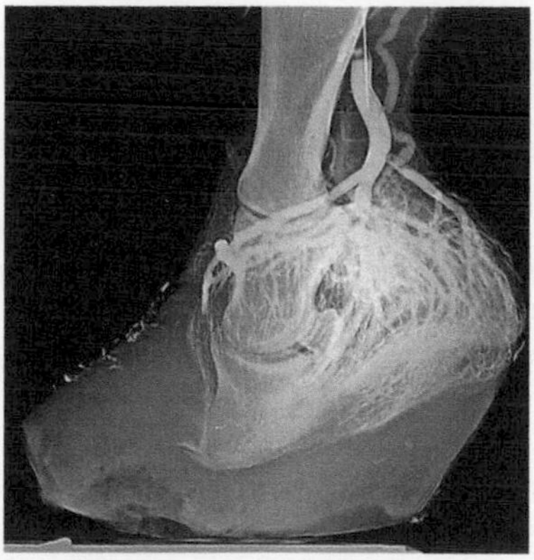

Fig. 8. Chronic laminitis with osteitis and bone resorption exposing the terminal arch. This lame foot has a sole depth of 23 mm and chronic osteitis of the DP. The palmar angle is 30°, and the pastern is vertical, secondary to contracture of the superficial and deep-digital-flexor tendons. Contrast is reduced in the coronary plexus, terminal arch, and circumflex vessels. There is diffuse contrast in the sublamellar vascular bed, and the lamellar-circumflex junction is repositioned around the fractured DP apex. The coronary plexus is elongated, and the papillae are oriented in the plane of the dorsal hoof wall.

of the DP is recognized within 24 to 48 hours of its development and treated aggressively. The author performs a deep digital flexor tenotomy, with or without transfixation pin casting of the limb, and total wall resection.

ACKNOWLEDGMENTS

The author wishes to thank her mentor, Dr Ric Redden, for teaching her these techniques. The author also conveys her thanks to Howard Wilson for help with the formatting of the digital images.

REFERENCES

1. Redden RF. The use of venograms as a diagnostic tool. In: Proceedings. Bluegrass Laminitis Symposium. Lexington (KY); 1993. p.1–6.
2. Redden RF. A technique for performing digital venography in the standing horse. Equine Vet Educ 2001;3(3):172–8.
3. Rucker A, Redden RF, Arthur EG, et al. How to perform the digital venogram. In: Proceedings. Am Assoc Equine Pract. San Antonio (TX), 2006; (52). p. 526–30.
4. Earl N, Wilson DA, Rucker A. Evaluation of the affects on vasculature perfusion in the equine hoof caused by corrective shoeing with a wedged heel using digital venography. University of Missouri-Columbia, MU Chapter of Phi Zeta-Poster Presentation. Columbia, 2004.
5. Baldwin G. Retrograde venous angiography (venography) of the equine digit during experimentally induced laminitis. In: Proceedings. International Equine Conference on Laminitis and Diseases of the Foot. Palm Beach (FL), November 4–6, 2005;(3). p. 359–60.
6. Arthur E, Rucker A. The use of digital venography for assessment of perfusion deficits in chronic laminitis. In: Proceedings. International Equine Conference on Laminitis and Diseases of the Foot. Palm Beach (FL), November 10–11, 2003;(2). p. 319.
7. Rucker A. The digital venogram. In: Floyd AD, Mansmann RA, editors. Equine podiatry. St Louis (MO): Saunders; 2007. p. 328–46.
8. Lyle BE. Venography as a tool for guiding surgery to the foot. In: Floyd AD, Mansmann RA, editors. Equine podiatry. St Louis (MO): Saunders; 2007. p. 284–93.
9. Rucker A. Key points of the digital venogram. In: Proceedings. 16th Bluegrass Laminitis Symposium. Lexington (KY), January 16–18, 2003. p. 105–09.
10. Rucker A. Aspects of the normal digital venogram: anatomy, parameters and variations. In: Proceedings. 16th Bluegrass Laminitis Symposium. Lexington (KY), January 16–18, 2003. p. 27–32.
11. Rucker A. Interpreting venograms: normal or abnormal and artifacts that may be misinterpreted. In: Proceedings. 16th Bluegrass Laminitis Symposium. Lexington (KY), January 16–18, 2003. p. 97–101.
12. Redden RF. Using venograms in laminitic cases. In: Proceedings. Dr. Redden's in-depth podiatry symposium. Versailles (France), January 16–18, 2009. p. 46–55.
13. Floyd AD. An approach to the treatment of the laminitic horse. In: Floyd AD, Mansmann RA, editors. Equine podiatry. St Louis (MO): Saunders; 2007. p. 347–58.
14. Hunt RJ. Equine laminitis: practical clinical considerations. In: Proceedings. Am Assoc Equine Pract. San Diego (CA), 2008;(54). p. 347–53.
15. Redden RF. Possible therapeutic value of digital venography in two laminitic horses. Equine Vet Educ 2001;13(3):128–34.

16. Hertsch B, Madeiczyk V. Diagnostic results of the angiographic and micro-angiographic examination of the digit of horses with acute and chronic laminitis. In: Proceedings. International Laminitis Symposium. Berlin (Germany), November 11–13, 2008.
17. D'Arpe L, Moreau X, Coppola LM, et al. Equine digital venogram in relation to the biomechanics of the foot. In: Proceedings. International Laminitis Symposium. Berlin (Germany), November 11–13, 2008.
18. Lochner FK, Milne DW, Mills EJ, et al. In vivo and in vitro measurement of tendon strain in the horse. Am J Vet Res 1980;41(12):1929–37.
19. Pollitt C, van Eps AW. Present state of research on chronic laminitis. In: Proceedings. International Laminitis Symposium. Berlin (Germany), November 11–13, 2008.
20. Geyer H. Microscopic changes in hooves with laminitis. In: Proceedings. International Laminitis Symposium. Berlin (Germany), November 11–13, 2008.

The Lamellar Wedge

Simon N. Collins, PhD[a,*], Andrew W. van Eps, BVSc, PhD[b], Christopher C. Pollitt, BVSc, PhD[b,c], Atsutoshi Kuwano, DVM, PhD[d]

KEYWORDS

- Laminitis • Suspensory apparatus of the distal phalanx
- Distal phalanx • Stratum lamellatum

OVERVIEW

Lamellar (laminar) wedge formation is a pathognomonic sequela of progression into chronic-phase laminitis after dislocation of the distal phalanx (DP).[1–4] This anatomic feature (**Fig. 1**), which is evident in gross anatomic sagittal section as a wedge-shaped structure, is referred to as lamellar thickening.[5] The term lamellar wedge is used to describe the pathologic tissues that compose the lamellar region (stratum lamellatum) of the chronic laminitic foot. The lamellar wedge results from abnormal hoof horn production after lamellar damage. This pathologic horn has been variably described as scar horn[2] or a second[3] or ectopic[6] white line. Lamellar wedge formation maintains the functional integrity of the foot. However, the structural organization and material characteristics of this pathologic tissue is inferior to that of the unaffected foot, compromising normal foot biomechanics.[1,2,7]

The histologic appearance of the lamellar wedge varies considerably among individuals.[1,2,8] This difference in appearance is thought to relate directly to disease severity within the affected foot, reflecting the degree of lamellar degeneration and subsequent regeneration and the progression of these processes over time. Understanding the pathologic and pathomechanical processes associated with lamellar wedge formation is needed to ensure that effective supportive foot management is instigated to aid in recovery and return to previous performance levels.

PATHOGENESIS OF THE LAMELLAR WEDGE

Disease progression into chronic-phase laminitis is characterized by mechanical failure of the suspensory apparatus of the distal phalanx (SADP).[1–4,9] The SADP unites

[a] Orthopaedic Research Group, Centre for Equine Studies, Animal Health Trust, Lanwades Park, Kentford, Newmarket, Suffolk, CB8 7UU, UK
[b] Australian Equine Laminitis Research Unit, The School of Veterinary Science, The University of Queensland, Brisbane 4072, Australia
[c] The Laminitis Institute, University of Pennsylvania School of Veterinary Medicine, New Bolton Center, Kennett Square, PA, USA
[d] Clinical Sciences and Pathobiology Division, Sports Science Research Centre, Equine Research Institute, Japan Racing Association, Utsunomiya-shi, Tochigi 320-0856, Japan
* Corresponding author.
E-mail address: SIMON.COLLINS@aht.org.uk

Vet Clin Equine 26 (2010) 179–195
doi:10.1016/j.cveq.2010.01.004

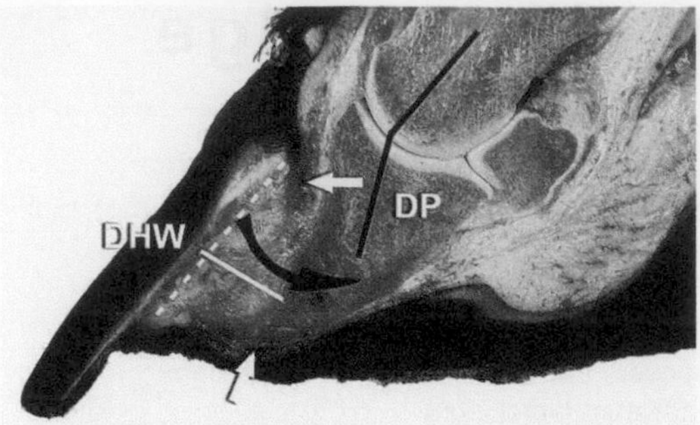

Fig. 1. Sagittal section of a foot with severe chronic laminitis showing presence of a large lamellar wedge. The attachment between the DP and the dorsal hoof wall (DHW) has failed, and hoof and bone are now widely separated. The dotted line shows the original position of the DP. The solid black line shows that the DP has rotated around the distal interphalangeal joint (*in the direction of the curved black arrow*) and is no longer in alignment with the pastern axis (longitudinal axis of the proximal and middle phalanges [phalangeal rotation]). The material now between the inner aspect of the hoof wall and the DP is abnormal and consists of hyperplastic epidermal tissue, which forms a weak, pathologic structure called the lamellar wedge (*yellow line*). The distal descent of the unsupported DP within the hoof capsule has affected the normal alignment of the dermal papillae, resulting in distorted growth of the proximal hoof wall tubules, and has caused the sole to become convex instead of concave (dropped sole). Two dark hemorrhagic zones (*white arrows*) show the sites of greatest pressure and trauma.

the DP and the hoof wall via the lamellar dermis and suspends the appendicular skeleton within the hoof capsule. The SADP is of major biomechanical importance because it enables these structures to act as a single functional entity to facilitate pain-free force transference between ground and skeleton.[1,2,4] This anatomic arrangement is unique to the ungulate foot, and in the horse, it constitutes the principle mechanism by which weight-bearing forces are accommodated and resisted.[9–12]

SADP damage due to laminitis directly affects this force transference process and results in excessive levels of DP movement within the affected foot during weight bearing.[1] This excess DP movement leads to increased levels of imposed strain and vascular damage within the lamellar and sublamellar dermis, which further compromise the SADP. Ultimately, these processes exceed the mechanical limits of the structure and lead to SADP failure.[1,2,4,9,13] Failure of the SADP results in permanent dislocation of the DP because damage to the lamellar interface is so extensive that the SADP can no longer maintain the normal anatomic relationship between the hoof capsule, dermis, and DP.[1,2,4] This dislocation, which has been described as structural failure and digital collapse,[2] leads to irreversible change of the anatomic interrelationships within the foot. These events collectively compromise normal biomechanical function during weight bearing, resulting in stance and gait alterations and debilitating foot pain.[1,2,4]

DP dislocation initiates several distinct reactive pathologies that further compromise foot function and alter the normal pattern of hoof horn production.[2,4,14] Most notable is the formation of the lamellar wedge. However, despite the pathologic and functional consequences associated with SADP failure, little is known of the specific etiopathophysiologic mechanisms that lead to its formation.

Considerable variation in the gross anatomic and histologic appearance of the lamellar wedge is reported.[2,3,8] This presumably reflects the severity of the underlying lamellar pathology, disease duration, and the progressive nature of the pathologic

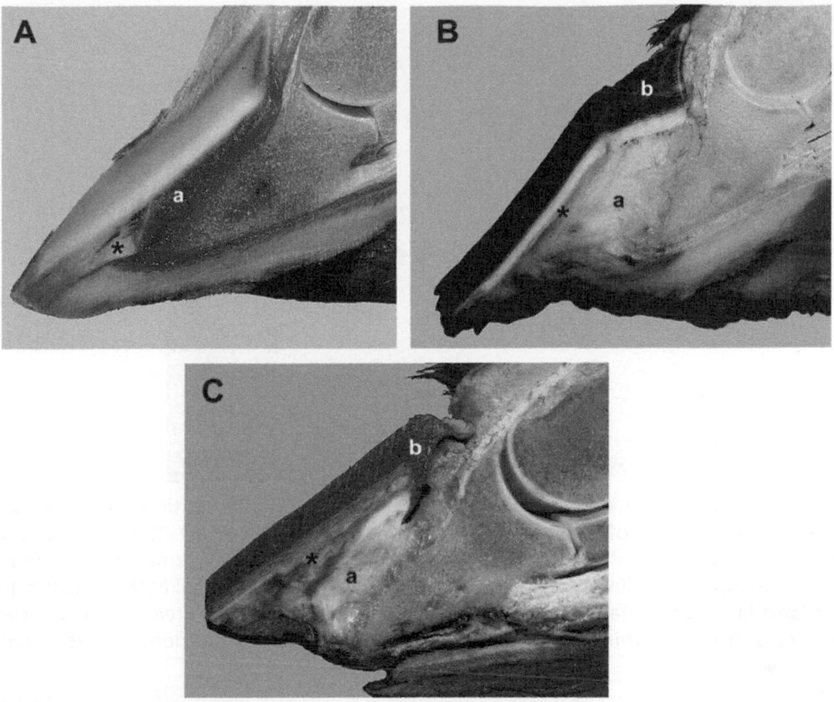

Fig. 2. Gross anatomic sections of the midline of the chronic laminitic foot showing the variable nature of lamellar wedge formation within the affected foot. (*A*) Modest changes with minimal epidermal dysplasia and keratinization within the lamellar wedge (a), apart from slight dysplasia occurring immediately proximal to the white line (*asterisk*). The lamellar wedge appears to be formed primarily of expanded dermal tissue. There is no visible distortion to the coronary papillae, and the orientation of hoof wall growth is unaffected, although the coronary dermis appears to be compressed between the hoof wall and the extensor process of the DP. There is no evidence of physical separation of the lamellar interface, and there is an absence of transudate/exudate within the dorsal region of the lamellar wedge. (*B*) Marked epidermal dysplasia and keratinization within the lamellar wedge (a), and a pronounced yellow horn mass (*asterisk*) indicating transudate/exudate formation after vascular trauma associated with physical lamellar separation. Note the disruption to the normal pattern of hoof horn production proximally (b) indicating reorientation of the coronary papillae associated with rotational dislocation of the DP. (*C*) Extensive epidermal dysplasia and ectopic white line formation within the lamellar wedge (a) along with extensive transudate/exudate formation throughout the keratinized lamellar wedge (*asterisk*) associated with vascular trauma. Note the pronounced distortion to the normal pattern of hoof horn growth within the hoof wall proximally. This is accompanied by physical separation along the coronary interface (shear lesion), with granulation tissue formation within the coronary dermis.

processes (degenerative and regenerative) that contribute to its formation over time. The appearance of the lamellar wedge is also affected by the success or failure of treatments aimed at stabilizing the DP, restoring the soft tissue and vascular deficits seen in the lamellar dermis by retrograde venograms and protecting any remaining regions of unaffected lamellae.[1]

Lamellar pathology initiated in acute phase laminitis can eventually lead to SADP failure. When SADP damage is minimal, the resultant lamellar wedge is characterized

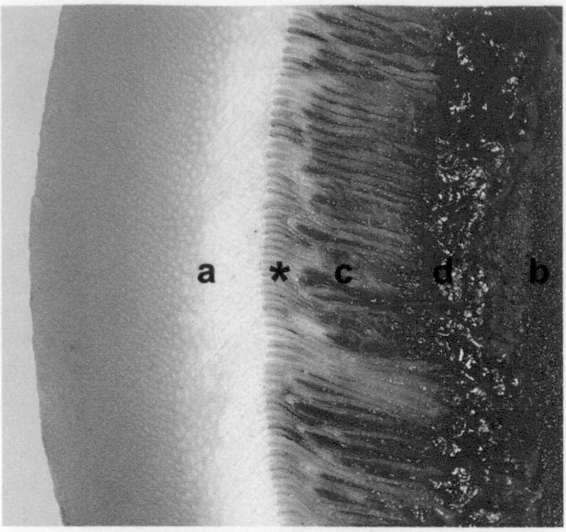

Fig. 3. Transverse section of the lamellar region of a chronic laminitic foot showing the macroscopic appearance of the lamellar wedge (hoof wall [a], DP [b]). The lamellar wedge displays extensive physical lamellar separation and dysplastic epidermal horn formation within the ectopic white line of the lamellar wedge (c); yellow material at the dorsal margin of the lamellar interface (*asterisk*) indicates the presence of transudate/exudate associated with vascular trauma within the lamellar circulation. The sublamellar dermis (d) is widened.

by elongation and attenuation of the normal lamellar architecture (**Fig. 2**A).[2,4] Conversely, when SADP damage is severe and extensive, physical separation occurs along the lamellar interface (**Fig. 2**B, C), characterized by lamellar fragmentation and a permanent reduction in the surface area of attachment.[1,15] In these severe cases, in which the resultant DP dislocation is pronounced, vascular trauma can occur, leading to fluid accumulation (sometimes referred to as a seroma) within the area of lamellar separation.[16] This fluid accumulation is usually seen between the apical tips of the primary dermal lamellae (**Fig. 3**) and the basal region of the primary epidermal lamellae (adjacent to the inner hoof wall). This zone can, occasionally, be discerned as a mild, linear reduction in radiopacity along the dermoepidermal junction on lateromedial radiographic views optimized for soft tissue visualization.[1]

Progressive lamellar separation and inspissation of the fluid results in the appearance of a radiolucent gasline (**Fig. 4**A, B) in a lateromedial radiographic view[1,4,14,16,17] (also referred to as a type 2 airline) or a series of fine, near-parallel radiolucent lines in the dorsopalmar radiographic view (**Fig. 4**C).[1] The appearance of radiolucency indicates that extensive lamellar separation has occurred within the affected foot. Urgent supportive foot management is therefore required to stabilize the foot, to protect the surviving lamellae from further mechanical failure, and to avert progressive DP dislocation.[1]

In the initial stages, the gasline rarely communicates with the exterior of the hoof capsule; however, with continued proximodistal hoof growth, the gasline moves distally and eventually becomes evident at the weight-bearing border of the foot, providing a potential portal for secondary, opportunistic bacterial and fungal infection.[1,2,17] The appearance of the gasline coincides with abnormal hoof horn production within the lamellar region. Epidermal tissues proliferate (**Fig. 5**) as part of a wound healing mechanism aimed at restoring the physical and mechanical integrity of the SADP.[1,6] It is suggested that physical separation removes the contact inhibition that normally limits and regulates mitotic activity within the basal keratinocytes of the

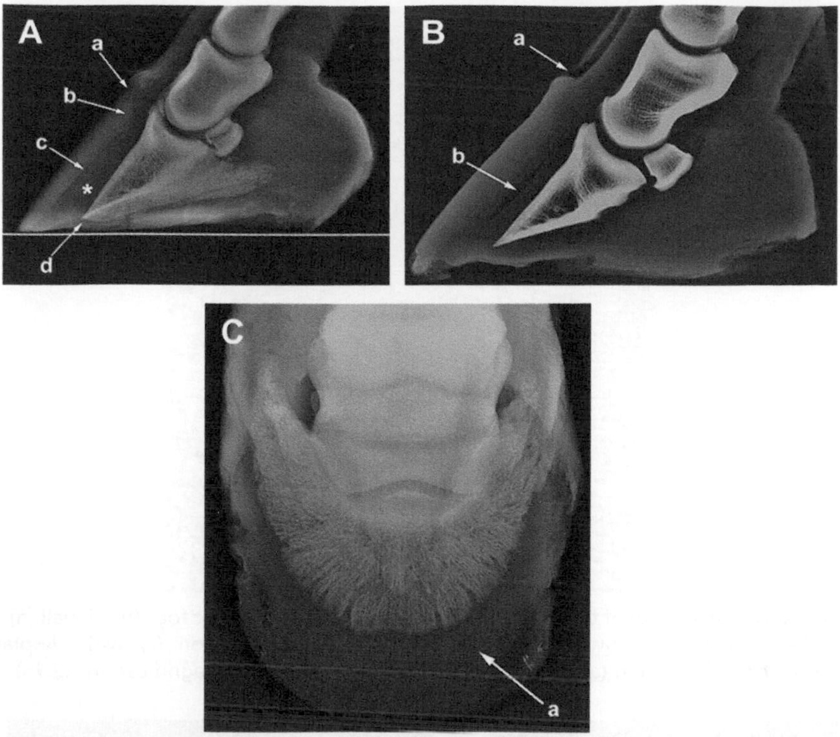

Fig. 4. (*A*) Lateromedial radiograph of a chronic laminitic foot showing a visible and palpable supracoronary depression (a) and compression and distortion of the coronary dermis between the hoof wall and the extensor process (b) after distal displacement of the DP. A visible radiolucent gasline (c) provides evidence of failure of the SADP and physical separation of the dermal and epidermal lamellae. The dislocation of the DP has resulted in lamellar wedge formation (*asterisk*) and penetration of the apex of the bone into the solear dermis (d). Note the modeling of the dorsodistal region of the DP and the associated loss of cortical bone density. (*B*) Thin-section radiograph of the midline of a chronic laminitic foot showing a pronounced supracoronary depression (a) after downward dislocation of the DP. A pronounced radiolucent gasline (b) indicates extensive failure of the SADP and physical separation of the dermal and epidermal lamellae extending distally from the coronary band. (*C*) Dorsopalmar radiograph of a chronic laminitic foot seen in **Fig. 2**B showing a fine near-parallel array of radiolucent lines (a), indicating failure of the SADP and physical separation of the dermal and epidermal lamellae. Note the asymmetric nature of the separation from the dorsal aspect toward the heels.

epidermal lamellae.[18] In the absence of contact inhibition, hyperplastic lamellar and tubular horn proliferation occurs, leading to abnormal, submural horn production (**Figs. 6** and **7**).[1–4,6,18,19]

The resultant dysplastic horn structure (**Fig. 8**) has been described as ectopic white line,[6] because the histologic appearance (a lamellated array of tubular and nontubular horn) resembles that of the white line, the sole-hoof wall junction, seen in the distal part of the hoof capsule. This ectopic white line occupies the space that results from the separation of the apex of the dermal lamellae and the adjoining bases of epidermal lamellae. Progressive dislocation of the DP is associated with the expansion of the lamellar wedge characterized by elongation and attenuation of the stratum lamellatum and epidermal hyperplasia within the primary and secondary lamellae (**Fig. 9**).[2,4,6]

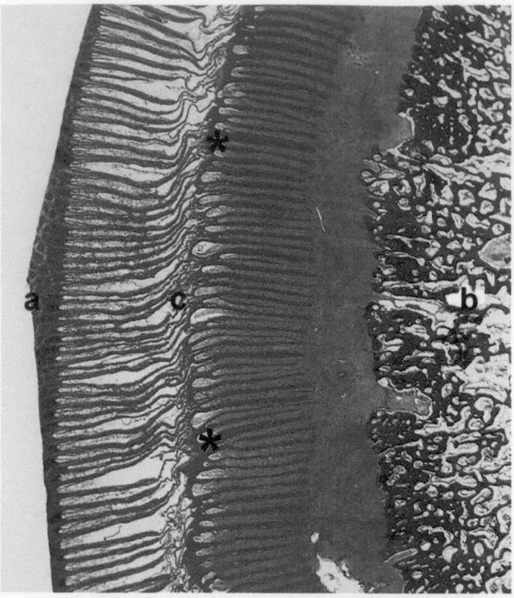

Fig. 5. Transverse section of the lamellar region of a chronic laminitic foot (hoof wall [a], DP [b]). The micrograph shows marked physical lamellar separation (c) with dysplastic epidermal horn formation (*asterisk*) (hematoxylin-eosin, original magnification ×2.75).

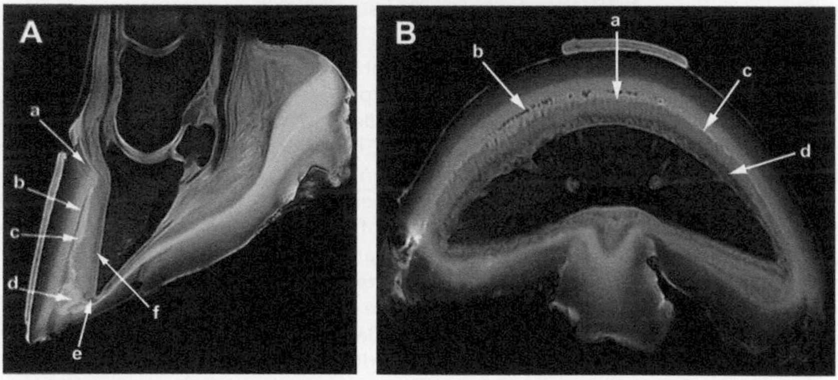

Fig. 6. (*A*) High-resolution sagittal 3-dimensional (3D) fat-saturated T1 spoiled gradient recalled (SPGR) magnetic resonance (MR) image of a chronic laminitic foot showing the following: (a) distortion of the proximal hoof wall; (b) linear hypointense MR feature at the dorsal margin of the lamellar interface, indicating lamellar separation; (c) development of the ectopic white line of the lamellar wedge (high MR signal intensity within the lamellar interface, indicating epidermal dysplasia and lamellar separation) and widened sublamellar dermis (moderate MR signal intensity); (d) distal expansion and inward encroachment of the dysplastic epidermal tissues; (e) circumflex junction of the lamellar and solear plexuses; (f) lamellar plexus (hypointense MR signal) within the sublamellar dermis. (*B*) High-resolution transverse 3D fat-saturated T1 SPGR MR image of a chronic laminitic foot showing (a) hyperintense MR signal of the ectopic white line of the lamellar wedge, indicating lamellar separation and epidermal dysplasia; (b) curvilinear hypointense MR signal of the airline after extensive lamellar separation; (c) hyperintense MR signal, indicating the presence of transudate/exudate within the region of lamellar separation, indicating vascular trauma within the lamellar circulation; (d) lamellar plexus within the expanded sublamellar dermis.

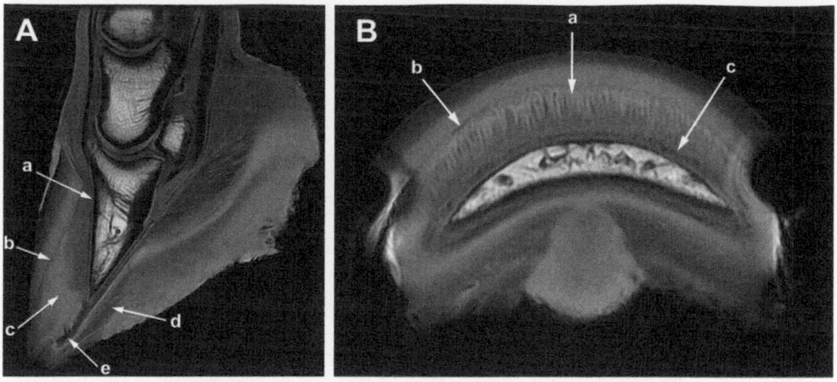

Fig. 7. (*A*) High-resolution sagittal 3D T1 SPGR MR image of a chronic laminitic foot showing (a) angular deviation between the dorsal surface of the hoof wall (viewed proximally) and the dorsal aspect of the DP; (b) extensive development of ectopic white line of the lamellar wedge (high MR signal intensity within the lamellar interface, indicating epidermal dysplasia and lamellar separation) and the widened sublamellar dermis proximally (moderate MR signal intensity); (c) linear hypointense feature at dorsal margin of the lamellar interface, indicating lamellar separation and/or vascular trauma; (d) double (false) sole; (e) track of solear abscessation passing through the widened white line at the hoof wall–sole junction. (*B*) High-resolution transverse 3D T1 SPGR MR image of a chronic laminitic foot showing (a) extensive development of the ectopic white line of the lamellar wedge (high MR signal intensity, indicating lamellar separation and epidermal dysplasia within the lamellar interface); (b) curvilinear hypointense MR feature at dorsal margin of the lamellar interface, indicating extensive lamellar separation; (c) lamellar plexus within the widened sublamellar dermis.

The precise pathogenic processes that cause metaplastic cap horn production are poorly defined. Wound healing mechanisms are thought to induce peripheral basal keratinocyte invagination from adjacent secondary epidermal lamellae into the apical region of affected dermal lamellae (**Fig. 10**).[9] These invaginations eventually unite to

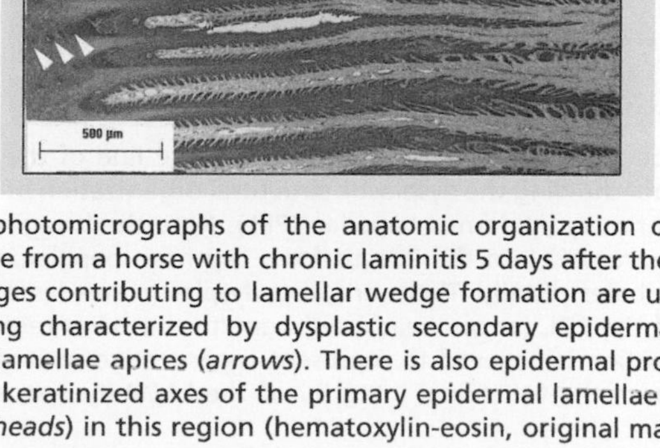

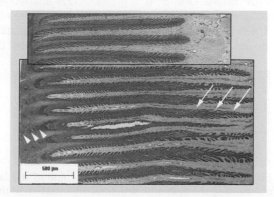

Fig. 8. Transverse photomicrographs of the anatomic organization of normal lamellae (*above*) and lamellae from a horse with chronic laminitis 5 days after the onset of lameness (*below*). Early changes contributing to lamellar wedge formation are underway, including lamellar lengthening characterized by dysplastic secondary epidermal lamellae at the primary epidermal lamellae apices (*arrows*). There is also epidermal proliferation adjacent to the bases of the keratinized axes of the primary epidermal lamellae and the formation of cap horn (*arrowheads*) in this region (hematoxylin-eosin, original magnification ×10).

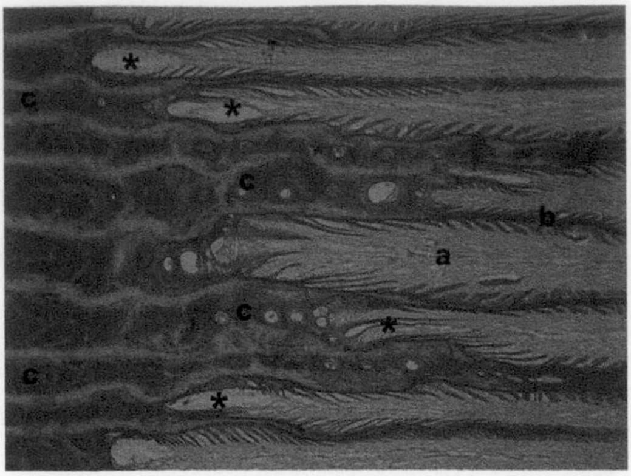

Fig. 9. Transverse photomicrographs of the ectopic white line of the lamellar wedge in a chronic laminitic foot showing disruption of normal regular anatomic organization of the dermal (a) and epidermal (b) lamellae. Note the elongation and attenuation of the secondary epidermal lamellae, separation of the lamellar interface adjacent to the base of the primary epidermal lamellae (*asterisk*), and marked development of dysplastic cap horn tubules (c). Collectively these changes contribute to the formation of the ectopic white line (hematoxylin-eosin, original magnification ×45).

form a series of dermal papillae (**Fig. 11**). Subsequent hyperproliferative hoof horn production, supported by these cap horn papillae, produces metaplastic cap horn tubules and intertubular arcades (**Fig. 12**). This abnormal ectopic horn production can ultimately fill the region of submural lamellar separation.[15] Hence, over time, the radiolucent zone may decrease in size, and in some cases, it can become completely filled by this aberrant hoof horn. This can be seen in gross section as a linear region of yellow abnormal horn, with or without the presence of hemorrhage, immediately adjacent to the inner aspect of the hoof wall.[6] Presumably, the yellow coloration of this horn mass, and indeed the associated hemorrhage that may be evident, relates to the initial phase of vascular trauma, transudate/exudate fluid accumulation, and inspissation after SADP failure. Over time, a gross wedge-shaped feature is formed in sagittal view as progressive capsular rotation occurs within the affected foot (see **Figs. 2**B, C and **3**). These changes may become evident as a progressive dorsopalmar widening of the white line on the solear aspect of the trimmed hoof capsule.[6,16,18]

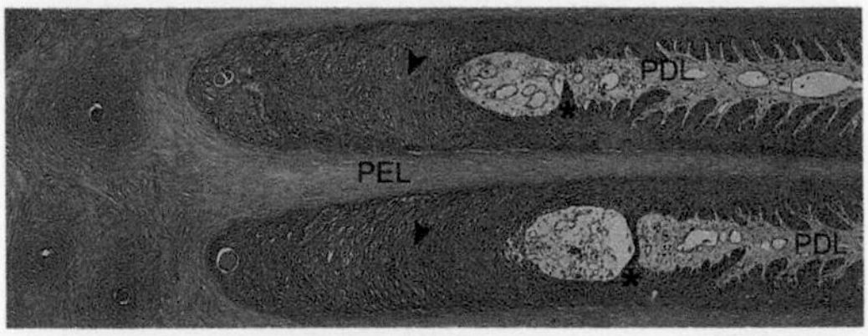

Fig. 10. Transverse photomicrographs of the ectopic white line of the lamellar wedge of a chronic laminitic foot showing the dysplastic structural organization of the primary dermal lamellae (PDL) and primary epidermal lamellae (PEL). Note the invagination of secondary epidermal lamellae (*asterisk*) into the PDL to form cap horn papillae, which are believed to form cap horn tubules distally. There are also dysplastic arcades of cap horn present within the apices of the PDL (*arrow heads*) adjacent to the basal region of the PEL. This dysplastic horn formation is believed to represent regenerative wound healing responses that attempt to restore the functional integrity of the SADP (hematoxylin-eosin, original magnification ×60).

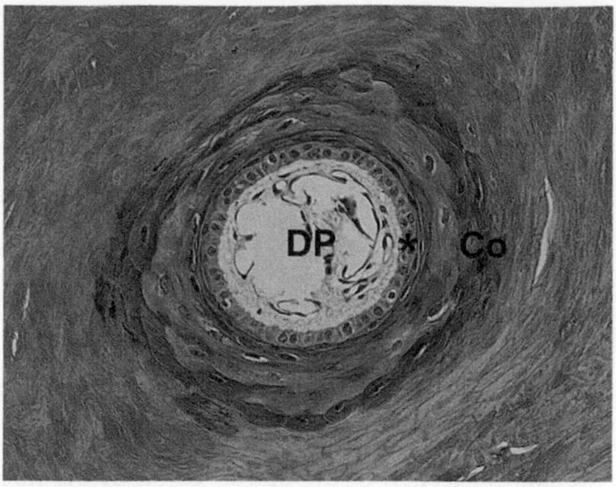

Fig. 11. Transverse photomicrograph of a dysplastic cap horn papillae within the ectopic white line of the lamellar wedge of a chronic laminitic foot formed by invagination of the secondary epidermal lamellae into the primary dermal lamellae (see **Fig. 13**). Basal epidermal cells (*asterisk*) surround the dermal cap horn papillae (DP) and the cortical cells of the resultant cap horn tubule (Co) at variable stages of keratinization (hematoxylin-eosin, original magnification ×200).

TEMPORAL DEVELOPMENT OF THE LAMELLAR WEDGE

Retrospective assessment of the gross morphometric characteristics of the lamellar wedge[6] (including proximodistal extent and cross-sectional area in the sagittal plane) suggests a marked and progressive expansion in the first 28 days after SADP failure. In the first 7 to 10 days, epidermal hyperproliferation can fill the areas of lamellar separation, thereby restoring, to varying degrees, the structural integrity of the SADP. During the next 26 days, there is rapid expansion of the wedge as DP dislocation progresses. At 36 days, dorsopalmar widening of the white line may become apparent.

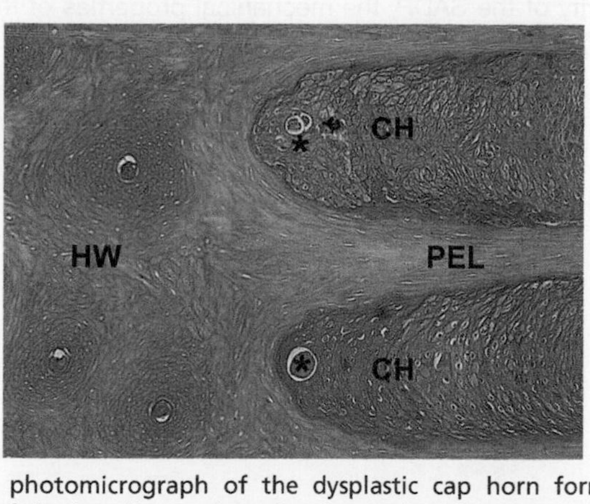

Fig. 12. Transverse photomicrograph of the dysplastic cap horn formation within the ectopic white line of the lamellar wedge of a chronic laminitic foot. There are arcades of cap horn present within the apical region of the primary dermal lamellae (CH) adjacent to the basal region of the primary epidermal lamellae (PEL) on the inner aspect of the hoof wall (HW). There are also small cap horn tubules (*asterisk*) present within these arcades, which are generated proximally from cap horn papillae formed by epidermal invagination of secondary epidermal lamellae into the primary dermal lamellae (see **Fig. 10**) (hematoxylin-eosin, original magnification ×60).

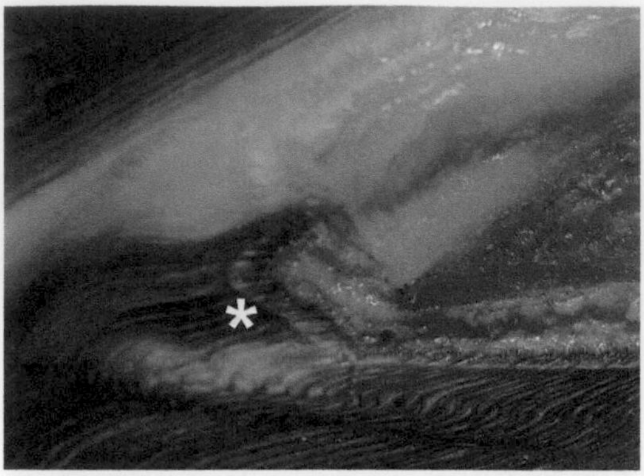

Fig. 13. Gross anatomic sagittal section of the apical region of the hoof at the midline of a chronic laminitic foot showing displacement of the solear dermis around the apex of the dislocated DP and the resultant distortion to the normal pattern of sole horn formation. This reorientation results in an inward growing mass of sole horn (*asterisk*).

These findings are consistent with other studies that have reported hyperproliferative wound healing responses within the stratum lamellatum after hoof wall stripping in the normal horse[19] and lamellar histopathology 7 days after experimental induction of laminitis.[20] Consistent with the histologic findings seen in 7-day laminitis is the aberrant nature of the resultant horn production and the abnormal lamellar architecture. Presumably, this relates to the loss of normal basement membrane organization during the acute phase of the disease, which precludes restoration of a normal lamellar structure within the affected foot.

BIOMECHANICAL CONSEQUENCE OF LAMELLAR WEDGE FORMATION

Although these hyperproliferative processes progressively restore, to varying degrees, the physical integrity of the SADP, the mechanical properties of the lamellar wedge

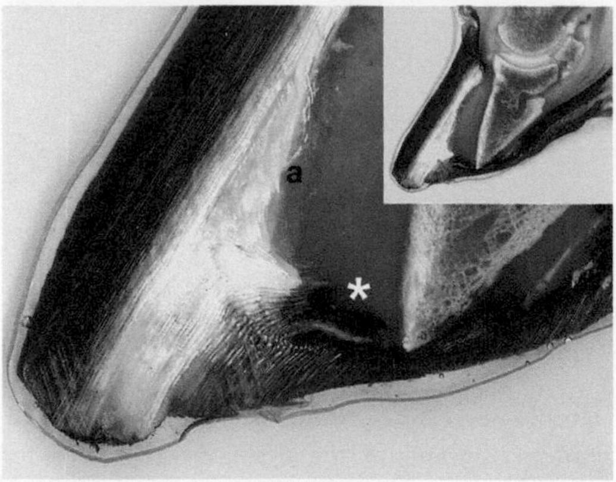

Fig. 14. Thin ground anatomic section of the apical region of the hoof at the midline of the chronic laminitic foot showing the inward growing mass of sole horn formed by reorientation of the solear dermis around the apex of the displaced DP (*asterisk*). This inward growing mass of sole horn is confined by the dysplastic ectopic white line of the lamellar wedge (a) and thereby encroaches on the apex of the DP. (*Courtesy of* Dr K.-D. Budras, Freie University, Berlin.)

differ significantly from that of the stratum lamellatum of the unaffected horse.[2,7] Hence the ability of the SADP of the laminitic horse to withstand the mechanical demands of weight bearing is reduced. These changes are of clinical importance because they directly affect the recovery prospects of the horse and limit return to previous performance levels. In particular, studies have shown that the rigidity of the regenerated SADP in the affected horse is significantly lower than that in the unaffected horse,[2,7] which results in increased movement of the DP during loading, causing mandatory solear weight bearing. This solear weight bearing can lead to vascular trauma and occlusion within the solear dermis of the foot. In addition, the failure strength of the SADP is reduced by up to 58%,[2,7] leaving the affected horse susceptible to recrudescent traumatic injury to the regenerated SADP.[1,2] These factors collectively contribute to the degree of locomotor impairment associated with chronic laminitis.

Various studies indicate an associative link between the size of the lamellar wedge and return to previous performance levels, with the likelihood of a successful return reducing as size of the lamellar wedge increases.[21,22] It has therefore been common treatment practice to resect the dorsal hoof wall and pare back the lamellar wedge. However, empiric evidence suggests variable success from this treatment approach. Another study[7] concluded a direct association between the material properties of the lamellar wedge and treatment success and suggested that these properties were critical in determining stability within the affected foot.

HIDDEN DANGERS: PATHOLOGIC CONSEQUENCES OF DP DISLOCATION

In cases in which DP dislocation causes minimal disturbance to the alignment of the coronary and solear dermis, conservative foot management can, over time, result in a near-normal recovery of the hoof capsule, as proximodistal hoof growth regenerates the hoof capsule. However, there are also specific hidden dangers associated with DP dislocation, which are only now being recognized fully.[1,4] These hidden dangers

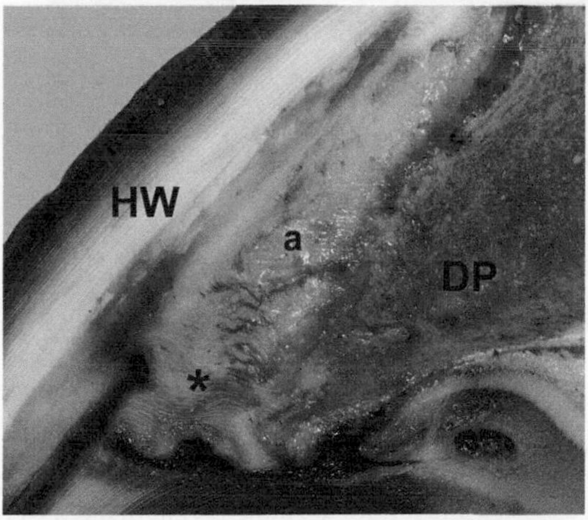

Fig. 15. Gross anatomic section of the apical region of the hoof at the midline of the chronic laminitic foot showing extreme degenerative changes to the normal anatomic organization of the foot after displacement of the solear dermis around the apex of the DP. The resultant sole horn production forms an inward growing mass that is confined by the hoof wall (HW) dorsally and the dysplastic ectopic white line of the lamellar wedge (a) proximally and encroaches directly on the apex of the DP.

prevent hoof capsule restoration without intervention. In particular, the solear dermis may become distorted around the distal margin of the DP, causing a reorientation of the dermal papillae in this region (**Fig. 13**).[1,4,10,11] This distortion changes the direction of sole horn production and leads to the development of an ingrowing mass of horn (**Figs. 14** and **15**).[1,4] This ingrowing horn mass progressively impinges on the lamellar dermis distally. Likewise, the horn mass impinges on the apex of the DP, leading to focal bone loss and modeling (**Fig. 16**).[1,4] In extreme cases, the progressive hyperproliferation of the lamellar wedge encroaches on the distodorsal aspect of the DP, leading to extensive bone lysis (**Fig. 17**) (see the article by Julie B. Engiles elsewhere in this issue for further exploration of this topic).[1,4]

DP dislocation can also result in elongation and encroachment of the coronary dermis into the lamellar dermis proximally.[1–4,23,24] Collectively, these pathologic processes distort the normal ordered lamellar array and decrease the proximodistal

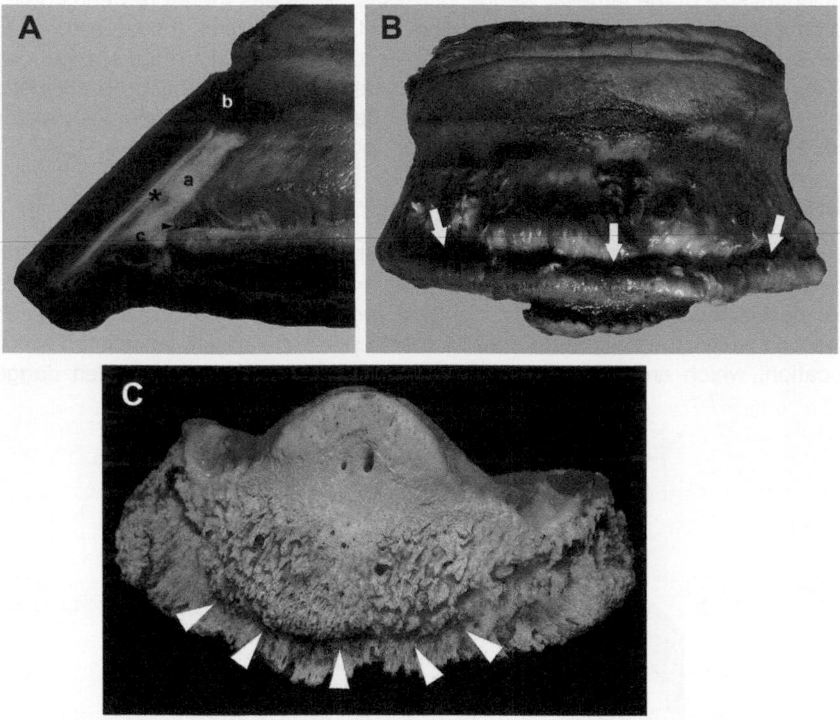

Fig. 16. The hidden dangers associated with lamellar wedge formation in the chronic laminitic foot. (*A*) Sagittal dissection of the midline of the hoof of a chronic laminitic foot showing (a) ectopic white line formation within the lamellar wedge of the affected foot and the yellow horn mass (*asterisk*), indicating the presence of transudate/exudate associated with vascular trauma within the lamellar region; (b) disorientation of the coronary papillae leading to a distorted and inward growing hoof horn mass; (c) reorientation of solear papillae around the apex of the DP, resulting in the development of an inward growing horn mass of sole horn that has encroached on the DP, resulting in the development of a marked depression in the lamellar dermis (*arrowhead*). (*B*) Disungulated foot showing the mediolateral extent of the dermal disruption associated with the inward growing distal horn mass encroaching on the apex of the DP (*arrows*). (*C*) Prepared bone specimen showing extensive bone modeling and lysis associated with the inward growing distal horn mass.

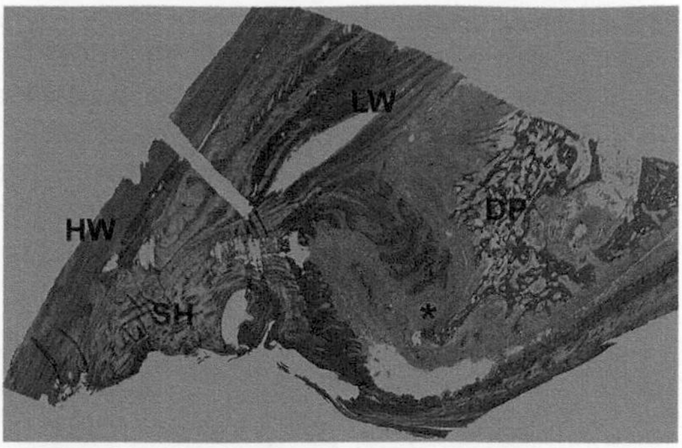

Fig. 17. Sagittal photomicrograph of the lamellar region of a chronic laminitic foot showing the anatomic interrelationship between the hoof wall (HW), the ectopic white line of the lamellar wedge (LW), the DP, and the inward-growing distal horn mass. Note that the inward-growing horn mass is formed by reoriented and distorted sole horn (SH) and also by dysplastic lamellar horn (*asterisk*). Indeed it would appear that the dysplastic lamellar horn is intimately associated with the region of pronounced bone loss.

length of the lamellar interface (**Fig. 18**). This intuitively reduces the effective area available for DP suspension[1,2,4] and further inhibits accommodatory DP movement during weight bearing. Elongation of the coronary dermis can result in a reorientation of the dermal papillae.[2,4,23,24] This alters the normal pattern of hoof wall production, which ultimately leads to the development of a highly distorted hoof capsule and to further expansion of the lamellar wedge (see **Figs. 2**B, C and **16**C).

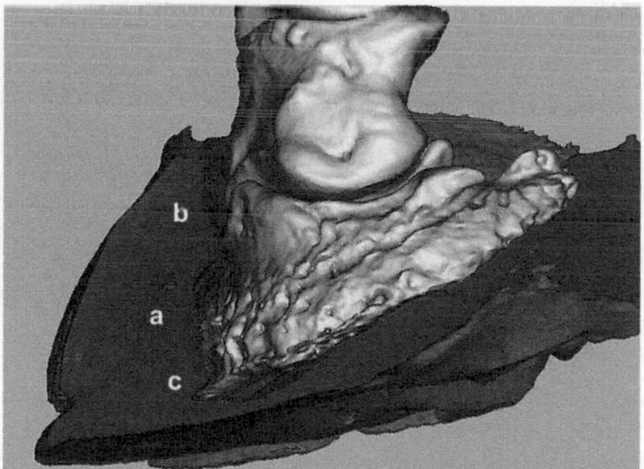

Fig. 18. Three-dimensional model of a chronic laminitic foot from computed tomography images, to show the hidden dangers associated with lamellar wedge formation. (a) Dysplastic ectopic white line on the inner aspect of the hoof wall. (b) Inward growing horn mass within the coronary region of the foot after papillae reorientation associated with the rotational dislocation of the DP. Note the elongation and encroachment of the coronary dermis, which reduces the proximodistal length of the lamellar interface. (c) Onward-growing distal horn mass resulting from displacement of the solear dermis around the apex of the dislocated DP. Note the associated modeling and lysis of the apex of the DP. For visualization purposes the dermal tissues have been excluded and the hoof capsule shown in sagittal section. (*Courtesy of* Don Walsh, Homestead Equine Hospital, Pacific, MO.)

Foot treatments should therefore be instigated to reduce the risk posed by these hidden dangers.[1,4] Specifically, timely resection of the proximal and distal dorsal hoof wall is required to allow reorientation of the dermal papillae of the sole and realignment of the coronary dermis.[1,4,23–26] This intervention facilitates restoration of normal pattern of hoof horn production. In addition, treatment shoes and sole inserts should support the palmar/plantar aspect of the foot and spare (relieve) any sole pressure beneath the dorsal margin of the dislocated DP. Shoe breakover should align with

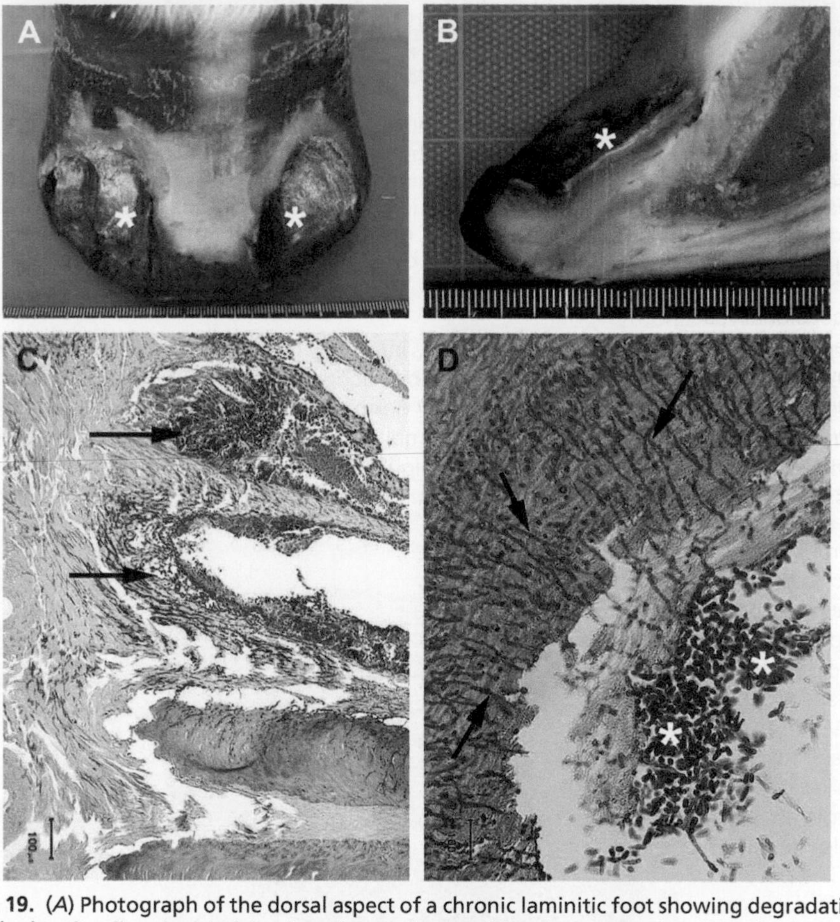

Fig. 19. (*A*) Photograph of the dorsal aspect of a chronic laminitic foot showing degradation of the hoof wall and underlying lamellar wedge resulting from secondary fungal infection - Onychomycosis (white line disease) of the ectopic white line (*asterisk*). (*B*) Sagittal section of the same foot showing fungal degradation of the horn tissue forming the lamellar wedge (*asterisk*) which extends proximally from the bearing border of the hoof capsule. (*C*) Photomicrograph of the transverse section of the lamellar wedge showing keratinophylic fungal degradation of the epidermal tissues forming the ectopic white line (*arrows*) (Periodic Acid Schiff, original magnification ×60). (*D*) Photomicrograph of a transverse section of the lamellar wedge showing *Scedosporium apiospermum* fungal infection of epidermal tissues. 'Yeast-like' organisms (*asterisks*) are seen inside the fissured cavity of the lamellar wedge, suggesting aerobic conditions, whilst 'mould-like' structures (hyphal/filamentous forms) are present within the horn tissues (*arrows*), suggesting anaerobic conditions. Note both are dimorphic forms of the same fungal species (Periodic Acid Schiff, original magnification ×1000).

the dorsodistal margin of the DP to minimize strain levels within the lamellar wedge and thereby protect the weakened SADP.

THE LAMELLAR WEDGE IN THE PASTURE-INDUCED LAMINITIC HORSE

It is generally accepted that the gross anatomic extent of the lamellar wedge relates directly to the severity of the initiating lamellar pathology within the affected foot. The greater the lamellar pathology the greater the degree of DP dislocation and therefore the greater the expansion of the lamellar wedge. More recent work has questioned this underlying assertion, indicating that cause of the disease itself may also be a contributory factor in the pathogenesis of the lamellar wedge. In particular, hyperinsulinemia, commonly associated with pasture-induced laminitis, has been shown to have a mitogenic effect on secondary lamellae keratinocytes, leading to basal cell hyperproliferation.[27] This insidious process results in elongation and attenuation of the lamellae and a progressive reduction in the ability of the SADP to suspend the DP in its normal anatomic position, leading to the development of a lamellar wedge.

SUSCEPTIBILITY TO ONYCHOMYCOSIS

Occasionally, soil-borne fungi may invade the dysplastic tissues of the lamellar wedge via the widened and pathologically altered white line, leading to the development of onychomycosis (white line disease) within the chronic laminitic foot (**Fig. 19**).[28] In particular, the fungal species *Scedosporium apiospermum* and its teleomorph, *Pseudallescheria boydii*, have been observed and isolated as a single cultivation colony from the lamellar wedge.[29] The reason for the particular susceptibility of the lamellar wedge to opportunist saprophytic fungal infection is unclear. However, it is possible that these fungal species have a strong affinity for damaged and/or pathologic altered keratinized tissues and produce enzymes with a specific keratinolytic activity that facilitates opportunistic secondary infection of hoof tissues.[30,31] In addition, the damaged and highly fissured nature of the lamellar wedge and white line likely permits rapid and extensive infection of these tissues in the chronic laminitic foot. This secondary infection can result in extensive hoof wall separation that further compromises the structural integrity of the hoof capsule and the functional integrity of the SADP. Onychomycosis can prove extremely difficult to treat, with various management approaches having been adopted with variable success. These treatments include complete resection of the lamellar wedge,[31–36] local cauterization, and topical application of antifungal agents with high horn affinity, for example, terbinafine hydrochloride, an allylamine antifungal drug.

The possibility of the fungal infection being passed to other animals through the use of farriery tools remains untested. However, appropriate disinfection of all tools after treatment of an infected hoof is strongly advised[28] to safeguard against any potential cross-infection.

SUMMARY

Lamellar wedge formation, in association with laminitis, represents a pathognomonic sequela to the failure of the SADP and anatomic dislocation of the DP within the hoof capsule. The lamellar wedge displays a variable structural organization that reflects the nature and extent of the lamellar separation and the healing responses within the affected foot. The lamellar wedge adversely affects normal biomechanical function within the foot and contributes further to pain and locomotor dysfunction of the chronically affected laminitic horse. There are hidden dangers associated with lamellar wedge formation, and inward growing horn masses that arise as a consequence of DP dislocation can lead to extensive bone modeling and lysis. The lamellar wedge also leaves the foot susceptible to secondary fungal infections. Treatment therefore needs to be instigated at the earliest opportunity to prevent and/or minimize lamellar wedge formation within the chronic laminitic foot and to counter the potential threat posed by its formation.

REFERENCES

1. Pollitt CC, Collins SN. Chronic laminitis. In: Ross M, Dyson SJ, editor. Lameness in the horse. 2nd edition, in press.
2. Hood DM. The mechanisms and consequences of structural failure of the foot. Vet Clin North Am Equine Pract 1999;15:437.
3. Marks G. Makroskopische, licht- und elektronenmikroskopische Untersuchungen zur Morphologie des Hyponichiums bei der Hufrehe des Pferdes. Diss med vet. Berlin: Freie Univ; 1984.
4. Pollitt CC. Equine laminitis; current concepts. Canberra (Australia): Rural Industries Research and Development Council; 2008.
5. Kameya T, Kiryu K, Kaneko M, et al. Histopathogenesis of thickening of the hoof wall laminae in equine laminitis. Jpn J Vet Sci 1980;42:361.
6. Kuwano A, Katayama Y, Kasashima Y, et al. A gross and histopathological study of an ectopic white line development in equine laminitis. J Vet Med Sci 2002;64:893.
7. Burnt NW, Baker SJ, Wagner, et al. Digital instability as a potential prognostic indicator in horses with chronic laminitis. In: Hood DM, Wagner IP, Jacobson AC, editors. Proceedings of the hoof project. College Station (TX): Private Publishers; 1997. p. 105.
8. Mostafa MB. Studies on experimental laminitis in the horse [PhD thesis]. Cairo University; 1986.
9. Pellmann R. Struktur und Funktion des Hufbeinträgers beim Pferd. Diss med vet. Berlin: Freie Univ; 1995.
10. Collins SN. A materials characterisation of laminitic donkey hoof horn [PhD thesis]. De Montfort University, Leicester; 2004.
11. Budras K-D, Bragulla H, Pellmann R, et al. Das Hufbein mit Periost und Insertionszone des Hufbeinträgers [The coffin bone with periosteum and insertion zone of the suspensory apparatus]. Wien Tierarz Monats 1996;84:241 [in German].
12. Budras K-D, Hinterhofer C, Hirschberg R, et al. [The suspensory apparatus of the coffin bone - part 1: the fan-shaped re-inforcement of the suspensory apparatus at the tip of the coffin bone in the horse]. Pferdeheilkunde 2009;25:96 [in German].
13. Budras K-D, Hinterhofer C, Hirschberg R, et al. [The suspensory apparatus of the coffin bone - part 2: clinical relevance of the suspensory apparatus and its fan-shaped reinforcement in chronic equine laminitis with coffin bone or hoof capsule rotation]. Pferdeheilkunde 2009;25:192 [in German].
14. Morgan SJ, Grosenbaugh DA, Hood DM. The pathophysiology of chronic laminitis. Vet Clin North Am Equine Pract 1999;15:395.
15. Marks G, Budras K-D. Zusammenhangstennung im corium und der epidermis bei der chronischen hufrehe des pferdes [Connection separation in the corium and the epidermis of chronic laminitis in horses]. Anat Histol Embryol J Vet Med Ser C 1985;14:187 [in German].

16. Linford RL. Laminitis (founder). In: Smith BP, editor. Large animal internal medicine. St Louis (MO): C.V. Mosby; 1996. p. 1300.
17. Wagner IP, Hood DM. Cause of airlines associated with acute and chronic laminitis. In Proceedings of the Annual Meeting American Association of Equine Practitioners. Phoenix (AZ), December 7–10, 1997. p. 363.
18. Budras K-D, Hullinger RL, Sack WO. Light and electron microscopy of keratinization in the laminar epidermis of the equine hoof with reference to laminitis. Am J Vet Res 1989;50:1150.
19. Pollitt CC, Daradka M. Hoof wall wound repair. Equine Vet J 2004;36:236.
20. Van Eps AW, Pollitt CC. Equine laminitis model: lamellar histopathology 7 days after induction with oligofructose. Equine Vet J 2009;41:735–40.
21. Kameya T. Clinical studies on laminitis in the racehorse. Exp Rep Equine Health Lab 1973;10:19.
22. Stick JA, Lann HW, Scott EA, et al. Pedal bone rotation as a prognostic sign in laminitis of horses. J Am Vet Med Assoc 1982;180:251.
23. Goetz TE. Anatomic, hoof, and shoeing considerations for the treatment of laminitis in horses. J Am Vet Med Assoc 1987;190:1323.
24. Eustace RA, Caldwell MN. The construction of the heart bar shoe and the technique of dorsal wall resection. Equine Vet J 1989;21:367.
25. Peremans K, Verschooten F, DeMoor A, et al. Laminitis in the pony: conservative treatment vs dorsal hoof wall resection. Equine Vet J 1991;23:243.
26. Eustace RA, Emery SL. Partial coronary epidermectomy (coronary peel), dorsodistal wall fenestration and deep digital flexor tenotomy to treat severe acute founder in a Connemara pony. Equine Vet Educ 2009;21:91.
27. De Laat M, McGowan CM, Sillence MN, et al. Equine laminitis: induced by 48 h hyperinsulinaemia in standardbred horses. Equine Vet J 2009;41(1), in press. DOI:10.2746/042516409X475779.
28. Budras K-D, Schiel C, Mulling C. Horn tubules of the white line: an insufficient barrier against ascending bacterial invasion. Equine Vet Educ 1998;10:81.
29. Kuwano A, Oikawa M, Takatori K. Pathomorphological findings in a case of onychomycosis of a racehorse. J Vet Med Sci 1996;58:1117.
30. Friedman DS, Schoster JV, Pickett JP, et al. *Pseudallescheria boydii* keratomycosis in a horse. J Am Vet Med Assoc 1989;195:616.
31. Davis PR, Meyer GA, Hanson RR, et al. *Pseudallescheria boydii* infection of the nasal cavity of a horse. J Am Vet Med Assoc 2000;217:707.
32. Redden RF. White line disease. Equine Pract 1990;12:14.
33. Ball D, Evans A. Needed: a more effective white line disease treatment. Am Farriers J 1992;18:30.
34. Gallenberger MR. Forget the yeast infection-it's a hoof fungus! Am Farriers J 1994;20:48.
35. Chapman B. The outbreak of equine onychomycosis. Swiss Vet 11-S/1993 Proceedings 3rd Geneva Congress of Equine Medicine and Surgery - 3rd Congress of the World Equine Veterinary Association (WEVA). Geneva; 1993. p. 42.
36. Chapman B. Onychomycosis. In: Proceedings of the 25th An Conv of Am Farriers Assoc. Missouri; 1996. p. 58.

Chronic Laminitis: Strategic Hoof Wall Resection

Amy Rucker, DVM

KEYWORDS

• Laminitis • Venogram • Foot • Distal phalanx • Wall resection

Historically, coronary band grooving and dorsal wall resection in conjunction with supportive shoeing was advocated as a treatment for laminitis.[1–8] This article describes a different technique: removing only a focal area of the proximal wall when the capsule is impinging on the coronary corium.[9–15] If the wall is stripped from a healthy foot, islands of epidermal lamellar tips are left behind along with the laminar basement membrane.[16] These epidermal cells proliferate and reconstruct the epidermal laminae. In the laminitic foot, destruction of the basement membrane and more complete epidermal separation make it difficult for repair to secure a functional connection of the wall to the dermis and the distal phalanx (DP).[16–18] Displacement of the DP results in compromise of circulation to the coronary, lamellar, and solar corium.[19] Most light breed horses load the medial aspect of their fore feet more than the lateral (as evidenced by slower medial wall growth and medial crushed heel). Laminitis follows this loading pattern and further compromises medial foot tissues. The palmar rim of the DP can become septic due to inadequate circulation, trauma, and abnormal mechanical loading. This condition usually appears 6 to 8 weeks after the onset of laminitis. Sepsis-induced inflammation migrates proximally up the wall, causing painful coronary band swelling and ultimately exiting at the coronary band, similar to other foot abscesses.

Poulticing the coronary band encourages drainage and reduces swelling, which may be enough treatment for some cases (Animalintex Poultice, 3M Animal Care Products, St Paul, MN, USA). However, the area of devitalized bone along the palmar margin is often large, encompassing the entire medial quarter and palmar process as the abscess migrates proximally. Extensive inflammation and separation causes the coronary band to bulge over the sharp edge of the proximal wall. The wall cuts into the swollen tissue, resulting in edema and further damage. Without wall resection the coronary corium can become necrotic and horn growth can be permanently damaged, preventing future growth of tubular horn.

Alternatively the dorsal coronary band may be affected by coronary corium compression between the extensor process and coronary groove. The dorsal coronet

MidWest Equine, PO Box 30520, Columbia, MO 65205, USA
E-mail address: ruckeramy@hotmail.com

Vet Clin Equine 26 (2010) 197–205
doi:10.1016/j.cveq.2009.12.009 **vetequine.theclinics.com**
0749-0739/10/$ – see front matter

can blow-out from sepsis on the palmar rim or also from compression/displacement. If the swollen coronary band is not responsive to an Animalintex Poultice and continues to bulge out over the horn wall, an upper wall resection is indicated.

Slow-onset cases of medial wall coronary-band impingement can result from slow growth of the medial quarter relative to the opposite quarter. Venographic studies indicate that the reason for extremely slow or no horn growth is compression of the coronary band growth zone. Most laminitic horses load the medial wall more heavily than the lateral wall, and are slower to develop a strong attachment between the laminae and medial wall. A severe medial listing of the DP can develop and compress the medial coronary and laminar corium. Once the foot grows a strong lamellar attachment from coronet to sole, the radiographic medial-lateral imbalance can be addressed. However, farriers often prematurely balance the foot by lowering the lateral heel and quarter, which can be counterproductive. Because the medial wall is not anchored to the corium or DP, the horn is all that moves, further compressing the medial coronary corium. These horses are mildly or moderately lame, but the lameness can become acutely painful when bone sepsis develops. At first the coronary band may appear normal, or may begin to bulge slightly over the hoof wall. The venogram reveals reduced or absence of contrast in the medial coronary and sublamellar vasculature. Severe cases show a stark loss of contrast along the circumflex vessels. Shoeing strategies (with or without a deep digital flexor tenotomy) may shift the internal load away from the compressed area. If shoeing does not restore medial growth on the slow coronary band impingement case, a venogram is indicated as an aid to better understand why there is no growth. These cases should be monitored closely as they often develop acute, painful swelling weeks later that can become a severe complication if not dealt with in a timely fashion.

Wall resection success is improved if performed while the laminar and coronary corium is still relatively healthy. The digital venogram helps identify the need for a wall resection before the foot indicates that it is not doing well. Most normal horses may have a slight reduction in contrast in the medially loaded coronary plexus. Injecting an inadequate volume of contrast also results in reduction in contrast filling on the venogram (**Fig. 1**).

Genuine lack of loss of contrast filling, due to pathology, alters the venogram in a way that differs from inadequate contrast dose or uneven normal foot loading (**Fig. 2**).

With wall impingement found in medial sinker syndrome secondary to laminitis, a contrast void is evident at the affected coronary and sublamellar vascular beds as well as along the circumflex vessels and sole corium (**Fig. 3**). Removing the upper horn wall before the germinal tubular horn center has sustained irreversible damage enhances the healing environment, and can save the quarters and the life of the horse.

PERFORMING THE WALL RESECTION

The horse is sedated and the foot is locally anesthetized by abaxial sesamoid nerve blockade. A tourniquet can be applied over the fetlock area; however, there is normally limited hemorrhage as the circulation is moderately or entirely compromised. The wall is removed from an area that extends slightly beyond either side of the swelling or coronary rupture. Distally the resection extends approximately halfway down the lamellar wall in a sweeping “smiley-face” arch. There is a strong tendency to be too conservative. Removing a very small area does not satisfy the demands for the procedure because the lamellar corium continues to swell outward along the lower margin of the resection.

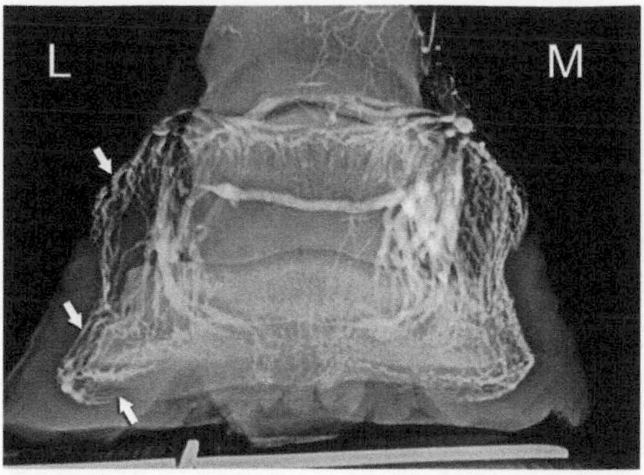

Fig. 1. Venogram using inadequate volume of contrast (13 mL). This horse is sound, with a rotational limb deformity and fractures of the solar margin. For the venogram, 13 mL of contrast has been injected into the medial (M) palmar digital vein. Lateral (L) vessels are narrowed and tapering. There is a load-induced reduction of contrast in the lateral coronary and laminar plexus and circumflex vessels (*arrows*).

A 1-cm wide groove is cut through the stratum medium using quarter-inch half-round nippers, a rotating high-speed burr, a rasp, or a sharp hoof knife (**Fig. 4**).

The border of the remaining wall is cut perpendicular to the face of the DP with a smooth margin void of fragments of stratum medium, which can further traumatize the laminae (**Fig. 5**). A sharp hoof knife is used to hook into the cornified tissue and pull away from the corium. Cutting the corium or causing heat necrosis with the high-speed burr can leave a permanent scar that will be evident in the new wall. Careful dissection is needed at the coronary band to avoid injuring the dermal papillae.

A scalpel blade is used to incise the final layer of stratum lamellatum. Half-round nippers are used to grasp the edge of the wall to be resected. The upper wall is slowly

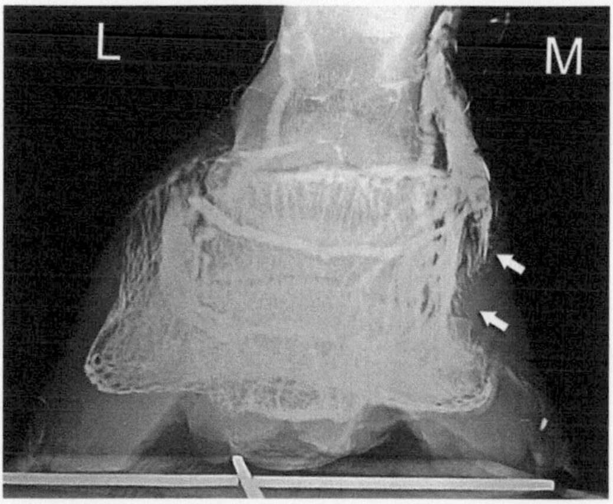

Fig. 2. Chronic wall impingement, medial sinker. One year after laminitis onset, this horse did not grow medial wall and became acutely lame after the foot was incorrectly balanced by lowering the lateral quarter and heel. Contrast is reduced at the coronet and is absent in the medial sublamellar vascular bed (*arrows*).

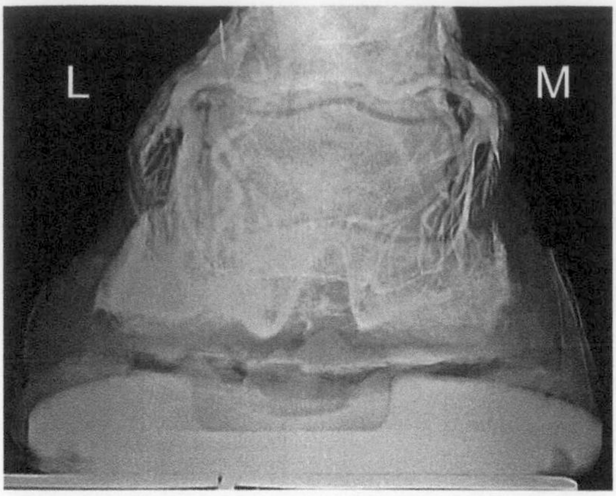

Fig. 3. Chronic laminitis of 2 months' duration. Contrast is greatly reduced at the medial coronet and truncated at the wall. Minimal contrast is evident in the widened medial sublamellar vascular bed. Contrast is void in the medial circumflex vessel and sole corium. The lateral sublamellar vascular bed is widened and homogeneous with contrast, indicating complete separation of the dermal and epidermal lamellae. (Note: Fig. 7 in the article by Amy Rucker elsewhere in this issue is the lateral view of this foot.)

peeled away en masse from the corium and coronary plexus in a smooth motion (**Fig. 6**).

If the stratum lamellatum remains intact it will prevent a smooth peel. Once the wall has been peeled, the margin of the remaining wall is again checked for any sharp areas. The corium is gently massaged using light digital pressure to induce hemorrhage. When massaging the exposed laminae, the often-distorted coronary papillae are directed in a distal direction before application of the pressure bandage.

The exposed corium varies in appearance in accordance with its pathology. Relatively healthy corium is pink or red and bleeds profusely when the wall is removed. Edematous corium is light in color and is slow to bleed, even with firm pressure massage. Granulation tissue is often seen in more chronic cases with extensive

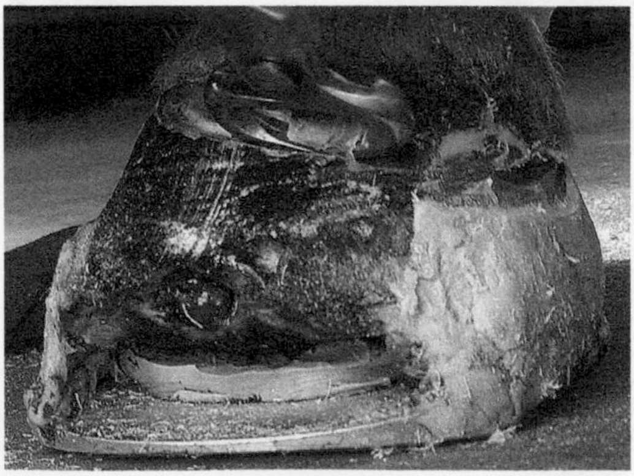

Fig. 4. The extent of wall to be resected is determined by the venogram in **Fig. 3**. A 1-cm wide curve is extended beyond the border of the separated coronary band of the dorsal and medial wall. The stratum externum and stratum medium are removed using half-round nippers.

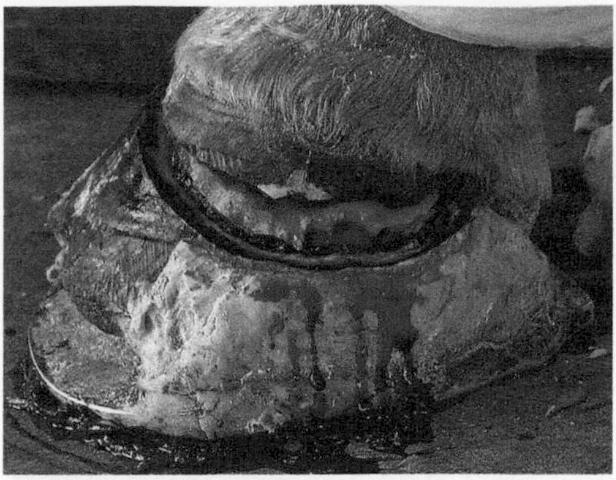

Fig. 5. The stratum internum is sharply dissected using the hooked end of a hoof knife. Care is taken not to damage the corium. Note the lack of hemorrhage in areas where the lamellar corium has been exposed.

vascular damage. The tissue appears shiny or pale and may drip serum, but does not hemorrhage readily. Severely compromised corium is dark red or purplish, and may have a ribbon of necrotic tissue at the coronet. The ribbon is the growth zone of the tubular horn. When the corium is dark or gray it is often no longer attached to the underlying bone, the result of terminal arch occlusion.

A piece of surgical quarter-inch felt is precut to the shape of the wall removed. The felt is soaked in betadine solution (Povidine 1%, Agripharm Products, Westlake, TX, USA) and applied to fit snug along the border of the wall defect (**Fig. 7**).

Elastic tape 5 cm wide is applied (Elastikon, Johnson & Johnson, New Brunswick, NJ, USA) to secure the felt and provide positive pressure to the exposed laminae. Pressure bandaging prevents exuberant granulation tissue from forming, and is an important aspect of the treatment. Loose-fitting bandaging over the exposed area invariably causes complications and increased pain as the tissue continues to swell. Preventing prolapse of the corium speeds cornification and helps create a tight, more uniform, new wall. Proximally, the felt can extend onto the skin. Alternatives to Betadine-soaked felt include placing amniotic membrane or wound-care products

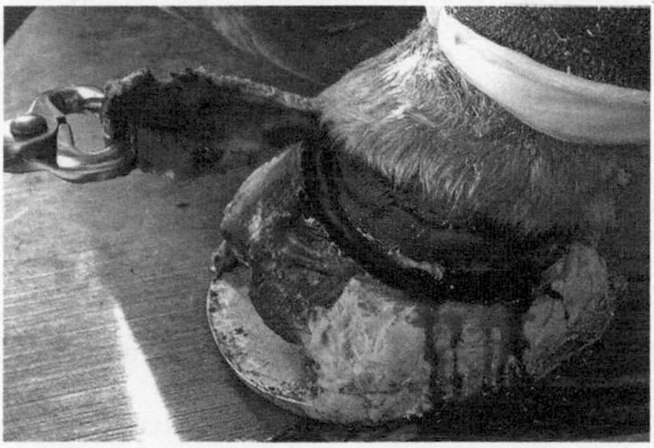

Fig. 6. Half-round nippers are used to grasp the area of wall to be resected. The wall is slowly peeled away from the coronet, allowing time for the papillae to separate from the hoof capsule.

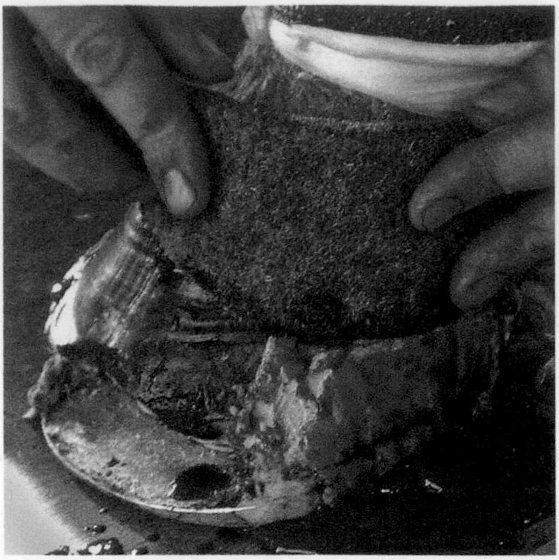

Fig. 7. Betadine soaked felt is pushed distally to orient the coronary papillae. The border of the felt is identical to the margin of the wall. The felt is firmly taped in place to prevent the corium from swelling and prolapsing over the wall, which delays healing.

(Lacerum Equine Platelet Rich Plasma, PRP Technologies, Roanoke, IN, USA) on the compromised coronary band before bandaging.[10,16] Additional bandage is placed over the foot to prevent trauma to the area and to keep it clean.

When large areas of horn wall (eg, from center of toe to heel) are removed, a short leg cast, can help to restrict motion and reduce pain. Butterfly catheters (Winged Infusion Set, Abbott Laboratories, Abbott Park, IL, USA) can be placed in the felt and brought out to the top of the cast for daily treatment with betadine solution. The felt is taped in place and covered with a breathable cast liner (PROCEL Cast Liner, WL Gore & Associates, Flagstaff, AZ, USA). If the corium was healthy when the cast was applied, the betadine felt may be left in place several weeks without the tubing for betadine infusion. A window may be cut into the cast to assess epithelialization and cornification, if it is suspected that the area requires additional treatment. Another option is to cast over a bandaged limb. To facilitate cast removal, a release membrane such as soft roll cast padding prevents the casting tape from adhering to the bandage. 4 to 5 days after application the cast can be cut along both sides and used as a bivalve splint for as long as required.

AFTERCARE

The Betadine-felt bandage is changed daily unless a cast is placed on the limb. If the felt is adhered to the tissue, it is loosened by soaking with saline to prevent further tissue trauma. When the corium has not been heavily damaged it may cornify rapidly over a period of a few days. This is the desired result. As healing occurs, islands of epithelium appear that are yellow in color and soon have a dry texture as they cornify and harden (**Fig. 8**).

The islands of epithelium spread across the corium, hardening as they cornify, and a new stratum medium develops. The entire wall resection should be cornified within 14 days unless serious vascular compromise has occurred. If a laminitic case is not responding to therapy, a venogram can be performed to assess vascular and soft

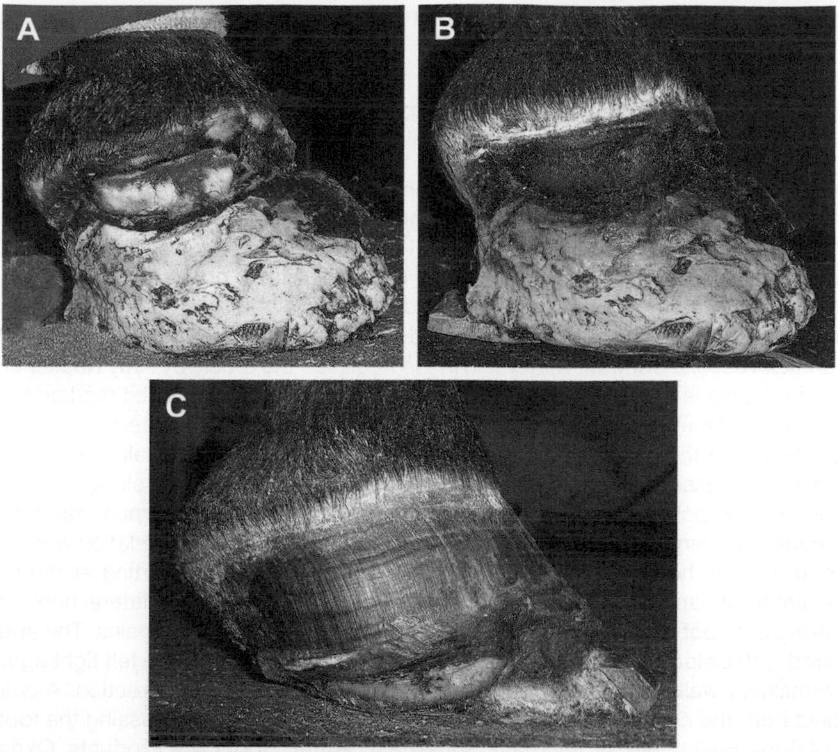

Fig. 8. (*A*) Waxy yellow islands of epithelium are evident within 6 days of wall resection. (*B*) Cornification of the resected wall with new growth of tubular horn at 6 weeks post resection (*C*) Six months after wall resection, new wall has grown to the ground surface.

tissue improvement. If performed before cornification, the contrast runs from the exposed corium.

Once the area has cornified, bandages may be changed every 3 to 5 days. Organized tubular horn begins at the coronary band and gradually grows to the ground surface. The new white line will be distinct and the wall strong. If a large area has been resected, stall rest is indicated for several weeks. Once the area is cornified and horn tubules have replaced most of the horn defect, the patient can be released into a small half-acre paddock. The regrown hoof capsule will be stronger and hold up to nailing and exercise.

COMPLICATIONS

In advanced chronic cases, necrotic bone may be identified on 65° dorsopalmar or 65° dorsopalmar/45° oblique radiographs. Soft bone fragments that are palpable once the wall is resected are removed by curettage.

Cornification does not occur when sepsis is present. Septic soft tissue and bone may be controlled by regional limb perfusions, local antimicrobials, or curettage of septic bone. Bandaging the tissue with amniotic membrane or other wound-care products (Lacerum, PRP Technologies, Roanoke, IN, USA) may improve healing.[10,20] The health of the DP, whether a focal area is necrotic, or whether the entire bone is compromised should be considered. This evaluation can be confirmed by the venogram. If the terminal arch is not evident on the venogram, the entire bone is in jeopardy and the prognosis is grave.

COMPLETE WALL RESECTION WITH DISTAL DISPLACEMENT

Transfixation pin casting of the metacarpus, with complete wall resection, is a salvage procedure when severe vascular compromise (confirmed by venograms) occurs within the first 24 to 48 hours of laminitis onset.[21] Typical cases have had dystocia or retained placenta, present with bilateral or quadrilateral laminitis, Obel grade 4 lameness, and edema in all 4 limbs, and are unresponsive to nonsteroidal anti-inflammatory drugs. Radiographs may be inconclusive, but venograms exhibit stark lack of contrast filling along the dorsal, medial, and lateral sublamellar vascular bed and the circumflex vessels. Contrast will remain in the heel (see the article by Amy Rucker elsewhere in this issue for Fig. 3). Cases with extensive early damage exhibit marked lameness that is difficult to block with local anesthetics. Separation and serous exudation may develop at the coronary band within hours of onset. Paradoxically, as ischemic necrosis progresses, comfort may improve until the hoof capsule is sloughed.

Two quarter-inch transcortical pins are placed in the distal metacarpus/metatarsus. The patient is generally anesthetized or standing in a sling, with sedation and local anesthesia. The hoof is detached from the sole using nippers. Starting at the heel, the entire hoof capsule is slowly peeled in one piece, from medial to lateral heel. After removing the hoof capsule, only a small portion of the caudal heel remains. The area is covered with betadine-soaked felt, again with exact placement of the felt tight against the remaining wall while orienting the coronary papillae in a distal direction. A cast is applied from the metacarpus/metatarsus over the pins and encompassing the foot. A ball of SuperFast acrylic (Equi-Thane SuperFast, Vettec Hoof Care Products, Oxnard, CA, USA) or a forged aluminum bowl is placed beneath the foot to prevent torque on the pins.

The casts are replaced over a period of 1 to 3 months, and a deep flexor tenotomy is usually indicated after the first cast. This procedure can be a life-saving one in achieving pasture soundness for a horse turned out in a small paddock. Soundness is increased if the DP does not develop osteitis and the wall is able to grow attached tubular horn. Cases of horses returning to work if treated promptly have been reported.[22]

ACKNOWLEDGMENTS

I would like to thank my mentor, Dr Ric Redden, for teaching me these procedures and reviewing this article. I would also like to thank Dr Roger Shaw, Dr Steve Tornberg, Dr Justin Berger and Howard Wilson for assistance with the images.

REFERENCES

1. Parks AH, O'Grady SE. Chronic laminitis: current treatment strategies. Vet Clin North Am 2003;19(2):412–3.
2. Parks AH, Balch OK, Collier MA. Treatment of acute laminitis: supportive therapy. Vet Clin North Am 1999;15(2):369.
3. Peremans K, Verschooten F, DeMoor A, et al. Laminitis in the pony: conservative treatment vs dorsal hoof wall resection. Equine Vet J 1991;23(4):243–6.
4. Redden RF. Hoof wall resection as a treatment in laminitis. In: Proceedings, American Association of Equine Practitioners; 1987. p. 647–56.

5. Eustace RA, Caldwell MN. Treatment of solar prolapse using the heart bar shoe and dorsal hoof wall resection technique. Equine Vet J 1989;21(5):370–2.
6. Moyer W, Redden RF. Chronic and severe laminitis: a critique of therapy with heart bar shoes and hoof wall resection. Equine Vet J 1989;21(5):317–8.
7. Curtis S, Ferguson DW, Luikart R, et al. Trimming and shoeing the chronically affected horse. Vet Clin North Am 1999;15(2):472–9.
8. Ritmeester AM, Ferguson DW. Coronary grooving promotes dorsal hoof wall growth in horses with chronic laminitis. In: Proceedings, American Association of Equine Practitioners. Denver (CO); 1996. p. 212–3.
9. Redden RF. Understanding laminitis. Lexington (KY): The Blood-Horse; 1998. p. 67.
10. Long CG, Schultz LA. How to use hoof-wall resection and amniotic membrane as a treatment for coronary-band prolapse. In: Proceedings, American Association of Equine Practitioners. San Antonio (TX); 2006. p. 501–4.
11. Morrison S. Foot management. Clin Techn Equine Pract 2004;3(1):71–82.
12. Floyd AE. An approach to the treatment of the laminitic horse. In: Floyd AE, Mansmann RA, editors. Equine podiatry. St. Louis (MO): Saunders; 2007. p. 347–58.
13. Rucker A. The digital venogram. In: Floyd AE, Mansmann RA, editors. Equine podiatry. St. Louis (MO): Saunders; 2007. p. 339–45.
14. Morrison S. Rehabilitating the laminitic foot. In Proceedings: North American Veterinary Conference—Large Animal; 2008. p. 186–9.
15. Eustace RA, Emery SL. Partial coronary epidermectomy (coronary peel), dorsodistal wall fenestration and deep digital flexor tenotomy to treat severe acute founder in a Connemara pony. Equine Vet Educ 2009;21(2):91–9.
16. Pollit CC, Daradka M. Hoof wall wound repair. Equine Vet J 2004;36(3):210–5.
17. Geyer H. Microscopic changes in hooves with laminitis. In: Proceedings, International Laminitis Symposium. Berlin, November 11–13, 2008.
18. Pollit CC. Laminitis pathophyslology. In: Floyd AE, Mansmann RA, editors. Equine podiatry. St. Louis (MO): Saunders; 2007. p. 313–9.
19. Hood DM, Grosenbaugh DA, Slater MR. Vascular perfusion in horses with chronic laminitis. Equine Vet J 1994;26(3):191–6.
20. Redden RF. How Lacerum has improved the progress of high scale foot damage. In: Proceedings, 17th Annual Bluegrass Laminitis Symposium. Lexington (KY), January 15–17, 2004.
21. Redden RF. How to treat high scale laminitis with wall ablation and transcortical cast. In: Proceedings, 16th Annual Bluegrass Laminitis Symposium. Lexington (KY), January 16–18, 2003.
22. D'Arpe L. Case reviews of high risk scale laminitic cases treated in Europe. In: Proceedings, International Laminitis Symposium. Berlin, November 11–13, 2008.

The Use of the Wooden Shoe (Steward Clog) in Treating Laminitis

Micheal L. Steward, DVM

KEYWORDS

• Laminitis • Wooden shoe • Steward Clog • Chronic laminitis • Therapeutic shoes

In cases of chronic laminitis, the wooden shoe (Steward Clog) reduces pain and enhances healing. Because the shoe offers a variety of benefits, it is being accepted and used throughout the horse industry. The full roller motion and solid base of the shoe (**Fig. 1**) bestow a range of mechanical and physical advantages[1] that stabilize and protect the distal phalanx by reducing shear and other forces to the damaged lamellae. These features create mechanical advantages that promote hoof regeneration and healing while enhancing vascular health and function to the compromised hoof. The wooden shoe enables realignment of the distal phalanx and has all the mechanical advantages of shoes previously advocated for the treatment of laminitis. Because of it's flat solar surface, the shoe concentrates weight bearing evenly over a specified section of the foot.[2] One of the major advantages of the shoeing system is its nontraumatic application process, which makes it possible to adjust the shoe while keeping the patient comfortable. Common wood screws can be applied distally through the hoof wall and into the wooden shoe with the horse standing on the shoe. A minimum of two screws (one through each quarter) is recommended to secure the shoe after sole impression material has been added to the palmar/plantar region of the hoof (**Fig. 2**). More screws can be added to the perimeter of the heel region for strut support. Hoof glue or fiberglass casting material can be added to further secure the shoe and provide wall stabilization.

Readily available materials (eg, plywood) can be easily modified using normal carpentry or farrier tools to provide dorsopalmar and mediolateral breakover to reduce the effective "lever arm" relating ground force to torque.[3] The hoof capsule (during the stance phase) exerts these forces on the distal phalanx via the laminar interface (wall–lamellae–third phalanx). The flat solar surface of the shoe protects the sole area, which is often damaged, and helps recruit and support the palmar structures of the hoof for

1509 North Kickapoo, Shawnee, OK 74804, USA
E-mail address: doxmls@aol.com

Vet Clin Equine 26 (2010) 207–214
doi:10.1016/j.cveq.2009.12.002 **vetequine.theclinics.com**
0749-0739/10/$ – see front matter

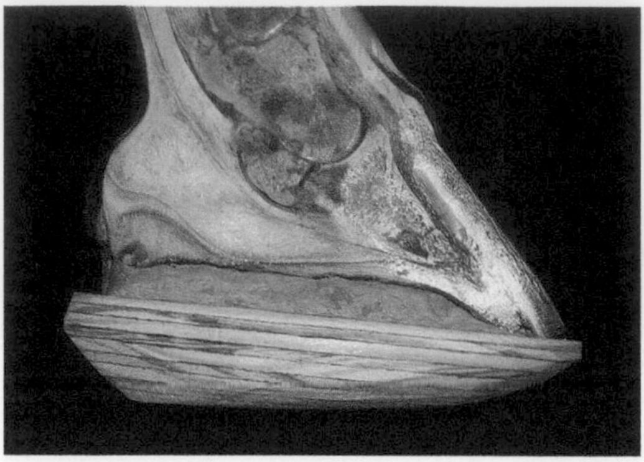

Fig. 1. This hoof model shows the full roller motion design of the wooden shoe with wedging sanded into the ground surface. The pink solar impression material is visible on the cut-away model.

weight bearing to reduce the laminar share of load. The shoe can be easily modified. For example, by recessing the shoe's solar surface, painful areas of the sole can be unloaded (**Fig. 3**). To reduce pain due to hoof laminar damage, sole impression material can be used in the palmar region of the foot to help load this area.

In cases of laminitis, wood (particularly plywood) has a variety of properties[4] that can aid in reducing pain and enhancing healing. The wood is strong enough to provide solar protection needed to enhance distal phalanx stabilization. Wood can be easily modified to add shoe height for enhanced shoe mechanics. The absorption properties of wood and sole impression material, cushions the impact with the ground, thus reducing pain. The addition of a second material (eg, sintered ethylene vinyl acetate [EVA]) to the ground surface can further cushion the impact. A shoe made with a combination of plywood and EVA provides stabilization and concussion-absorption properties superior to those of any system tried to date. The EVA, applied to the ground surface (**Fig. 4**), provides selective stabilization, a very desirable feature for critical cases on hard surfaces. Selective stabilization is achieved when the horse

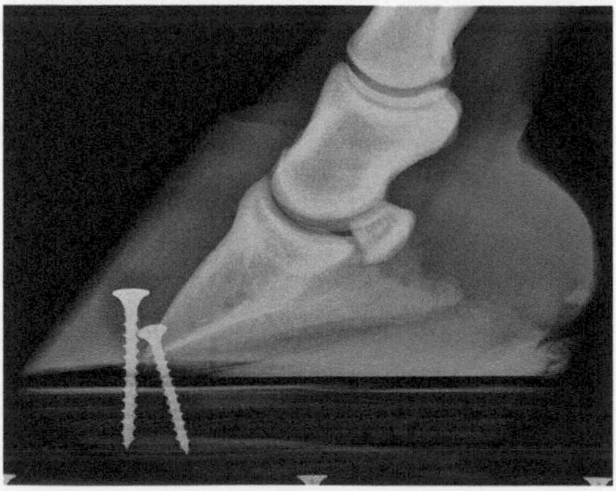

Fig. 2. Two screws penetrating the hoof wall (in the quarter regions) accommodate shoe adjustments during shoe placement. Additional screws need not penetrate the wall, but can be used as strut supports to further aid in shoe attachment.

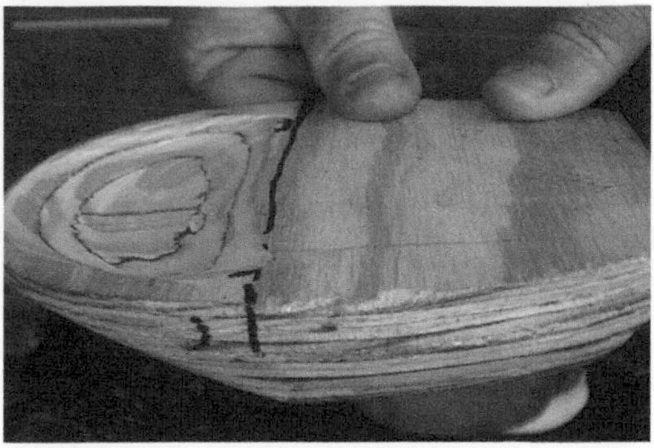

Fig. 3. The toe area of the laminitic hoof is often painful and in need of unloading. Unloading is accomplished by recessing (via sanding) the solar surface of the shoe in the toe region.

can determine (with relative stability) where to apply the stance forces on the solar surface of the shoe and, thus where to apply some of the hoof forces. Commercially available composite shoes (eg, Steward Clog, Equine Digit Support System, Inc., Penrose, CO, USA) are used in cases that need extra traction/durability and don't require the enhanced concussion-absorption properties.

Shoe modifications are easily added or subtracted (eg, rasping the applied shoe to adjust breakover). The wooden shoe is self-modifying by normal wear and this feature further enhances the comfort of the patient. Normal farrier and carpentry tools and techniques are easily mastered to apply wedge features and to layer materials for greater strength and more concussion relief.

Radiographs (lateral-medial and dorsopalmar views) are essential to determine optimum shoe prescription. Radiographs are taken post-shoeing to ensure the best shoe fit and to provide sole and wall growth references for assessing healing rates before the next shoeing.

Therapeutic shoeing in laminitis is aimed at reducing deleterious forces on the injured laminar region, enhancing vascular flow, and stabilizing the distal phalanx. Static weight bearing, as well as locomotion, produce shear and various tension

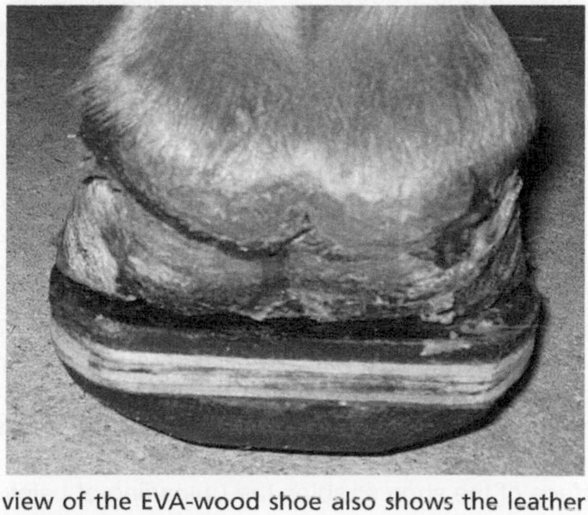

Fig. 4. The palmar view of the EVA-wood shoe also shows the leather wedge pad on the solar surface of the roller-motion shoe.

and compressive forces on the damaged laminae. The proper modification and distribution of these forces can enhance healing after laminitis.

Ameliorating the ongoing deleterious force of the horse's weight on the injured laminae is a very challenging problem in laminitis. The upward ground force and the downward weight interact primarily at the laminar interface when the horse is standing or walking on a hard, smooth surface (primarily wall support). By transferring a portion of the horse's weight to an unaffected (or less affected, less painful) area of the foot, the affected laminae can at least be partially unloaded, resulting in a significant reduction in pain. The flat, solid base of the wooden shoe enables the easy recruitment of the soft structures of the palmar (plantar) foot for weight sharing. This portion of the foot is well adapted to energy dissipation and load support and is less likely than the dorsal wall to be affected in laminitis.

The use of sole impression material increases the surface area the palmar/plantar hoof can provide for weight sharing. The conforming material, when properly applied, provides a passive loading of the sole, digital cushion, and frog (including the sulci regions) in the palmar/plantar region of the hoof and may massage the vascular system within the foot. Venospasm may play a significant role in the pain of the laminitic case.[5] Massage may be helpful in relieving the pain. The conformation of the palmarly placed impression material mimics the internal architecture of the foot and may provide, compared to other systems, a less traumatic, more structurally (ergonomically) correct way of applying additional load to the palmar region of the foot. The impression material may also provide a benefit by serving as an energy-dispersing medium to the palmar/plantar foot. The application of too much impression material may destabilize the distal phalanx and cause active loading of the sole by compressing solar and laminar blood vessels. Passive loading is accomplished by loading the hoof/sole impression material before the "curing" process and allowing the excess material to exit palmarly, via the frog sulci, before it has cured. Passive loading enables gentle compression to the sole impression material and the soft, extremely vascular structures of the palmar/plantar foot during hoof loading.

The hoof trim, impression material, and solid base of the wooden shoe act together in support of the opposing forces (upward ground force vs downward weight) as they are dispersed over the wall, sole, bars, frog, digital cushion, and distal phalanx. The load is distributed as evenly and atraumatically as possible.

The proper application of the wooden laminitis shoe begins, as with any shoeing system, with the proper hoof trim. The proper trim is aimed at realignment of the distal phalanx with the ground surface. This should also recruit more surface area of the palmar foot for weight redistribution and may help to reduce the compressive forces on solar vessels, especially at the distal margin of the distal phalanx.

The trim is started at the apex of the frog and continues into the heel regions, maintaining the solar plane of support to the widest part of the frog, if atraumatically possible. Normal farrier practices should not be violated in the trim. Trimming should result in a significant increase in contact surface area, characterized by increased uniformity of wall contact, increase in the contact of the peripheral sole,[6] and full contact of the frog and bars with the sole impression material. The trim facilitates palmar/plantar shoe placement and maximizes palmar/plantar distribution of load to an increased surface area of the palmar/plantar foot (**Fig. 5**). A foot load with a small surface area will produce higher compressive force in the underlying tissues than an identical load applied to a greater surface area.[7]

The solid, flat surface of the shoe enables the unloading of painful areas (generally the toe region) by excavating shoe material beneath the painful area. Sole impression

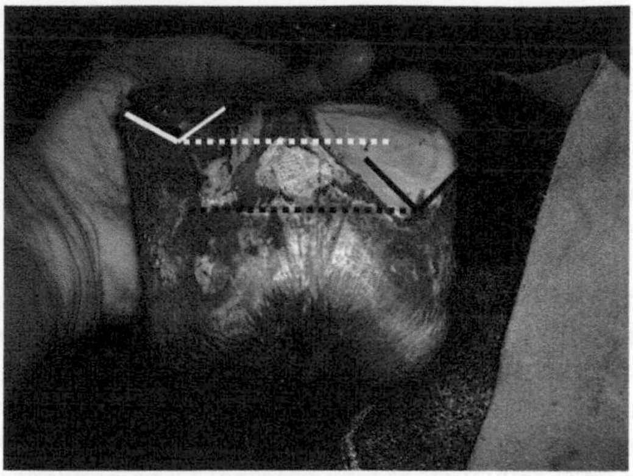

Fig. 5. The untrimmed heel/bar area (*yellow lines*) shows shoe placement (*yellow dotted line*) when heels are allowed to grow. Properly trimmed heels (*black lines*) allow for more palmar shoe (weight) application and different shoe placement (*black dotted lines*).

material should not be applied beneath painful areas. The solid surface area of the shoe protects the bottom of the foot from external injury.

The characteristics of the sole impression material are important in applying weight to the palmar digit in as nontraumatic a way as possible. A two-part hand-mixed impression material with a Shore durometer reading (hardness/softness) that closely mimics the consistency of the digital cushion, the frog, and the sole is usually superior to pour-in mixes (**Fig. 6**). In critical cases, sole packing materials, such as Venice turpentine–impregnated cotton, can be used for palmar hoof support. Pour-in impression materials presently available adhere to the sole in a manner that may trap abscesses and tend to harden over time (ie, the durometer reading changes from week to week).

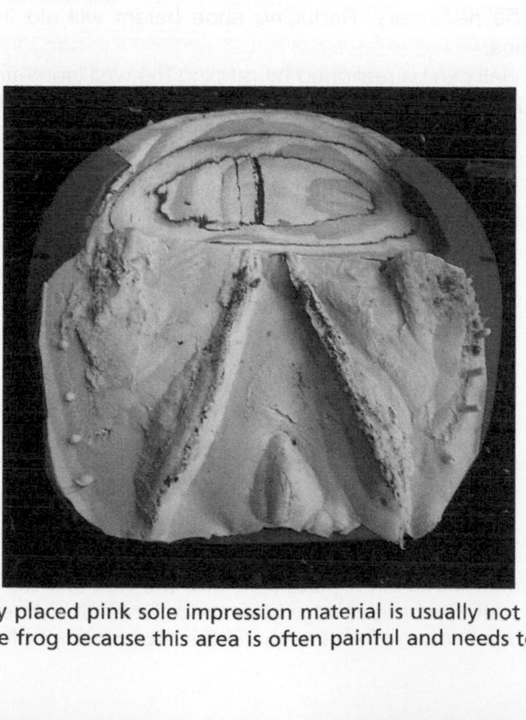

Fig. 6. The palmarly placed pink sole impression material is usually not allowed to extend past the apex of the frog because this area is often painful and needs to be unloaded.

The full roller motion of the wooden shoe reduces the forces between the laminar region of the hoof wall and the distal phalanx. The dorsal wall laminae undergo radial tension, compression, and shear forces during the stationary stance phase. Dorsal laminar torque forces are significantly increased as the unshod horse walks. Turns increase the torque forces to the wall quarters by 40%.[8] The full roller motion (wooden) shoe reduces laminar torque force (the distance from the point of force application to the resulting moment rotational center) by shortening the moment arm between wall and laminae.

The force that the deep digital flexor tendon (DDFT) exerts on the dorsal hoof wall laminae is further reduced via heel wedging and more palmar placement of breakover. The shoe mechanics shorten moment arm forces and may also reduce the time these forces affect the damaged dorsal lamellar interface. In experimental models, a 1° wedge reduces the force the DDFT exerts on the navicular bone by 4% (thus, 6° wedging leads to a 24% reduction of these forces).[9] The application of heel wedges may also reduce the force on the laminar interface, although no data currently exist to confirm this.

The unique (variable) height of the shoe enables placement of a continuous bevel around the perimeter of the shoe to further enhance breakover (dorsopalmar and mediolateral) and reduce leverage on the lamellar interface. Reducing the force required for breakover encourages stabilization of the distal phalanx–lamellar interface.

Caution should be exercised in adding excessive shoe height to a horse that may travel at a pace faster than a walk. The roller-motion shoe (**Fig. 7**) increases mobility to the foot, but does so at the expense of hoof capsule stability because the shoe makes it possible for smaller than usual forces to cause movement. Breakover placed within the perimeter of the base of the distal phalanx will cause excessive instability to the foot and is usually detrimental. When breakover is placed too far palmarly (radiographically palmar to the dorsal margin of the distal phalanx), the laminitic patient will immediately exhibit distress by knuckling forward at the fetlock. As soundness in the laminitic patient increases and the horse becomes more active, restricting the space for exercise may be necessary. Reducing shoe height will aid in limb stability as soundness increases.

The dorsal hoof wall can be realigned by rasping the wall (sometimes to the level of the white line, and often into the damaged, stretched laminae), leaving a potentially

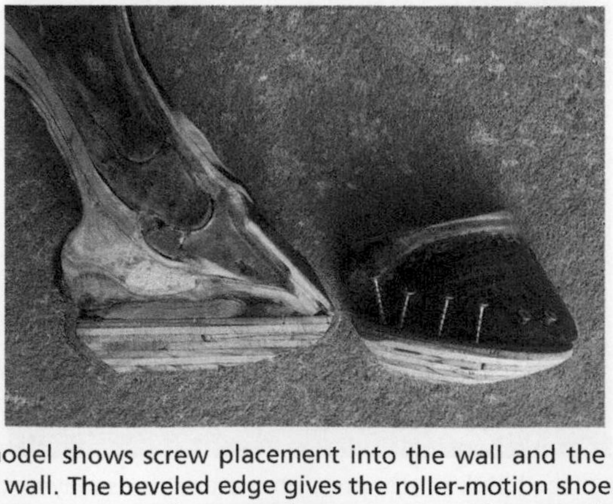

Fig. 7. This hoof model shows screw placement into the wall and the strut placement to contain the palmar wall. The beveled edge gives the roller-motion shoe mechanical advantages in shortening moment arm forces to the entire circumference of the hoof capsule.

unstable hoof wall structure (**Fig. 8**). Screws are used to attach the wooden shoe, and they can substantially aid in wall stabilization. Most of the screws are not set into the wall, but are just outside the wall, acting as strut supports. These help to attach and stabilize the lateral and medial heel walls to the shoe.

Hoof wall stabilization is further accomplished by applying fiberglass casting material (eg, Equicast, Equicast, Inc, Aberdeen, NC, USA). Ground reaction forces in the palmar hoof cause heel expansion on initial heel impact in the normal hoof (particularly at speed). Due to their painful condition, foundered horses are relatively immobile and, therefore, wall expansion is unnecessary. Wall glue is often applied to the heel wall/strut–screw/shoe interface. This is to provide added support in cases that are going to be overly mobile, or when shoe loss would be devastating. Lateral/medial (perimeter) wall glue alone does not provide the stabilization to the entire hoof structure that properly applied casting affords.

Stabilization of the distal phalanx occurs when a properly designed and fitted wooden shoe is applied. The reduction in laminar leverage moments and the redistribution of weight are the likely mechanisms behind the beneficial effect. The less movement the distal phalanx experiences, the faster healing occurs in most situations.

High-frequency impact forces are the forces of stance most damaging to the normal foot.[10] Distal concussion is dampened primarily by the laminar interface of the hoof.[11] In cases of severe laminitis, the painful response to high-frequency impact is exaggerated—especially when a horse is walking on concrete instead of grass. Reducing the high frequency impact with a properly applied wooden shoe (wood-EVA shoe) can significantly reduce the pain of walking on hard surfaces and therefore enhance soundness. To ensure greater patient comfort, screws should be positioned so they do not penetrate the ground surface of the shoe. This is especially important for horses walking on concrete because screws act as conductors of those high frequency impacts.

Success rates for treatment of dorsal capsular/phalangeal rotation with the wooden shoe are higher than those for treatment of distal displacement of the third phalanx ("sinkers"). The shoe has been used successfully to treat unilateral palmar/plantar displacement of the third phalanx.[2] No matter the therapy, cases of severe distal displacement rarely return to acceptable soundness levels.

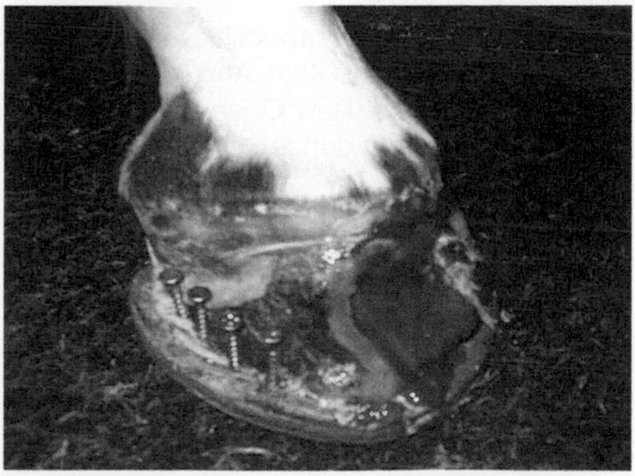

Fig. 8. The detached dorsal hoof wall was resected because the dead wall was creating torque forces on the new wall growth and creating a potential trap for pathogens, which could cause further complications.

Whatever the therapeutic shoeing system, successful treatment of chronic laminitis is dependant on the amount of irreversible lamellar/vascular damage that occurred in the acute stage. The wooden shoe (Steward Clog) provides the veterinarian/farrier a practical, atraumatic, orthotic device that, by incorporating currently available mechanical and physical attributes, provides the laminitic hoof an opportunity to heal.

REFERENCES

1. Steward ML. How to construct and apply atraumatic therapeutic shoes to treat acute or chronic laminitis in the horse. American Association of Equine Practitioners 49th Annual Convention. New Orleans (LA), November 21–23, 2003. p. 337–46.
2. O'Grady SE, Steward ML, Parks A. How to construct and apply the wooden shoe for treating three manifestations of chronic laminitis. 53rd Annual Convention of the American Association of Equine Practitioners. Orlando (FL), December 1–5, 2007. p. 423–29.
3. Craig JJ. Introduction to robotics: mechanics & control. 3rd edition. New Jersey: Prentice Hall; 2004.
4. Reid SR. Impact energy absorption mechanisms in the crushing and indentation of wood. In: Proceedings of IUTAM Symposium on Impact Dynamics, 1993. Beijing (China): Peking University Press; 1994. p. 390–406.
5. Peroni JF, Moore JN, Noschka E, et al. Predisposition for venoconstriction in the equine laminar dermis: implications in equine laminitis. J Appl Phys 2006;100: 759–63.
6. Hood DM, Taylor D, Wagner IP. Effects of ground surface deformability, trimming, and shoeing on quasistatic hoof loading patterns in horses. Am J Vet Res 2001; 62:895–900.
7. Bowker RM. Contrasting structural morphologies of 'good' and 'bad' footed horses. 49th Annual Convention of the American Association of Equine Practitioners. New Orleans (LA), November 21–23, 2003.
8. Thomason J, Bignell W, Batiste D, et al. Effects of hoof shape, body mass and velocity on surface strain in the wall of the unshod forehoof of Standardbreds trotting on a treadmill. Equine Comp Exerc Physiol 2004;1:87–97.
9. Willemen MA, Savelberg H, Barneveld A. The effect of orthopaedic shoeing on the force exerted by the deep digital flexor tendon on the navicular bone in horses. Equine Vet J 1999;31:25–30.
10. Bowker RM. The growth and adaptive capabilities of the hoof wall and sole: functional changes in response to stress 49th Annual Convention of the American Association of Equine Practitioners. New Orleans (LA), November 21–23, 2003.
11. Pollitt CC. Equine laminitis—current concepts. Canberra: RIRDC; 2008.

Home Care for Horses with Chronic Laminitis

James A. Orsini, DVM*, Jennifer Wrigley, CVT, Patrick Riley

KEYWORDS

• Laminitis • Home care • Management • Nursing

Home care for horses with chronic laminitis has been discussed rarely in the veterinary literature even though, at any given time, most of us have at least 1 chronic laminitis case in our care that is being managed at home by the owner. Almost all of our knowledge on this aspect of laminitis treatment has been gleaned through experience, by individually working through the medical, ethical, financial, and emotional challenges these cases can present. Much has already been presented on the medical management of the laminitic horse and on strategies for trimming and shoeing the laminitic foot. This article focuses on the other challenges so often faced when directing the home care of a horse with chronic laminitis.

A good outcome in all but the mildest of cases takes a team of dedicated people: veterinarian, farrier or trimmer, horse owner (or other daily caretaker), and perhaps a physical therapist or other licensed animal therapist. Even so, the horse owner is usually the principal caregiver and therapist when the case is managed at home. It is particularly important that the owner is well informed about the disease process in general and their horse's case in particular, what is involved in recovery, whether recovery is likely to be complete, how long it is likely to take, and what challenges may be encountered. Without the owner's continued commitment and care, a good outcome is next to impossible.

PAIN MANAGEMENT

For humane reasons, owner compliance, and perhaps also for optimal tissue repair, pain management is a crucial component of the home treatment plan. Pain management is of chief concern to most horse owners, and owners often gauge the success or failure of the treatment and rehabilitation plan based on their perception of the horse's comfort. In this Internet age, owners often go outside the team for help if they perceive that their horse's pain is not being adequately managed. Good communication and an effective pain management plan are important in dealing with these cases.

University of Pennsylvania, Department of Clinical Studies, New Bolton Center, 382 West Street Road, Kennett Square, PA 19348, USA
* Corresponding author.
E-mail address: orsini@vet.upenn.edu

Vet Clin Equine 26 (2010) 215–223
doi:10.1016/j.cveq.2009.12.012

When devising a treatment plan for the chronically laminitic horse, the first step is to determine the extent of the disease process and why the horse remains painful. Is the persistent foot pain simply the result of displacement of the distal phalanx (P3) and its consequences? Or might there also be ongoing insult to the feet, such as could occur with poorly regulated pituitary pars intermedia dysfunction (PPID) or hyperinsulinemia associated with obesity (equine metabolic syndrome)? Are you dealing simply with the aftermath of acute laminitis or does this particular case represent a chronic active process? Distinguishing between these 2 possibilities is important in devising a comprehensive treatment plan, including a safe and effective pain management strategy.

Pain management has been a focus of clinical and experimental laminitis research in recent years. As a result, a multimodal approach has emerged as the optimal pain management strategy in moderate to severe cases.[1–4] When the hospitalized laminitis case has recovered sufficiently to return home, and in less severe cases of laminitis that can be managed entirely at home, nonsteroidal antiinflammatory drugs (NSAIDs) such as phenylbutazone may provide sufficient pain relief on their own. Care should be taken with chronic NSAID use to monitor the horse for signs of gastric or colonic ulceration, and to ensure that the horse is drinking well.

The newer NSAIDs of the selective cyclooxygenase type 2 (COX-2) inhibitor class, such as firocoxib, are showing promise for effective and safe pain management in the horse.[5,6] It has recently been suggested that a nonselective COX inhibitor may be best in the developmental and acute stages of laminitis, when the lamellar microvasculature is activated or inflamed, as selective COX-2 inhibitors in humans have caused the most serious problems in patients with vascular disease (eg, rofecoxib [Vioxx] associated with heart attack or stroke). The COX-2 selective drugs may therefore be more appropriate in the treatment of chronic laminitis, when vascular inflammation has subsided, but a safe NSAID may be needed for long-term use.[5]

Some veterinarians have been using doxycycline for pain management, on the premise that its effect as a matrix metalloproteinase (MMP) inhibitor renders it a useful antiinflammatory and thus analgesic agent. Although anecdotal reports are encouraging, no clinical studies have yet been published to validate these observations or to determine the optimal dosage for this purpose. In 1 recent study, neither doxycycline nor oxytetracycline sufficiently inhibited MMP production to prevent the development of Obel grade 3 lameness in experimentally induced laminitis caused by carbohydrate overload.[7]

This approach to pain management has several potential adverse effects. One is disruption of the body's normal microflora; another is the development of resistance to this class of antimicrobial drugs. A third is the potential for nonspecific MMP inhibition to impede tissue repair. As destructive as these enzymes can be when unleashed from their normally tight regulation, MMPs also have essential roles in normal tissue turnover and in tissue repair. Similar in this regard to the cyclooxygenases, the MMPs as a class have essential constitutive roles in normal physiologic processes.[8] Recent research indicates that the timing of MMP-2 upregulation in experimentally induced laminitis suggests a greater involvement in tissue repair than in tissue damage.[9,10] Although MMP regulation is undoubtedly important in the treatment and prevention of laminitis, it is too soon in our understanding of the molecular mechanisms of laminitis to know how best to restore MMP regulation in the laminitic foot.

Other substances that have been tried with some clinical success include opioids (eg, fentanyl, tramadol), gabapentin, acetyl-L-carnitine.[11,12] Various medicinal herbs, such as turmeric, ginger, devil's claw, salicylate-containing plants (meadowsweet, white willow bark, and so forth), and *Gynostemma pentaphyllum* (jiaogulan) have also been included in pain management regimens; however, the safety and efficacy of many of these substances are little studied in the horse,[13] so broad recommendations cannot be made at this time.

Appropriate hoof care and footing are as important as medical therapy for pain management. Phenylbutazone is a poor substitute for proper hoof care and comfortable footing. If a horse continues to require daily NSAIDs or other pain medications several weeks or months beyond the laminitic event, then the case may need to be reviewed. Perhaps the trimming, shoeing, and/or footing needs to be adjusted in some way; or maybe there is a concurrent medical issue that is not being adequately addressed.

Pain medications can interfere with our ability to accurately evaluate the horse's current condition and needs. Although the horse's comfort is important, an equally important goal of the treatment plan should be to get the horse off pain medication as soon as possible. It is a milestone in the recovery when the horse can comfortably move around without needing pain medication.

CONCURRENT MEDICAL ISSUES

Any medical conditions that could have caused or contributed to the laminitic event or that might now be impeding recovery must be addressed. Most common are PPID, obesity, and the systemic inflammatory response triggered by endotoxemia or other microbial toxins. The medical management of these conditions is discussed elsewhere.

The prompt identification and management of infection within the compromised foot is also important. With any laminitic horse, the owner must be warned of the potential for infections to develop within the laminitic foot, even months after the laminitic event. Foot abscesses are common in the months following the laminitic episode, but they can usually be dealt with successfully as for any subsolar or submural infection. More severe infections such as osteomyelitis of distal phalanx are less common. These cases generally require debridement of the diseased bone and systemic or regional antimicrobial therapy. Such therapy is best provided in a hospital setting.

NUTRITION

Feeding the chronically laminitic horse can be a challenge. The diet must meet the body's needs for maintenance and repair, while addressing any special issues. For example, if there are metabolic issues that render the horse particularly sensitive to starches and simple sugars, then care must be taken to feed a diet that meets the horse's daily caloric needs while keeping the amount of nonstructural carbohydrates (NSC) low. An NSC content of 10% or less is recommended for these horses.[14] At the other end of the spectrum is the late-term pregnant or lactating broodmare, whose greater caloric needs may necessitate the inclusion of some carbohydrate-rich foods, although digestible fiber sources such as beet pulp (without molasses) and fats can safely be used to make up some of the shortfall in these mares. In general, a diet that is low in NSC and high in fiber is appropriate for most horses with chronic laminitis. Safe grazing and hay selection for horses needing a low NSC diet is discussed in detail elsewhere and at http://www.safergrass.org.

Protein, Amino Acids

Little clinical research has been conducted on the other nutritional needs of the laminitic horse. It would seem reasonable to ensure that the protein intake is moderate but not excessive (eg, a crude protein content of 10%–12% overall for most nonpregnant, nonlactating adult horses), of high biologic quality, and from species-appropriate sources (ie, grasses and legumes primarily).

Individual amino acids have been studied in the context of various medical conditions in other species. For example, arginine has been reported to be useful in vasoconstrictive conditions because it is a nitric oxide precursor and thus theoretically useful in improving blood flow. However, studies involving L-arginine supplementation have shown inconsistent effects on endothelial function in other species.[15] It is not yet known if it is worthwhile supplementing this or any other specific amino acid beyond what is found in the horse's natural diet of grasses, legumes, and various other herbage.

Vitamins, Minerals, Essential Fatty Acids

The horse's daily vitamin, mineral, and essential fatty acid requirements must be met. A body cannot recover fully without all of the building blocks needed for tissue repair. A diet that consists of nothing but inferior quality hay will likely be marginal for protein, frankly deficient in vitamin E, omega-3 fatty acids, and probably other antioxidant complexes, and possibly some of the essential primary and trace minerals.[16] This commonly used diet is incomplete and should be considered substandard in the care of the chronically laminitic horse. No horse ever recovered fully on such a diet.

In 2007 the National Research Council (NRC) published its revised guidelines for feeding horses.[16] However, some equine nutritionists consider these guidelines too conservative and advise supplementing vitamins and minerals at a rate of NRC+50% for special-needs horses, such as those with chronic laminitis.

Antioxidants

Antioxidants have received much attention in the lay press and on the Internet in the fields of human and animal health. Although a diet that contains ample antioxidant substances seems to be important for health, there is a lot of hype and very little science on what constitutes ample antioxidants in any species, including the horse. Recent research suggests that oxidative stress plays a limited role in laminitis. Treiber and colleagues[17] reported that there was no difference in the serum levels of 3 markers of antioxidant function (glutathione, glutathione peroxidase, and superoxide dismutase) or increased oxidative pressure between ponies with a history of pasture-associated laminitis and those that had never had laminitis. Belknap[5] found that in the black walnut extract and carbohydrate overload models of laminitis, oxidative stress is minimal and does not seem to be primarily involved in causing lamellar injury and failure.

Many different substances can act as antioxidants or reducing agents, including several of the vitamins and trace minerals. Feeding a species-appropriate diet of high-quality forages, with supplemental vitamins, minerals, and essential fatty acids as needed, should provide the chronically laminitic horse with ample antioxidants. Fresh species-appropriate plant material is an especially good source of antioxidant substances for the horse. However, this benefit must be tempered with concerns about the NSC content of improved grass varieties, in particular, when managing carbohydrate-susceptible horses. In these cases, pasture turnout time should be limited or simply hand-graze the horse along the edges of meadows, paths, and hedgerows, where there is nongrass herbage on which the horse can forage.

Gut Health

Restoring and maintaining gut health is an aspect of overall health that has yet to be studied extensively in the laminitic horse, but the authors believe it is a crucial component of hoof health, particularly in cases of laminitis caused by carbohydrate overload. The gut barrier is compromised in these cases, potentially allowing substances normally confined to the lumen to enter the systemic circulation and trigger a cascade of biochemical events that culminate in laminitis.[18] The severity and duration of this greater intestinal permeability remain to be fully studied and are probably case specific, but it would seem prudent to include restoration of gut health in the list of nutritional goals for the laminitic horse.

What is required for gut health in this species will likely prove to be a diet that mimics the horse's natural diet, which is high in fermentable fiber and generally low in NSC. In some cases the addition of soil- or pasture-based microbial species might prove beneficial, but the colonic microflora is by nature highly adaptable and self-replenishing, so it may well be that providing suitable substrate (ie, fermentable fiber), along with judicious grazing (hand-grazing or hand-picking suitable plant materials if necessary), is all that is required to restore a healthy microbial population in most cases. Feeding a good quality, low NSC grass hay at a rate of 1.5% to 3% of ideal body weight per day, according to the horse's caloric needs (ie, less for the fat ones, more for the thin ones), should meet the need for suitable microbial substrate. The amino acid L-glutamine is considered conditionally essential for enterocyte health in other species,[19] and presumably also in the horse, but it remains to be seen whether supplemental glutamine would be helpful in most chronic cases of laminitis.

One other aspect of gut health that receives too little attention is gut motility. A healthy gut is one that has healthy peristaltic activity. Two management practices that encourage restoration of healthy gut motility are to mimic the natural feeding pattern of horses (ie, feed little and often if free-choice feeding is not advisable for the individual), and to encourage movement throughout the day.

REHABILITATION

Movement is essential to the physical and psychological health and well-being of the horse. In our experience, it is also a crucial component of recovery from laminitis. Daily activity should be introduced as soon as the horse can safely be walked without causing further damage to the digital tissues. It is important to stay within the current constraints of the individual's digital pathology, but it is just as important to get the horse moving as soon as it is safe and comfortable.

At one end of the spectrum is the horse who is so stiff and sore that slow hand walking on a forgiving surface for just a few minutes at a time is all the system can cope with at first. At the other end is the horse that is now off NSAIDs, is walking and perhaps even trotting comfortably and spontaneously, and is ready to resume light work. Regardless of the starting point, the goal is to gradually increase the duration and intensity of activity as comfort and mobility improve; otherwise, recovery is slow and likely to be incomplete. No horse ever recovered fully by just standing around in a dry lot.

Horses with even mild to moderate laminitis are often stiff and sore throughout the body, but particularly through the muscles and connective tissues of the shoulder girdle, back, and hindquarters. These patterns reflect the chronic attempt to relieve some of the load on the painful feet. In addition to daily activity, physical therapy can improve the horse's comfort, mobility, willingness to exercise, and capacity to exercise, which speeds the overall recovery. A trained physical therapist or licensed animal therapist (if state law allows) can be a valuable asset to the team.

If such a trained and licensed individual is not available, then there are some simple exercises that can be taught to the horse owner and added to the horse's daily routine. One is a forelimb stretch in which the horse's forelimb is lifted and gently drawn forward to extend all of the joints in the limb and to stretch the myofascial tissues along the palmar and caudal aspects of the forelimb all the way up to the trunk. This stretch is particularly useful because chronic tension in the muscles of the shoulder girdle increases the tension in the deep digital flexor tendon, by virtue of the strong interconnections among muscles and connective tissues throughout the limbs and trunk.[20]

Performing this stretch 3 to 5 times on each forelimb, twice a day initially, can improve the horse's comfort and mobility after even just a couple of sessions. However, the stretch must be performed gently, by slowly and softly drawing the limb forward rather than pulling on it. Being too forceful or pushing the limits of a stretch can cause muscle soreness,[21] which is counterproductive. The caretaker should also be instructed to keep the hoof in line with the shoulder, keep the hoof close to the ground, make the entire stretch fluid and pleasurable, stay within the horse's comfortable limits, and be content with small gains each day. When done correctly, there is minimal risk of harm in unskilled hands.

Another exercise that can be easily taught to the owner carries even less risk of harm. Based on the work of Milton Trager, MD, it involves simple weight shifting: standing beside the horse and gently shifting the horse's weight from side to side, front to back or back to front, and even diagonally. The horse's feet do not move, but rather the body sways slightly on the static feet. The movements should be gentle, slow, and of small amplitude, working with the elastic recoil of the tissues.

The owner is instructed to gently push on the horse's body and then let the body roll back toward the person, at which time it can be gently moved away again to create a slow, rhythmic rocking or swaying motion. With as much pressure as it takes to gently throw a beach ball to a small child, and working with the rhythm and rate of the horse's tissues, chronic myofascial tension can be greatly relieved and a more healthy stance restored even in one session.

Another often-overlooked element of physical activity for the recovering horse is play. Not only is play important for mental health, but it can also be remarkably useful for physical rehabilitation, particularly if the play becomes spontaneous and self-directed. In general, it is best to encourage play with other horses, rather than with the owner. If play is not possible or advisable in the current circumstance, then it can be sufficient for the moment to bring a playful attitude to the horse's physical therapy and other daily management.

NURSING CARE

In many cases, nursing care for the chronically laminitic horse is not much different from good basic horse management. If the horse spends much of his time lying down, then extra care to prevent or treat pressure sores, muscle compression, and other consequences of excessive recumbency is needed.[22] For ambulatory cases, nursing care may simply involve some extra tender-loving care for the horse's mental health and whatever daily activity and physical therapy are advised.

HOUSING AND FOOTING

There are several elements to housing and footing for the chronically laminitic horse. The aim is to ensure that the horse's environment is safe and conducive to repair and rehabilitation. The housing should be warm, dry, comfortable, safe, and spacious. In particular, there should be ample opportunity for the horse to lie down and rest. It is important for tissue repair that the body gets plenty of rest and deep restorative sleep. The bedding or footing must be comfortable and the horse must feel safe. There must also be plenty of room for the horse to get up and down without risk of being cast or otherwise caught up.

Compatible company is important for the sense of safety and security. Horses generally feel safer in the company of others, so a sense of safety often necessitates keeping at least one other horse nearby. Healthy social interactions can facilitate recovery. The importance of good mental health in these chronic cases cannot be overemphasized. No horse ever recovered fully by standing around on his own, isolated to a stall or a dirt lot. The company of healthy horses can greatly speed recovery.

The footing requirements often change as healing progresses. Initially, while the feet are still sore, the footing should be soft and supportive, but not so deep that it increases the work of moving. Clean sand or fine gravel is ideal; deep sawdust, shavings, or other soft stall bedding can also be suitable. Later, as the horse becomes more comfortable and more mobile, the horse can tolerate a wider range of footing materials. Footing that is comfortable but which engages the hoof and encourages the growth of a healthy hoof capsule is best. Such footing can include typical arena surfaces, wood-chip covered pens or paddocks, grassy pastures (with all the usual caveats about limiting the NSC intake), coarser gravel, and loose dirt.

Regardless of the type of material, the chosen footing should be dry and kept clean of manure and urine. Although mud is soft underfoot, and may even be useful during the acute phase of laminitis, standing in mud or mucky footing greatly increases the potential for foot abscesses in the chronically laminitic hoof.

HOOF CARE

Management of the chronically laminitic foot is discussed at length elsewhere. It is essential to trim the hoof to optimize blood flow within the digital circulation and normalize the biomechanical forces on the compromised digit. That generally requires trimming to restore the normal orientation of the distal phalanx in relation to the other phalanges, to the normal portion of the hoof capsule, and to the ground.

Communication

The interpersonal element of hoof care is important, that is, working closely with the farrier or trimmer, and having frequent dialog about the horse's progress and current needs. It is equally important to include the horse owner in the discussion. With the explosion of information available to horse owners on the Internet and in magazines, it is understandable that they may be confused about the plan of care at times. Teamwork and good communication are crucial in these cases.

Frequent reassessment, with repeated radiographs or venograms as needed, is essential to success. This aspect of home care is where many veterinarians are weakest. A "call me if you need me" approach may work well with some horse owners, but with many others it places too great a responsibility on someone with too little knowledge of this disease process. The team leader must direct the management of the horse. That involves frequent monitoring of the horse, factoring in the farrier's perspective and the horse owner's daily observations, and charting the course accordingly. Trying to save the owner money by not arranging revisits on a schedule that is appropriate for the case may not be in the horse's best interest.

Sole Protection

Whether to use a shoe, glue-on pad (wood, leather, plastic, and so forth), pour-in material, or removable boot to protect the compromised hoof depends on many factors, including the owner's wishes. An increasing number of clients want to keep their horses barefoot. This approach does not necessarily compromise the horse's comfort or recovery. There are now many different kinds of hoof boot on the market.

All have the benefit of providing sole protection to the vulnerable or sensitive-soled foot. Some are designed specifically for the painful foot, and they generally include a cushioned insole with or without frog support. Others are designed primarily for the healthy horse, to be used during exercise, but they can be suitable for use in the chronically laminitic horse.

When managing the barefoot laminitic horse, boots should be used as much as necessary to protect the damaged sensitive sole and ensure that the horse is comfortable. The horse must be comfortable enough to move around at will, and if that necessitates the use of boots during turnout, then so be it. However, no one has yet designed a boot that fits every horse perfectly and that can be used without issue all day, every day. If boots are used instead of shoes, glue-on pads, or some other form of sole protection, then it is important to ensure the best possible fit, and advise the owner to check daily for rubbing. Although it is important to use the boots when needed, it is equally important to leave them off for as much of the day and night as possible, relying instead on clean, dry, comfortable footing. The newer pour-in sole protection products such as Sole Guard (Vettec, Inc, Oxnard, CA, USA) are useful in some cases, but they are not as effective in the flat-soled horse as in those with normal concavity to the sole.

ENSURING OWNER COMPLIANCE

The owner's active and ongoing participation in home care is important. Owner compliance problems are minimized by discussing at the outset the time and financial commitments required in these cases and by setting realistic goals, expectations, and protocols. Equally important is providing frequent assessment, feedback, and encouragement. Celebrate even the small measures of progress, but remain the voice of reason, particularly with regard to expectations for return to athletic function.

It is easy for the owner, who sees the horse every day, to miss small but significant changes, and to become discouraged by persistent or recurrent foot pain or by common sequelae such as foot abscesses, white line disease, and vulnerability to sole bruising. Most horse owners are willing to put in the time and money, as long as they have sufficient support and realistic expectations. These cases can turn out well, but it takes considerable commitment by everyone on the treatment team, most especially the horse owner.

REFERENCES

1. Driessen B. Review of equine pain medications in laminitis. In: Orsini JA, editor. Proceedings, 4th international equine conference on laminitis and diseases of the foot. Palm Beach (FL); 2007. p. 66.
2. Hubbell JAE. Systemic pain therapy in the horse with laminitis. In: Orsini JA, editor. Proceedings, 4th international equine conference on laminitis and diseases of the foot. Palm Beach (FL); 2007. p. 91.
3. Jones E, Vinuela-Fernandez I, Eager RA, et al. Neuropathic changes in equine laminitis pain. Pain 2007;132:321–31.
4. Yaksh T. Pain management I and II. In: Orsini JA, editor. Proceedings, 5th international equine conference on laminitis and diseases of the foot. Palm Beach (FL); 2009. p. 84–7.
5. Belknap JK. Pharmacology: is there a scientific basis for anti-inflammatory therapy in laminitis? In: Orsini JA, editor. Proceedings, 5th international equine conference on laminitis and diseases of the foot. Palm Beach (FL); 2009. p. 88–9.

6. Doucet MY, Bertone AL, Hendrickson D, et al. Comparison of efficacy and safety of paste formulations of firocoxib and phenylbutazone in horses with naturally occurring osteoarthritis. J Am Vet Med Assoc 2008;232:91–7.
7. Eades SC. Laminitis research: Louisiana State University. In: Orsini JA, editor. Proceedings, 5th international equine conference on laminitis and diseases of the foot. Palm Beach (FL); 2009. p. 34–5.
8. Clutterbuck AL, Harris P, Allaway D, et al. Matrix metalloproteinases in inflammatory pathologies of the horse. Vet J 2010;183:27–38.
9. Black SJ. Enzymes: what role do they play? In: Orsini JA, editor. Proceedings, 5th international equine conference on laminitis and diseases of the foot. Palm Beach (FL); 2009. p. 82–3.
10. Pollitt CC. Laminitis research: University of Queensland. In: Orsini JA, editor. Proceedings, 5th international equine conference on laminitis and diseases of the foot. Palm Beach (FL); 2009. p. 26–7.
11. Orsini JA, Moate P, Kuersten K, et al. Pharmacokinetics of fentanyl delivered transdermally in healthy adult horses – variability among horses and its clinical implications. J Vet Pharmacol Ther 2006;29:539–46.
12. Orsini JA, Galantino-Homer H, Pollitt CC. Laminitis in horses: through the lens of systems theory. J Equine Vet Sci 2009;2:105–14.
13. Tinworth KD, Harris PA, Sillence MN, et al. Potential treatments for insulin resistance in the horse: a comparative multi-species review. Vet J 2009. [Epub ahead of print].
14. Geor R. Nutritional management of the prelaminitic and laminitic horse. In: Proceedings, 5th international equine conference on laminitis and diseases of the foot. Palm Beach (FL); 2009. p. 48–9.
15. Jahangir E, Vita JA, Handy D, et al. The effect of L-arginine and creatine on vascular function and homocysteine metabolism. Vasc Med 2009;14:239–48.
16. Anon. Nutrient requirements of horses. In: National research council, committee on nutrient requirements of horses. 6th revised edition. Washington, DC: The National Academies Press; 2007.
17. Treiber K, Carter R, Gay L, et al. Inflammatory and redox status of ponies with a history of pasture-associated laminitis. Vet Immunol Immunopathol 2009;129: 216–20.
18. Weiss DJ, Evanson OA, Green BT, et al. In vitro evaluation of intraluminal factors that may alter intestinal permeability in ponies with carbohydrate-induced laminitis. Am J Vet Res 2000;61:858–61.
19. Bergen WG, Wu G. Intestinal nitrogen recycling and utilization in health and disease. J Nutr 2009;139:821–5.
20. King C. Equine anatomy in perspective: an integrative view of equine musculoskeletal anatomy. In: Proceedings, 3rd international symposium on rehabilitation and physical therapy in veterinary medicine; 2004. p. 89–93.
21. Rose NS, Northrop AJ, Brigden CV, et al. Effects of a stretching regime on stride length and range of motion in equine trot. Vet J 2009;181:53–5.
22. Floyd AE. Environmental management of the severely laminitic horse. In: Floyd AE, Mansmann RA, editors. Equine podiatry. St. Louis (MO): Saunders; 2007. p. 359–67.

Index

Note: Page numbers of article titles are in **boldface** type.

Vet Clin Equine 26 (2010) 225–232
doi:10.1016/S0749-0739(10)00017-9 vetequine.theclinics.com

S

T

V

Printed and bound by CPI Group (UK) Ltd, Croydon, CR0 4YY
03/10/2024
01040448-0004